NEURODEVELOPMENTAL DISEASES - LABORATORY AND CLINICAL RESEARCH

PROGRESSIVE COGNITIVE IMPAIRMENT AND ITS NEUROPATHOLOGIC CORRELATES

NEURODEVELOPMENTAL DISEASES - LABORATORY AND CLINICAL RESEARCH

Additional books in this series can be found on Nova's website
under the Series tab.

Additional e-books in this series can be found on Nova's website
under the eBooks tab.

NEURODEVELOPMENTAL DISEASES - LABORATORY AND CLINICAL RESEARCH

PROGRESSIVE COGNITIVE IMPAIRMENT AND ITS NEUROPATHOLOGIC CORRELATES

GEDIMINAS PETER GLIEBUS
EDITOR

NOVA BIOMEDICAL
New York

Library of Congress Cataloging-in-Publication Data

ISBN: 978-1-63485-221-0
Library of Congress Control Number: 2016939079

Published by Nova Science Publishers, Inc. † New York

CONTENTS

Foreword	*Carol F. Lippa*	**vii**
Introduction	*Gediminas Peter Gliebus*	**ix**
Chapter 1	Neuropathology of Neurodegenerative Disorders *Esther N. Bit-Ivan and Eileen H. Bigio*	**1**
Chapter 2	Imaging and Cerebrospinal Fluid Biomarkers in Alzheimer's Disease and Lewy Body Spectrum Disorders *Usman Saeed, Sandra E. Black and Mario Masellis*	**17**
Chapter 3	Function and Dysfunction of the Prefrontal Lobes in Neurodegenerative Diseases *Alexandre Henri-Bhargava, Donald T. Stuss and Morris Freedman*	**51**
Chapter 4	Action-Intentional Disorders in Neurodegenerative Diseases *Kenneth M. Heilman, Arash Salardini and Adam D. Falchook*	**69**
Chapter 5	Emotional Processing and Neurodegenerative Diseases *Peter Pressman and Elliott Ross*	**85**
Chapter 6	Memory Disorders in Neurodegenerative Diseases *Gediminas Peter Gliebus*	**127**
Chapter 7	Language Disorders in Neurodegenerative Diseases *Borna Bonakdarpour*	**155**
Chapter 8	Neurovisual Impairment in Neurodegenerative Diseases *Christian Schenk and Alan J. Lerner*	**193**
Chapter 9	Introduction to Combined Cognitive and Movement Disorders *Jill M. Farmer*	**261**
About the Editor		**277**
Index		**279**

FOREWORD

Carol F. Lippa, MD
Professor,
Department of Neurology
Drexel Neurosciences Institute
Drexel University College of Medicine, Philadelphia, PA, US

Dr. Gediminas (Peter) Gliebus wondered, "What is needed the most, if anything, in a textbook on dementia?"

The brain is more complicated than other organs because every convolution has different functions, and the different brain regions are highly interconnected. This added layer of complexity makes learning about neurological problems challenging. If you picked up this textbook, you probably are probably looking for a comprehensive, clinically useful source of information on the diagnosis and management of Alzheimer's disease, the related dementias and other conditions impacting thinking and memory. "A Practical Approach to Establishing a Diagnosis of Progressive Cognitive Impairment and its Neuropathological Correlation" is just that. Gliebus' textbook provides clinically relevant guidance on how to approach progressive cognitive disorders in the outpatient setting. By understanding the basic brain circuitry for the various cognitive functions, and applying that information in the patient care setting, the reader can gain a better understanding of which cognitive domains are affected and what underlying pathologies are likely. Practicing physicians in neurology, primary care specialties, geriatrics, internal/family medicine and psychiatry, as well as fellows, residents, medical students, and allied health professionals will all benefit from this approach.

As a cognitive disorders specialist, I have a professional fondness for Gliebus' approach of study. As my training involved geriatric neurology and neuropathology, I soon learned that specific cognitive profiles can be caused by several underlying pathological processes. For example, impaired executive function can be observed in frontotemporal degeneration due to abnormal (conformational) alterations in a number of brain-specific proteins, but it may also be caused by traumatic brain injury, and may even be seen, to some extent in depression, vascular cognitive syndromes, and Alzheimer's disease. The reverse is also true; one pathological brain protein can underlie a variety of clinical neurological syndromes when it is expressed in different brain regions. For example, hyperphosphorylation of the protein tau in a common abnormality that underlies the symptoms in corticobasal degeneration, progressive supranuclear palsy and some types of frontotemporal degeneration.

Understanding the anatomical connections or networks is a critical basic layer of understanding that we need in order to understand the underlying pathophysiological processes. The available links between a specific cognitive impairment profile, its anatomic substrate, and the potential underlying neuropathology's are provided in this book. This information will help with understanding the diagnosis, and will be critical for our selection of disease modifying interventions as they are developed. The material may also serve the reader a translational bridge to help understand the rationale behind diagnostic biomarker development and use.

Carol F. Lippa, MD
Professor and Interim Chair, Department of Neurology
Drexel Neurosciences Institute
Director, Memory and Cognitive Disorders Program
Drexel University College of Medicine
Philadelphia, PA 19102

INTRODUCTION

Gediminas Peter Gliebus, MD
Drexel Neurosciences Institute
Drexel University College of Medicine, Philadelphia, PA, US

Recent decades represent a very exciting time for the neurosciences and neurology. Fundamental discoveries in basic neurosciences and advancements in imaging techniques have led to understanding how nerve cells from anatomically separate brain regions function in cohesive networks. Discoveries in biochemistry and advancements in pathology detection have provided increasing information on known neuropathological processes and have uncovered new neuropathological entities. These fundamental advancements in basic sciences have enabled us to elucidate anatomical - functional entities that were previously unknown. For example, brain regions that become active and work in concert during task-free states are now recognized. In short, recent decades have significantly shifted our understanding of how the brain functions.

This knowledgc sheds more light on brain function and dysfunction; however, it also increases the depth of knowledge that practitioners will be expected to understand. Neurology as a specialty is becoming very complex and now necessitates the creation of subspecialties.

Exciting advancements in medicine have contributed to longer life expectancy. However, due to an aging population, the prevalence of age-related neurodegenerative diseases has begun to increase. This has resulted in increased interest in understanding and treating these conditions in research and clinical settings.

Information on neurodegeneration is increasing at an exponential rate. These rapid changes could leave practicing physicians at a loss. The majority of new discoveries increase our understanding of these conditions; however, new discoveries sometimes contradict previous discoveries. It may also be difficult for practitioners who do not closely follow these changes to understand where these discoveries fit into the larger puzzle of neurological normality and abnormality.

Classical teachings stated that selected brain regions are responsible for set functions. New teachings have moved away from a regional approach and now consider brain functions to be rooted in neuronal networks. These neuronal networks consist of interconnected brain regions that are simultaneously activated during the performance of specific activities. These brain regions may be distal from each other anatomically. Furthermore, the same brain regions could also be activated during different functional tasks. This concept demonstrated why lesions in different parts of the brain could present with the same or similar symptoms.

Several other concepts of brain function have become apparent. First, the data supports the notion that clinical disease presentation frequently depends more on the location of the pathology than its nature. Second, certain pathological conditions, especially neurodegenerative conditions, affect particular regions or networks. For example, initial pathological changes in typical Alzheimer's disease frequently occur in the regions associated with memory function: neurofibrillary tangles begin to accumulate in the neurons of medial temporal lobe structures, whereas fibrillary amyloid plaques are deposited in the regions overlapping with the posterior regions of the default mode network. This principle is sometimes referred to as selective regional vulnerability. The exact mechanism explaining why certain brain regions are more vulnerable to certain pathologies is not completely understood. Third, the same brain regions and networks may be vulnerable to several pathological processes. In other words, different pathological processes can present with similar symptoms. This complicates the diagnostic process and necessitates more definitive tests to pinpoint the underlying pathology.

Terminology represents another confusing factor in cognitive neurology. Similar terminology can be used by pathologists to describe a specific underlying neuropathological process but by clinicians to describe a clinical syndrome. For example, corticobasal degeneration refers to a specific neuropathological process in the brain, whereas corticobasal syndrome refers to a specific clinical syndrome. Corticobasal syndrome could be caused by various underlying pathological processes; corticobasal degeneration represents only one of these processes.

Patients presenting with cognitive disorders present very complex cases. After careful evaluation, clinicians usually establish a cognitive impairment profile and the time frame of its development. The identification of a cognitive profile usually leads to the question of which conditions are causing it. This can be answered after the careful selection and execution of specific tests. This book helps to bridge the gap between clinical presentations and underlying pathology.

The book begins with chapters describing common neuropathological entities that are responsible for progressive neurodegenerative conditions. The following chapter describes currently available biomarkers tests for neurodegenerative conditions such as Alzheimer's disease and Lewy Body Spectrum disorders and research about possible disease-specific diagnostic measures. The tests of Frontotemporal spectrum and primary language disorders are discussed separately in cognitive domain specific chapters. The subsequent chapters describe abnormal cognitive profiles according to cognitive function. Each chapter explains the current understanding of the function and functional anatomy of each cognitive domain and then goes on to discuss the tests that are used to evaluate these cognitive functions. Each chapter then overviews the underlying pathology.

Cognitive neurology cannot be viewed separately from other neurology subspecialties, especially movement disorders. Many cognitive disorders develop a component of movement impairment. The last chapter reviews provides an introduction to the conditions that present with both cognitive and movement impairments.

This book is geared towards those who evaluate and treat patients with cognitive disorders, including students, residents, fellows, practicing physicians and allied health care providers. The book approaches cognitive neurology in the same way that clinicians approach it daily when examining their patients: utilizing tools to identify the clinical-pathological syndrome, generating a differential diagnosis and obtaining knowledge of the possible underlying neuro-pathological processes. This creates a system for integrating knowledge on (1) a given pathological clinical syndrome, (2) the underlying pathologies affecting relevant networks and (3) biomarker studies to identify the abnormal biochemical process.

A targeted approach to cognitive disorders is very important for improving diagnostic accuracy and avoiding unnecessary testing. The increasing epidemiological burden of individuals affected by these diseases enhances the importance of addressing this emerging issue.

In: Progressive Cognitive Impairment …
Editor: Gediminas Peter Gliebus

ISBN: 978-1-63485-221-0

Chapter 1

Neuropathology of Neurodegenerative Disorders

Esther N. Bit-Ivan[1] and Eileen H. Bigio[2,*]
[1]Southern Illinois University School of Medicine, Springfield, IL, US
[2]Northwestern University Feinberg School of Medicine, Chicago, IL, US

Abstract

Advances in clinical detection and assessment of patients with neurodegenerative disease are assisting clinicians in the diagnosis and treatment of their patients; however, there are many diseases that cause progressive cognitive impairment and many of them have overlapping clinical features. It is also common for patients to have concurrent primary diseases of the brain or concomitant systemic diseases that cause cognitive decline. As such, postmortem neuropathologic evaluation is still the gold standard for the diagnosis of neurodegenerative disease. This chapter will review current autopsy procedures, and gross and microscopic neuropathologic evaluation of the most common neurodegenerative diseases that cause progressive cognitive impairment.

Brain Examination and Sections

At autopsy, gross examination is performed noting cerebral atrophy, edema and herniation, vascular atherosclerosis and anatomic variances of the circle of Willis, as well as any other abnormalities that can be seen on the surface of the brain such as infarcts or contusions. The intact brain is weighed and then typically undergoes formalin fixation for approximately 10 days before sectioning and sampling. Some protocols; however, call for sectioning first and then brief cold paraformaldehyde fixation followed by cryopreservation in sucrose before histologic sampling. Normally, coronal sections of the cerebrum, sagittal and parasagittal or transverse sections of the cerebellum, and transverse sections of the brainstem

* Corresponding author: E-Bigio@northwestern.edu.

and spinal cord (when available) are performed. Again, inspection for abnormalities in anatomy, color, texture, and gross lesions is performed.

The United States National Institute on Aging-Alzheimer's Association (NIA-AA) currently recommends a minimum of 13 brain sections for the histologic study of Alzheimer disease neuropathologic change, Lewy body disease, and other conditions such as vascular brain injury, microvascular lesions and hippocampal sclerosis [1]. The same 13 initial brain sections can also be used for the evaluation of frontotemporal lobar degeneration. The sections include the middle frontal gyrus, superior and middle temporal gyri, inferior parietal lobule, occipital cortex, anterior cingulate gyrus, amygdala, hippocampus with dentate gyrus and entorhinal cortex, basal ganglia at the level of the anterior commissure to include the caudate putamen, globus pallidus and nucleus basalis of Meynert, thalamus and subthalamic nucleus, cerebellar cortex and dentate nucleus, midbrain with substantia nigra, pons with locus coeruleus, and medulla with dorsal motor nucleus of the vagus and hypoglossal nucleus (Figure 1). Sections are typically taken from the dominant hemisphere, which in most cases is the left hemisphere, but some protocols include bilateral neocortical sections, which are especially important in cases of asymmetric clinical findings such as primary progressive aphasia. Additional sections of any gross lesions and areas of interest are also taken.

Tissue blocks are composed of formalin fixed, paraffin embedded tissue. Thin sections (4-6 μm) are sliced from these blocks, routinely stained with hematoxylin and eosin (H & E), and are used for the assessment of neuronal loss and gliosis, superficial microvacuolation and gliosis, white matter rarefaction, vascular pathology, and other basic histologic findings. Some inclusions can also be seen on H & E, such as Pick and some Lewy bodies. Sections are secondarily evaluated with special stains (such as fluorescent thioflavin-S, Bielschowsky or Gallyas silver stains, and Luxol fast blue) and specific immunohistochemical stains including tau (AT8 or PHF, and sometimes antibodies to 3R and 4R tau), ubiquitin or p62, TDP-43, and FUS. Ultimately, an autopsy report with all of the observed pathologic findings is issued. The standard autopsy report includes gross and microscopic descriptions, a list of sections examined and final pertinent diagnoses.

Alzheimer Disease Neuropathologic Change

Alzheimer Disease (AD) is the most common clinical diagnosis of progressive dementia in older adults, and with onset younger than 65 in early onset cases. The corresponding pathology is called Alzheimer Disease Neuropathologic Change, or ADNC [1]. ADNC (Figure 2) is also implicated in primary progressive aphasia, where ADNC is seen in up to half the cases, and often affects the hemispheres asymmetrically [2].

The two major proteins implicated in AD are phosphorylated tau and beta amyloid (Aβ). Tau isomers, which are normally created by alternative splicing of *MAPT*, contain varying numbers of repeats within the microtubule-binding domain. Both 3-repeat (3R) and 4-repeat (4R) tau isomers are abnormally phosphorylated in AD aggregates [3, 4]. Aβ is derived from the cleavage of amyloid precursor protein by two enzymes: a protease called β-secretase activity enzyme (BACE) and γ-secretase enzymatic complex which creates two Aβ peptides, Aβ40 and Aβ42 [5].

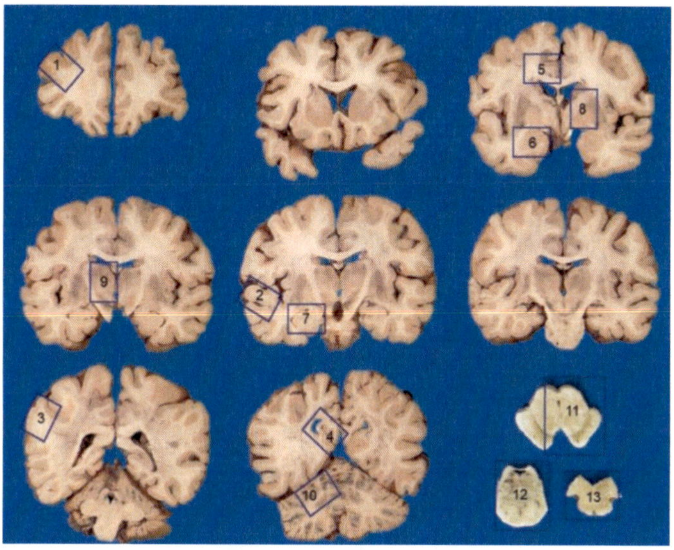

Figure 1. A minimum of 13 regions of the brain are examined including middle frontal gyrus (1), superior and middle temporal gyri (2), inferior parietal lobule (3), occipital cortex (4), anterior cingulate gyrus (5), amygdala (6), hippocampus with dentate gyrus and entorhinal cortex (7), basal ganglia at the level of the anterior commissure with caudate, putamen, globus pallidus, and the nucleus basalis of Meynert (8), thalamus with subthalamic nucleus (9), cerebellar cortex and dentate nucleus (10), midbrain with substantia nigra (11), pons with locus coeruleus (12), and medulla with dorsal motor nucleus of the vagus and hypoglossal nucleus (13).

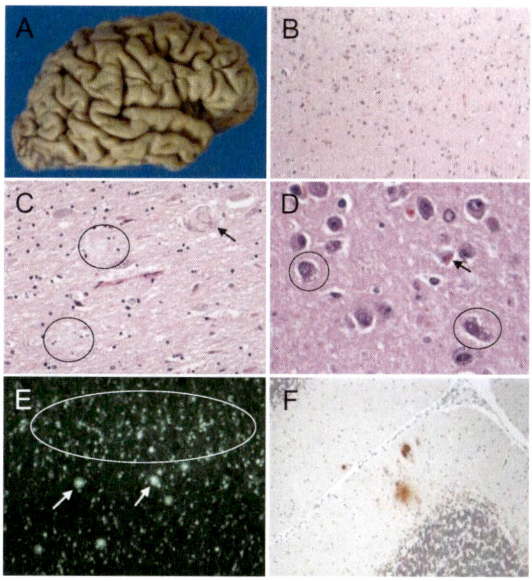

Figure 2. Global cerebral atrophy is seen in Alzheimer Disease Neuropathologic change (A). Neuronal loss and gliosis is observed on H & E in affected areas with entorhinal cortex shown here (B). H & E findings include neurofibrillary tangles (arrow) and ghost tangles (circled) seen here in the nucleus basalis of Meynert (C), granulovacuolar degeneration (circled) and Hirano bodies (arrows) (D). Thioflavin-S fluorescent stain highlights frequent neurofibrillary tangles (circle) and neuritic plaques (arrows) (E). Diffuse plaques are best seen on Aβ staining (F).

Postmortem examination of the AD brain, like antemortem imaging, reveals global cerebral atrophy affecting even the occipital lobes, with compensatory dilatation of the ventricular system, also called hydrocephalus ex vacuo. The mesial temporal lobe is usually most affected with involvement of the entorhinal cortex, hippocampus, and amygdala. Additionally, pallor of the locus coeruleus is typically seen and is usually greater than that of the substantia nigra [6].

Although cognitive decline correlates best with synapse loss [7], there is no efficient way to study synapse loss in postmortem tissue. Instead, microscopic examination reveals neuronal loss and gliosis, which is generally pronounced in the nucleus basalis of Meynert, entorhinal cortex, hippocampus, amygdala, and locus coeruleus, followed by neocortex. Neurofibrillary tangles (tangles, NFTs) can be seen as amphophilic, fibrillary/filamentous inclusions within neurons; many more tangles are seen with special stains and immunostains (see below). When affected neurons die, the faded tangles remain in the neuropil and are termed "ghost tangles." Neurons may also demonstrate granulovacuolar degeneration and associated eosinophilic, rod shaped inclusions called Hirano bodies. Amyloid plaques, seen in the neuropil, are composed predominantly of Aβ42. Some of the plaques have incorporated dystrophic neurites, microglia and astrocytic processes and are termed neuritic plaques (NPs). Vascular amyloid deposits (cerebral amyloid angiopathy, or CAA), composed predominantly of Aβ40, are often seen in AD. Both cortical neuronal loss with descending Wallerian degeneration, and vascular disease, including both CAA and arteriolosclerotic vascular disease, may contribute to underlying white matter rarefaction.

Silver stains such as Gallyas and Bielchowsky, immunohistochemical stains for phosphorylated tau, and the thioflavin-S florescent stain highlight accumulations of phosphorylated tau in NFTs. Silver stains and thioflavin-S also highlight NPs, and the amyloid accumulations in diffuse plaques (DPs). Congo-red and immunohistochemical stains for Aβ highlight the amyloid in DPs and NPs, and also CAA.

Through the years, the pathologic criteria and accepted grading schemas for Alzheimer Disease have evolved. In 2012, the National Institute on Aging/Alzheimer's Association (NIA/AA) Consensus Guidelines combined the Thal Phase for Aβ/amyloid plaques, Braak Neurofibrillary Tangle stage, the Consortium to Establish a Registry for Alzheimer Disease (CERAD) neuritic plaque score into the "ABC" algorithm for designating low, intermediate or high Alzheimer Disease Neuropathologic Change (ADNC) [1]. According to guidelines, a stepwise process for staining different brain regions is performed for assessing the Aβ/amyloid within the brain (cortical sections, followed by hippocampus/entorhinal cortex, basal ganglia, and lastly the brainstem and cerebellum). And at least three cortical regions (superior and middle temporal, middle frontal, inferior parietal lobule) are assessed for NFTs and NPs. It is important to know that NFTs and NPs accumulate with age, and that a threshold must be passed for their presence to cause dementia.

High ADNC is most often the pathology in end-stage clinical "probable Alzheimer disease," but sometimes intermediate ADNC can be seen. Low ADNC may or may not be significant, depending on whether or not there is additional pathology present. In 30 to 60% of cases ADNC is seen with Lewy Body Disease (see next section), work-up of which is also recommended by the Consensus Guidelines [1, 8, 9]. TDP-43 pathology is also seen in up to approximately 60% of cases with ADNC and is often associated with hippocampal sclerosis [10]. Vascular disease, especially CAA, is another frequent concomitant finding.

LEWY BODY DISEASE

Pathologically, Lewy Body Disease (Figure 3) is accumulation of abnormally phosphorylated, insoluble aggregates of α-synuclein (α-synucleinopathy), a pre-synaptic protein encoded by *SNCA*. α-synucleinopathies encompass Parkinson Disease (PaD), Parkinson Disease Dementia (PDD), Dementia with Lewy Bodies (DLB) and include other diseases such as multiple system atrophy (MSA). Parkinson Disease is a movement disorder, while PDD and DLB are two clinical categories of disease in which patients have cognitive impairment. PDD also has a movement disorder while DLB may or may not have an associated movement disorder [11, 12]. Grossly, PaD and PDD have pallor of the substantia nigra and locus coeruleus, with microscopic neuronal loss and gliosis as well as α-synuclein aggregates, while DLB may or may not have these brainstem findings. Both PDD and DLB generally have atrophy of the limbic system and mild cortical atrophy with microscopic superficial microvacuolation.

The α-synuclein aggregate within the neuronal soma is round, eosinophilic, and fibrillary and is called a Lewy body (LB). LBs within pigmented neurons of the substantia nigra have a halo of clearing around them, while cortical LBs are less conspicuous due to the lack of a halo, their presence in small cortical neurons, and the absence of cytoplasmic neuromelanin in cortical neurons to highlight them. Accumulations of α-synuclein within dendrites are also present and are called Lewy neurites (LNs). These findings are sometimes incidentally seen in non-impaired patients; however, if clinical manifestations were present during life, are the likely major contributor to neurocognitive and motor decline.

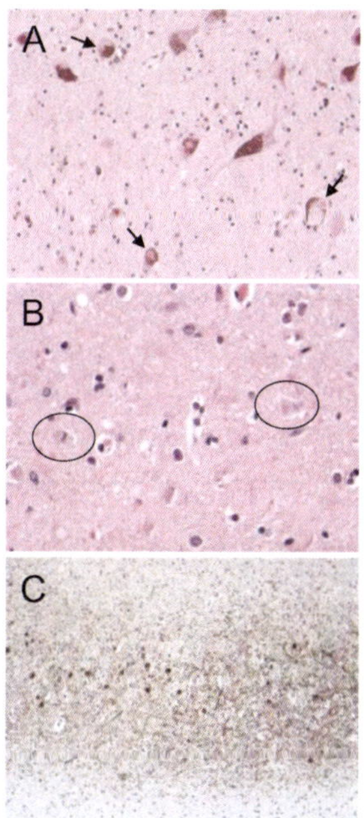

Figure 3. Lewy Bodies (arrows) are easily seen in the substantia nigra (A) and are less conspicuous in the cortex (circles, B). Immunohistochemical staining for α-synuclein highlights many cortical LBs and Lewy neurites seen here in the CA2 region of the hippocampus (C).

Lewy body disease is pathologically divided into four categories depending on the anatomic spread of disease [13]. The brainstem-predominant type demonstrates involvement of the substantia nigra in the midbrain, dorsal motor nucleus of the vagus nerve in the medulla, and locus coeruleus in the pons. Limbic or transitional type has α-synuclein inclusions in the brainstem plus the cingulate gyrus or entorhinal cortex or both. Disease that has spread to involve the brainstem, limbic system, and neocortex is called Neocortical or diffuse Lewy Body Disease (DLBD). The fourth subtype, often seen with other diseases like Alzheimer Disease, or even in non-cognitively impaired individuals, is Amygdala Predominant type. Immunohistochemical staining for α-synuclein highlights LBs and LNs, and is used for categorization of disease.

Frontotemporal Lobar Degeneration

Frontotemporal lobar degeneration (FTLD) is an "umbrella" term used for the pathology of a rapidly evolving group of diseases that now account for as many cases of dementia in patients under 65 years of age as Alzheimer Disease [14]. The clinical syndrome of frontotemporal dementia (FTD) includes both the behavioral variant (bvFTD) and several language disorders known in general as primary progressive aphasia (PPA). The pathologic entities underlying FTD include FTLD, (Figure 4), as well as AD, DLB, and even Creutzfeldt-Jakob disease [15]. The FTLDs include tau, TAR DNA binding protein of 43 kD (TDP-43), and fused in sarcoma (FUS) proteinopathies. There may also be as yet unidentified proteins to be discovered in FTLDs. In addition to the proteins for which FTLD-tau, FTLD-TDP and FTLD-FUS are named, at least a subset of their inclusions are also ubiquitin or p62 positive. Each of these proteinopathies is further subdivided into distinct pathologic "subtypes." FTLD-tau includes Pick Disease, Progressive Supranuclear Palsy (PSP), Corticobasal Degeneration (CBD), FTDP-17, Globular Glial Tauopathies (GGT), and others; FTLD-TDP is divided into Types A, B, C and D, and each of these subtypes is associated with characteristic clinical presentations and genetic mutations; and FTLD-FUS includes Neuronal Intermediate Filament Inclusion Disease (NIFID), Basophilic Inclusion Body Disease (BIBD), and atypical FTLD-U [15-17]. There are also rare categories with protein aggregates containing only ubiquitin or p62 (FTLD-UPS [ubiquitin proteasome system] and FTD-3, associated with CHMP2B mutation), and one that has no protein aggregates yet described called FTLD-ni (no inclusions) [15]. The following is a brief review of the most common pathologic types of FTLD.

Pick Disease (FTLD-tau, PiD)

Pick Disease (PiD, Figure 5), or FTLD-tau (PiD), was the first FTLD to be described pathologically, and is due to neuronal cytoplasmic and dendritic accumulation of 3-repeat tau. At gross examination, the frontal and temporal lobes exhibit severe atrophy with characteristic "dried walnut" or "knife-edge" gyral atrophy and severe ventricular dilatation. There is also atrophy of the corpus callosum, hippocampus, thalamus and caudate nuclei.

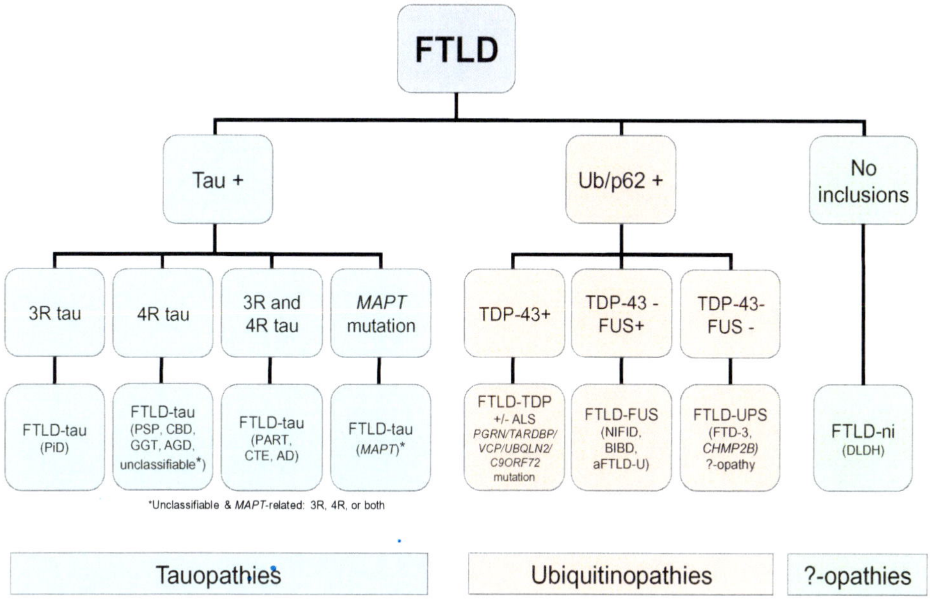

Figure 4. FTLD subtypes with or without amyotrophic lateral sclerosis (ALS) are subgrouped based on proteinopathy and associated genetic mutations. They include: AGD, argyrophilic grain disease; BIBD, basophilic inclusion body disease; CBD, corticobasal degeneration; CTE, chronic traumatic encephalopathy; DLDH, dementia lacking distinctive histology; FTD-3, frontotemporal dementia associated with chromosome 3; FTLD-FUS, frontotemporal lobar degeneration with fused in sarcoma proteinopathy; FTLD-ni, frontotemporal lobar degeneration with no inclusions; FTLD-tau, frontotemporal lobar degeneration with tauopathy; FTLD-TDP, frontotemporal lobar degeneration with TDP-43 proteinopathy; FTLD-UPS, frontotemporal lobar degeneration with involvement of the ubiquitin proteasome system; GGT, globular glial tauopathies; NIFID, neuronal intermediate filament inclusion dementia; PART, primary age-related tauopathy; PiD, Pick disease; PSP, progressive supranuclear palsy. Other abbreviations used include: TDP-43, transactive response deoxyribose nucleic acid binding protein of 43 kDa; FUS, fused in sarcoma protein; Ub, ubiquitin; 3R, tau isoforms with 3 microtubule-binding repeats; 4R, tau isoforms with 4 microtubule-binding repeats.

Histologic sections demonstrate marked neuronal loss and gliosis of the frontal and temporal lobes with rarefaction of the underlying white matter. The parietal lobes may also be affected, as well as the hippocampus, amygdala and substantia nigra. In the most severe cases of neuronal loss and gliosis, the cortex appears vacuolated and is called status spongiosis.

The hallmark inclusion in Pick disease is the Pick body, which is a cytoplasmic neuronal inclusion composed of hyperphosphorylated 3R tau. Pick bodies (PB) are easily identified on H&E sections in the granular neurons of the hippocampal dentate gyrus, which have expanded cytoplasm containing round, often basophilic fibrillary inclusions. PBs in the cortex are more difficult to see on H & E sections. Within the cortex, chromatolytic, ballooned neurons called Pick cells are also seen. PBs are easily identified by immunohistochemistry for phosphorylated tau and 3R tau. They are also positive on Bielchowsky silver stain and neurofilament, and are weakly positive for ubiquitin [18, 19].

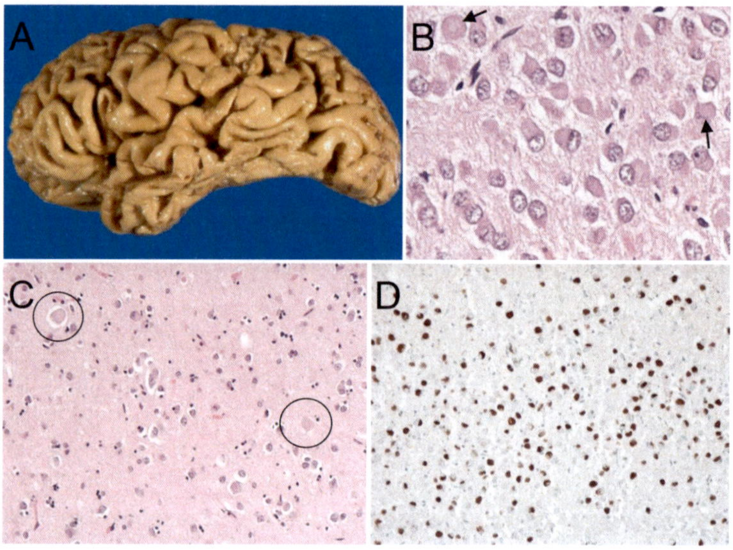

Figure 5. Severe frontotemporal atrophy is seen in FTLD-tau (PiD) (A). Pick bodies (arrows) are easily identified on H &E in the dentate gyrus (B). Ballooned neurons, also called Pick cells (circled), are seen (C). Pick bodies are positive for phosphorylated tau and 3R tau (3R tau, D).

Progressive Supranuclear Palsy (FTLD-tau, PSP)

Progressive Supranuclear Palsy (Figure 6), or FTLD-tau (PSP), like LBD, is a disease of cognitive decline or movement disorder or both. It classically presents with supranuclear ophthalmoplegia and symmetric parkinsonism-like features, but can also present as FTD. The most prominent gross findings in PSP include thinning/atrophy of the subthalamic nucleus, atrophy and greenish discoloration of the globus pallidus, and an indistinct cerebellar dentate nucleus. There may also be mild atrophy of the cerebral cortex and brainstem (particularly the substantia nigra, superior colliculus, red nucleus, periventricular gray matter, pontine tegmentum and locus coeruleus).

The MAPT gene H1 haplotype is found is virtually all cases of PSP, and microscopically, 4-repeat tau accumulates in neurons and glia that can be demonstrated with antibodies to phosphorylated tau and 4R tau. Tau pathology is present in atrophic areas. Astrocytes with perinuclear accumulations in their stellate processes are called tufted astrocytes and are a key pathologic feature in PSP. Oligodendrocytes have fibrillary inclusions which surround the nucleus and are called coiled bodies. Phosphorylated tau accumulation within neurons in the neocortex, subcortical gray matter and brainstem, take a round, whorled configuration and are called globose tangles. There are also tau-positive neuropil threads, predominantly in gray matter, but also present to a mild degree in white matter. In addition to neuronal loss and gliosis in the grossly atrophic areas described above, the cerebellar dentate nucleus (DN) demonstrates grumose degeneration, which on routine H & E staining, consists of eosinophilic granular material in place of DN neurons, thought to be derived from degeneration/collapse of axonal terminals. Grumose degeneration can be better demonstrated by synaptophysin immunohistochemical staining [19].

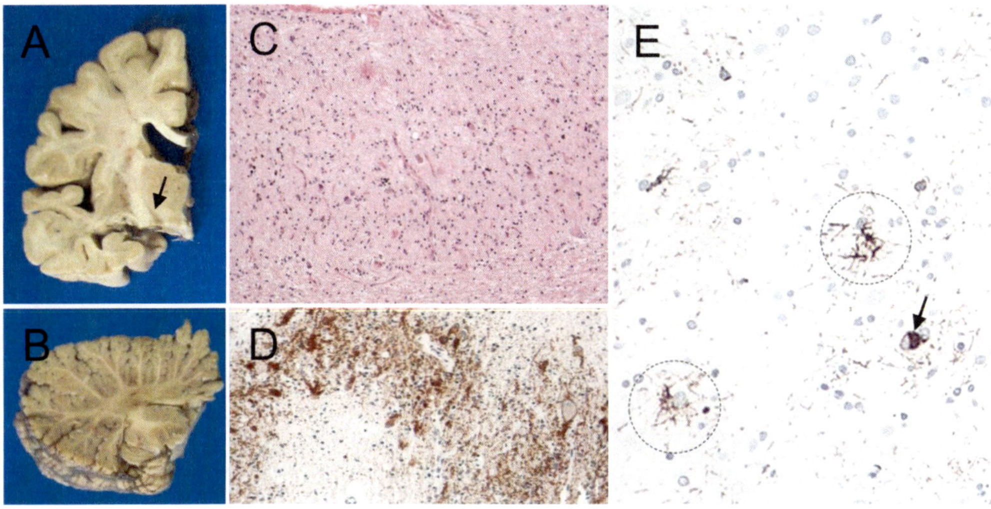

Figure 6. Grossly, atrophy of the subthalamic nucleus (arrow) is prominent in FTLD-tau (PSP) (A) as is an indistinct cerebellar dentate nucleus (B). Neuronal loss and gliosis in the dentate nucleus (C) is known as grumose degeneration, which is best highlighted by synaptophysin immunohistochemical stain (Normal perineuronal synaptic staining, bottom right; grumose degeneration, top left, D). Staining with tau reveals neuronal inclusions (arrow) and tufted astrocytes (circles) (E).

Corticobasal Degeneration (FTLD-tau, CBD)

Corticobasal degeneration (CBD, Figure 7), or FTLD-tau (CBD), is another disease of cognitive decline or movement disorder or both, presenting classically with progressive, asymmetric movement and upper motor neuron dysfunction with parkinsonism-like features, but can also present as FTD. The gross findings are often subtle and include atrophy of the superior frontal and parietal parasagittal regions, often asymmetric, with thinning of the corpus callosum and atrophy of the basal ganglia and substantia nigra.

Microscopically, there is neuronal loss and gliosis in the grossly affected areas as well as ballooned neurons in neocortex. Immunostaining with antibodies to phosphorylated tau or 4R tau highlights globose neurofibrillary tangles in the enlarged neurons, coiled bodies in oligodendrocytes, and threads in the gray and white matter. The threads in CBD are much more numerous than in PSP. The key histologic feature is the astrocytic plaque which is an accumulation of phosphorylated 4R tau within the distal astrocytic processes creating a void near the nucleus [19].

Frontotemporal Lobar Degeneration with TDP-43 Proteinopathy (FTLD-TDP)

The discovery that TAR DNA binding protein 43 (TDP-43, encoded by *TARDBP*) was the major protein component of the ubiquitinated inclusions in FTLD-U occurred in 2006 and FTLD-TDP (Figure 8) is now considered to be the most common type of FTLD [20, 21]. Grossly, FTLD-TDP brains have atrophy of the frontal and temporal lobes as well as the caudate nucleus, and pallor of the substantia nigra (usually greater than that of the locus coeruleus). Routine histologic examination demonstrates superficial microvacuolation with neuronal loss and gliosis of the cortex and associated white matter rarefaction.

TDP-43, which has roles in DNA/RNA processing, is normally transported back and forth between the nucleus and cytoplasm but is primarily found, on immunohistochemical staining of brains of normal subjects using an antibody to non-phosphorylated TDP-43, to be diffusely distributed in the nucleus. In FTLD-TDP, the protein is ubiquitinated and phosphorylated, and inclusions are found within neuronal cytoplasm, dendrites, and glia, and infrequently in neuronal nuclei as "cat-eye" or lentiform inclusions. It is unclear whether the pathology is due to loss of function of the protein's normal roles or a gain of function due to the insoluble aggregates of abnormal TDP-43 in cells and cellular processes [22].

The current harmonized classification system for FTLD-TDP divides the disease into four different types, A through D, depending on the inclusion location, morphology, and frequency [16]. The four different types are also commonly associated with characteristic clinical presentations and genetic aberrations.

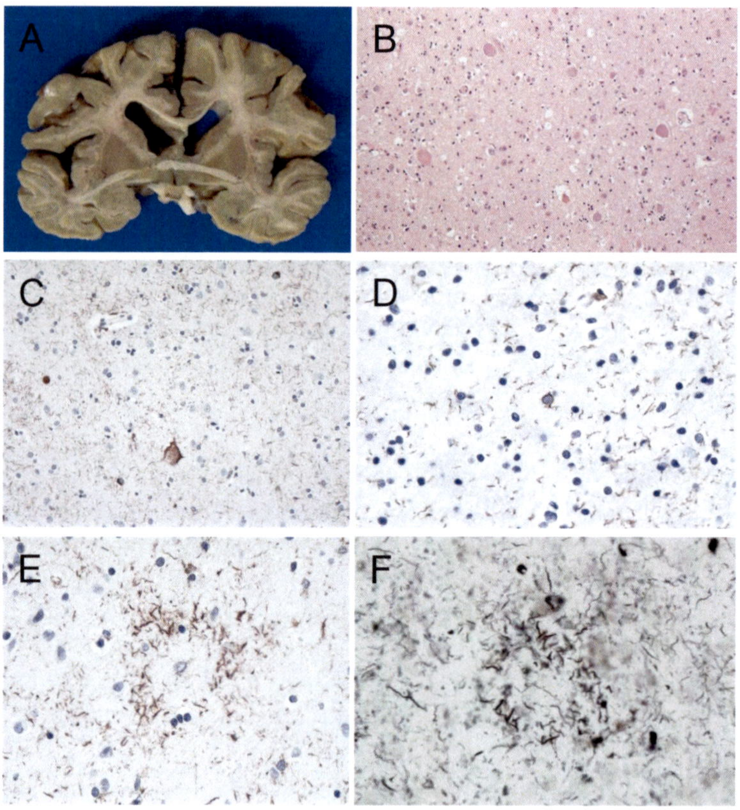

Figure 7. Cortical atrophy in FTLD-tau (CBD) is subtle but ventricular dilatation is often seen (A). Ballooned neurons are present in a background of neuronal loss and gliosis (B). Tau labels ballooned neurons and cortical threads (C) as well as white matter threads and glial inclusions (D), and astrocytic plaques (E). Silver stain also highlights astrocytic plaques (Gallyas, F).

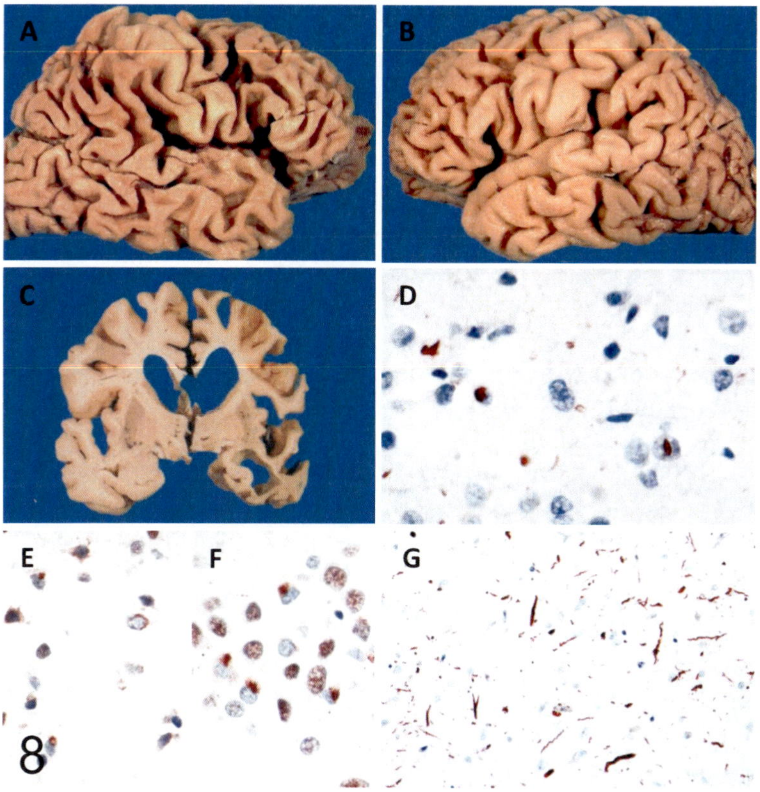

Figure 8. FTLD-TDP cases may have asymmetric cortical atrophy. This case has severe atrophy of the right hemisphere (A) and mild to moderate atrophy of the left hemisphere (B). The disparity is best appreciated on side to side comparison of coronal sections that also demonstrate variation in ventricular dilatation (C). TDP-43 positive inclusions consist of neuronal cytoplasmic (NCIs) and intranuclear inclusions (NIIs), and long or short dystrophic neurites (DNs) which vary by location and frequency in the four common types of disease. Type A cases (D) have NCIs, NIIs and short DNs. Type B cases may have granular cytoplasmic inclusions (E) and NCIs of the dentate gyrus (F). Type C cases have long DNs (G). Reprinted from EH Bigio, Making the Diagnosis of Frontotemporal Lobar Degeneration. *Arch Pathol Lab Med.* 2013; 137(3): 314-25 with permission from *Archives of Pathology and Laboratory Medicine*.

Type A has many neuronal cytoplasmic inclusions and many short dystrophic neurites, as well as sparse intranuclear inclusions, predominantly in layer 2 of the cortex. This type is associated with bvFTD and progressive non-fluent aphasia (PNFA), and familial cases may have *GRN* mutations [23, 24].

Type B has moderate neuronal cytoplasmic inclusions and few dystrophic neurites in all cortical layers. This type is most often seen in bvFTD and in motor neuron disease with frontotemporal degeneration. Familial cases are associated with an intronic mutation resulting in expansion of a GGGGCC hexanucleotide repeat in *C9ORF72* found on the short arm of chromosome 9 [25, 26].

Type C has many long dystrophic neurites and few neuronal cytoplasmic inclusions predominantly in layer 2 of the cortex. Patients often present with semantic dementia or occasionally with bvFTD. This type is usually sporadic.

Type D has many lentiform and round neuronal intranuclear inclusions, short dystrophic neurites, and few neuronal cytoplasmic inclusions in all cortical layers. This type is seen in Familial Inclusion Body Myopathy with Paget's Disease of Bone and Frontotemporal Dementia (IBMPFD) and virtually all cases are associated with VCP mutations [27].

FTLD-FUS

FTLD-FUS (Figure 9) is a rare group of pathologic diagnoses that include Neuronal Intermediate Filament Inclusion Disease (NIFID), Basophilic Inclusion Body Disease (BIBD), and atypical FTLD with ubiquitin-immunoreactive inclusions (aFTLD-U) [15, 17]. Each disease has slightly different gross and pathologic findings.

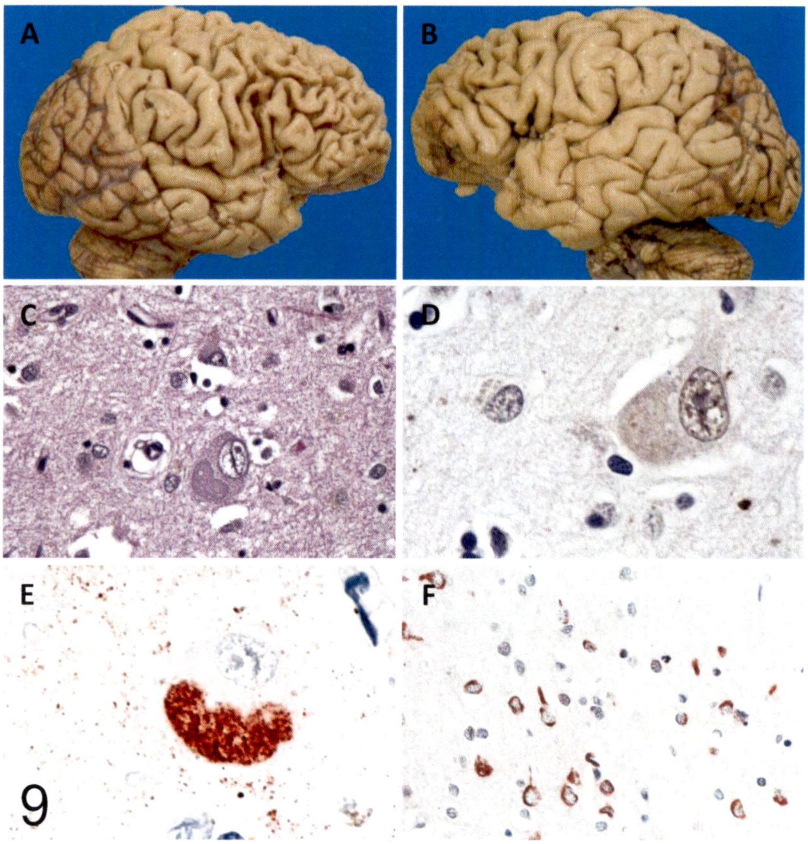

Figure 9. FTLD-FUS cases are rare. An example of BIBD type shows asymmetric atrophy of frontal cortex, which is moderate to severe on the right (A) and mild on the left (B). Basophilic inclusions can sometimes be seen on H & E (C) and are positive with ubiquitin (D) and FUS (E) immunohistochemical stains. Reprinted from EH Bigio, Making the Diagnosis of Frontotemporal Lobar Degeneration. *Arch Pathol Lab Med.* 2013; 137(3): 314-25 with permission from *Archives of Pathology and Laboratory Medicine*.

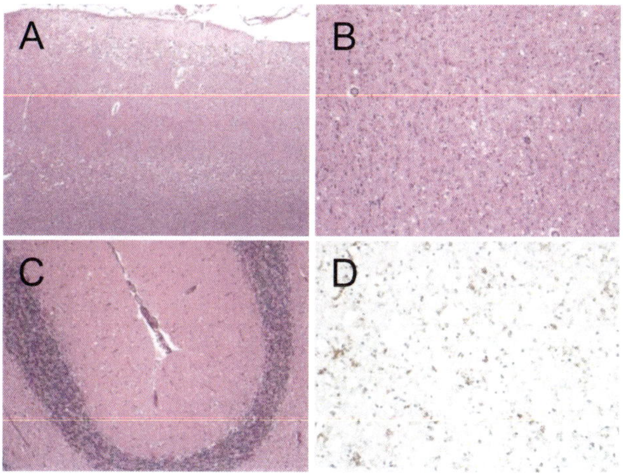

Figure 10. CJD has neuronal loss and gliosis with associated vacuoles in cortical gray matter called spongiform change, sometimes transcortical, and sometimes in a laminar distribution, as shown here in the occipital lobe (A). Spongiform change and gliosis can also affect the deep gray matter (thalamus shown here in B) and the cerebellum (C). Immunohistochemical stain for prion protein (PrPSc) highlights abnormal prion aggregates in a synaptic type perivacuolar pattern (D).

FTLD-FUS (NIFID) grossly shows frontotemporal atrophy with marked atrophy of the caudate nucleus and marked ventricular dilatation. Microscopically, in affected areas, there is neuronal loss and gliosis. Staining with antibodies to ubiquitin, p62, FUS and class IV intermediate filaments, as well as silver stains such as Bielchowsky highlight the neuronal cytoplasmic inclusions. FUS positive glial cytoplasmic inclusions and "vermiform" neuronal intranuclear inclusions (NIIs) are also seen.

FTLD-FUS (BIBD) also grossly demonstrates frontotemporal atrophy with involvement of the striatum, thalamus and amygdala. Again, neuronal loss and gliosis in the affected areas is seen, and may be severe. Basophilic inclusion bodies, for which the category is named, are also seen on routine H & E stains and are present in the cortex, striatum, subthalamic nucleus, nucleus basalis of Meynert, and gray matter of the midbrain and spinal cord. Many more cytoplasmic inclusions are seen with FUS immunostains, and vermiform NIIs may also be seen.

In atypical FTLD-U (aFTLD-U), the atrophy of the frontotemporal regions and striatum is severe corresponding to severe neuronal loss and gliosis. p62, ubiquitin, and FUS immunohistochemistry demonstrates neuronal cytoplasmic inclusions, and vermiform NIIs are seen with FUS.

PRION DISEASE

The most common cause of rapidly progressive dementia is prion disease. Prion protein, PrP, which is encoded in the *PRNP* gene, when misfolded is capable of altering the conformation of adjacent proteins to cause one of several diseases including sporadic diseases such as Creutzfeldt-Jakob Disease (CJD) and fatal sporadic insomnia, hereditary diseases such as Gerstmann-Straussler-Scheinker disease and fatal familial insomnia, and zoonotic disease such as bovine spongiform encephalopathy and scrapie [28]. Misfolded prion protein is considered infectious as it is transmissible between subjects of the same or different species. Some proteins involved in neurodegenerative disease such as TDP-43 are said to have prion-like domains, which may be involved in disease propagation [29].

The most common type of prion disease is sporadic CJD (Figure 10), which accounts for up to 95% of rapidly progressive dementia cases. When clinical suspicion is high, the pathology department should be alerted due to the potentially infectious quality of the disease. Special precautions for brain retrieval, and tissue transport and processing are used with the use of formic acid to "inactivate" prion protein [30]. Gross examination demonstrates a wide spectrum of findings from normal for the decedent's age to severe atrophy of the cerebrum and cerebellum. Microscopically, there is spongiform change of gray matter with associated neuronal loss and gliosis. Congophilic amyloid plaques may also be seen. Immunohistochemical stains are valuable in the diagnosis of CJD and other prion diseases, highlighting the abnormal protein deposition.

Summary

Our understanding of neurodegenerative disease is quickly evolving. Currently, many pathologic entities are seen in patients with cognitive impairment, each pathologic entity with its own unique distribution of abnormal protein aggregates, the most common of which have been discussed above. More than one concomitant neurodegenerative disease can also exist within a single patient. The prospect of future discoveries and further comprehension of the pathways in neurodegenerative disease is not only academically and clinically exciting, but will be necessary for the development of treatments and prevention of disease in our aging population.

References

[1] Montine, TJ; Phelps, CH; Beach, TG; Bigio, EH; Cairns, NJ, Dickson DW, et al. National Institute on Aging-Alzheimer's Association guidelines for the neuropathologic assessment of Alzheimer's disease: a practical approach. *Acta Neuropathol.*, 2012, 123(1), 1-11.

[2] Mesulam, MM; Weintraub, S; Rogalski, EJ; Wieneke, C; Geula, C; Bigio, EH. Asymmetry and heterogeneity of Alzheimer's and frontotemporal pathology in primary progressive aphasia. *Brain.*, 2014, 137(Pt 4), 1176-92.

[3] Jakes, R; Novak, M; Davison, M; Wischik, CM. Identification of 3- and 4-repeat tau isoforms within the PHF in Alzheimer's disease. *EMBO J.*, 1991, 10(10), 2725-9.

[4] Iqbal, K; Alonso, AC; Gong, CX; Khatoon, S; Singh, TJ; Grundke-Iqbal, I. Mechanism of neurofibrillary degeneration in Alzheimer's disease. *Mol Neurobiol.*, 1994, 9(1-3), 119-23.

[5] Huse, JT; Doms, RW. Closing in on the amyloid cascade: recent insights into the cell biology of Alzheimer's disease. *Mol Neurobiol.*, 2000, 22(1-3), 81-98.

[6] Bigio, EH. Making the diagnosis of frontotemporal lobar degeneration. *Arch Pathol Lab Med.*, 2013, 137(3), 314-25.
[7] Terry, RD; Masliah, E; Salmon, DP; Butters, N; DeTeresa, R; Hill, R; et al. Physical basis of cognitive alterations in Alzheimer's disease: synapse loss is the major correlate of cognitive impairment. *Ann Neurol.*, 1991, 30(4), 572-80.
[8] Parkkinen, L; Pirttila, T; Alafuzoff, I. Applicability of current staging/categorization of alpha-synuclein pathology and their clinical relevance. *Acta Neuropathol.*, 2008, 115(4), 399-407.
[9] Parkkinen, L; Soininen, H; Alafuzoff, I. Regional distribution of alpha-synuclein pathology in unimpaired aging and Alzheimer disease. *J Neuropathol Exp Neurol.*, 2003, 62(4), 363-7.
[10] Josephs, KA; Murray, ME; Whitwell, JL; Parisi, JE; Petrucelli, L; Jack, CR; et al. Staging TDP-43 pathology in Alzheimer's disease. *Acta Neuropathol.*, 2014, 127(3), 441-50.
[11] McKeith, IG; Dickson, DW; Lowe, J; Emre, M; O'Brien, JT; Feldman, H; et al. Diagnosis and management of dementia with Lewy bodies: third report of the DLB Consortium. *Neurology.*, 2005, 65(12), 1863-72.
[12] McKeith, IG. Consensus guidelines for the clinical and pathologic diagnosis of dementia with Lewy bodies (DLB): report of the Consortium on DLB International Workshop. *J Alzheimers Dis.*, 2006, 9(3 Suppl), 417-23.
[13] Alafuzoff, I; Ince, PG; Arzberger, T; Al-Sarraj, S; Bell, J; Bodi, I; et al. Staging/typing of Lewy body related alpha-synuclein pathology: a study of the BrainNet Europe Consortium. *Acta Neuropathol.*, 2009, 117(6), 635-52.
[14] Ratnavalli, E; Brayne, C; Dawson, K; Hodges, JR. The prevalence of frontotemporal dementia. *Neurology.*, 2002, 58(11), 1615-21.
[15] Mackenzie, IR; Neumann, M; Bigio, EH; Cairns, NJ; Alafuzoff, I; Kril, J; et al. Nomenclature and nosology for neuropathologic subtypes of frontotemporal lobar degeneration: an update. *Acta Neuropathol.*, 2010, 119(1), 1-4.
[16] Mackenzie, IR; Neumann, M; Baborie, A; Sampathu, DM; Du Plessis, D; Jaros, E; et al. A harmonized classification system for FTLD-TDP pathology. *Acta Neuropathol.*, 2011, 122(1), 111-3.
[17] Lashley, T; Rohrer, JD; Mead, S; Revesz, T. Review: An update on clinical, genetic and pathological aspects of frontotemporal lobar degenerations. *Neuropathol Appl Neurobiol.*, 2015.
[18] Dickson, DW. Neuropathology of Pick's disease. *Neurology.*, 2001, 56(11 Suppl 4), S16-20.
[19] Dickson, DW; Kouri, N; Murray, ME; Josephs, KA. Neuropathology of frontotemporal lobar degeneration-tau (FTLD-tau). *J Mol Neurosci.*, 2011, 45(3), 384-9.
[20] Neumann, M; Sampathu, DM; Kwong, LK; Truax, AC; Micsenyi, MC; Chou, TT; et al. Ubiquitinated TDP-43 in frontotemporal lobar degeneration and amyotrophic lateral sclerosis. *Science.*, 2006, 314(5796), 130-3.
[21] Arai, T; Hasegawa, M; Akiyama, H; Ikeda, K; Nonaka, T; Mori, H; et al. TDP-43 is a component of ubiquitin-positive tau-negative inclusions in frontotemporal lobar degeneration and amyotrophic lateral sclerosis. *Biochem Biophys Res Commun.*, 2006, 351(3), 602-11.

[22] Halliday, G; Bigio, EH; Cairns, NJ; Neumann, M; Mackenzie, IR; Mann, DM. Mechanisms of disease in frontotemporal lobar degeneration: gain of function versus loss of function effects. *Acta Neuropathol.*, 2012, 124(3), 373-82.

[23] Baker, M; Mackenzie, IR; Pickering-Brown, SM; Gass, J; Rademakers, R; Lindholm, C; et al. Mutations in progranulin cause tau-negative frontotemporal dementia linked to chromosome 17. *Nature.*, 2006, 442(7105), 916-9.

[24] Cruts, M; Gijselinck, I; van der Zee, J; Engelborghs, S; Wils, H; Pirici, D; et al. Null mutations in progranulin cause ubiquitin-positive frontotemporal dementia linked to chromosome 17q21. *Nature.*, 2006, 442(7105), 920-4.

[25] DeJesus-Hernandez, M; Mackenzie, IR; Boeve, BF; Boxer, AL; Baker, M; Rutherford, NJ; et al. Expanded GGGGCC hexanucleotide repeat in noncoding region of C9ORF72 causes chromosome 9p-linked FTD and ALS. *Neuron.*, 2011, 72(2), 245-56.

[26] Renton, AE; Majounie, E; Waite, A; Simon-Sanchez, J; Rollinson, S; Gibbs, JR; et al. A hexanucleotide repeat expansion in C9ORF72 is the cause of chromosome 9p21-linked ALS-FTD. *Neuron.*, 2011, 72(2), 257-68.

[27] Watts, GD; Wymer, J; Kovach, MJ; Mehta, SG; Mumm, S; Darvish, D; et al. Inclusion body myopathy associated with Paget disease of bone and frontotemporal dementia is caused by mutant valosin-containing protein. *Nat Genet.*, 2004, 36(4), 377-81.

[28] Head, MW; Ironside, JW. Review: Creutzfeldt-Jakob disease: prion protein type, disease phenotype and agent strain. *Neuropathol Appl Neurobiol.*, 2012, 38(4), 296-310.

[29] Prusiner, SB. Biology and genetics of prions causing neurodegeneration. *Annu Rev Genet.*, 2013, 47, 601-23.

[30] Brown, P; Wolff, A; Gajdusek, DC. A simple and effective method for inactivating virus infectivity in formalin-fixed tissue samples from patients with Creutzfeldt-Jakob disease. *Neurology.*, 1990, 40(6), 887-90.

In: Progressive Cognitive Impairment …
Editor: Gediminas Peter Gliebus
ISBN: 978-1-63485-221-0

Chapter 2

IMAGING AND CEREBROSPINAL FLUID BIOMARKERS IN ALZHEIMER'S DISEASE AND LEWY BODY SPECTRUM DISORDERS

Usman Saeed,[1,2] Sandra E. Black [1,2,3,4,5] and Mario Masellis[1,2,3,5,6,*]

[1]Institute of Medical Science, Faculty of Medicine, University of Toronto, Toronto, Canada
[2]L.C. Campbell Cognitive Neurology Research Unit, Sunnybrook Health Sciences Centre, Toronto, Canada
[3]Department of Medicine, Division of Neurology, Sunnybrook Health Sciences Centre, University of Toronto, Toronto, Canada
[4]Heart and Stroke Foundation Canadian Partnership for Stroke Recovery, Toronto, Canada
[5]Hurvitz Brain Sciences Research Program
[6]Cognitive and Movement Disorders Clinic, Sunnybrook Health Sciences Centre, Toronto, Canada

ABSTRACT

Alzheimer's disease (AD) and Lewy body spectrum disorders (LBD) are the most common incurable neurodegenerative morbidities in the elderly with momentous global health burden. Despite great advances in neurodegenerative research over the past decade, the definitive diagnosis of these disorders rests upon neuropathological examination. In clinical practice, however, an accurate early diagnosis is vital to accommodate differential prognostic and disease management approaches as well as to assess the efficacy of drugs in clinical trials. This goal can be challenging to achieve due

[*]Corresponding author: Dr. Mario Masellis, Cognitive & Movement Disorders Clinic, Sunnybrook Health Sciences Centre, 2075 Bayview Ave., Room A4-55, Toronto, Ontario, Canada, M4N 3M5, Tel.: 416-480-4661, ext. 89351 Mario.Masellis@sunnybrook.ca.

to substantial heterogeneity observed in these disorders in terms of disease presentation and progression. To aid in this quest, a range of imaging and cerebrospinal (CSF) biomarkers are actively being explored. Imaging biomarkers are exciting as they can allow a 'window' into the human brain and help visualize the structural or functional abnormalities. On the other hand, CSF biomarkers can be helpful in identifying the underlying mechanistic or dynamic biochemical alterations among the disorders. This chapter will present an overview of well-established and promising imaging and CSF biomarkers with emphasis on their distinguishing features in AD and LBD. Structural magnetic resonance imaging (MRI) will be explored to identify biomarkers of cerebral atrophy (cross-sectional volumetric patterns and longitudinal atrophy rates), medial temporal lobe and other subcortical structures as well as small vessel disease. The role of diffusion tensor imaging as a potential biomarker will be investigated to assess its utility in identifying white matter tract injury, integrity and microstructural abnormalities. Positron emission tomography will be examined along with a variety of different radiotracers to identify alterations in tissue glucose metabolism and cerebral amyloid loads. Biomarkers in single photon emission computed tomography will be presented to assess cerebral perfusion differences. Roles of proton magnetic resonance spectroscopy, resting-state and task-based functional MRI and myocardial scintigraphy techniques will also be highlighted. Finally, an overview of commonly implicated CSF biomarkers will be surveyed. Although imaging, fluid and other biomarkers have their respective strengths and weaknesses, a combination of different biomarkers to aid in the differential diagnosis seems promising. This 'multimodal approach' may eventually be able to provide powerful ways of measuring disease progression and therapeutic responses to drugs. More research is needed to further refine the measurement techniques, standardize research protocols and to understand the underlying pathological mechanisms in order to improve the diagnostic sensitivity and specificity of these devastating disorders.

GLOSSARY

$[^{123}I]$MIBG	$[^{123}I]$Metaiodobenzylguanidine
^{11}C-PIB	^{11}C-labelled Pittsburgh compound-B
^{123}I-FP-CIT	^{123}I-2β-carbometoxy-3β-(4-iodophenyl)-*N*-(3-fluoropropyl) nortropane
^{123}I-IMP	*N*-isopropyl-p-$[^{123}I]$iodoamphetamine
^{123}I-β-CIT	^{123}I-β-carbomethoxy-3ss-(4-iodophenyl) tropane
^{18}F-FDG	^{18}F-labelled fluorodeoxyglucose
^{1}H-MRS	Proton (^{1}H) magnetic resonance spectroscopy
^{99m}Tc-ECD	^{99m}Tc-ethyl cysteinate dimer
^{99m}Tc-HMPAO	^{99m}Tc-hexamethylpropyleneamineoxime
AD	Alzheimer's disease
ADC	Apparent diffusion coefficient
APOE ε4	Apolipoprotein-E ε4 allele
APP	Amyloid precursor protein
Aβ	Amyloid-beta
$A\beta_{40}$	Amyloid-beta, 40-residue peptide
$A\beta_{42}$	Amyloid-beta, 42-residue peptide
$A\beta_{42}^{*}$	Oxidized version of amyloid-beta, 42-residue peptide
BOLD	Blood-oxygen-level dependent

CA1	Cornu ammonis-1
CAA	Cerebral amyloid angiopathy
CBF	Cerebral blood flow
CIS	Cingulate island sign
Cr	Creatine
CSF	Cerebrospinal fluid
$\bar{D}$	Mean diffusivity
DLB	Dementia with Lewy bodies
DMN	Default mode network
DTI	Diffusion tensor imaging
FA	Fractional anisotropy
FC	Functional connectivity
FLAIR	Fluid-attenuated inversion recovery
fMRI	Functional magnetic resonance imaging
GM	Gray matter
H/M Ratio	Heart to mediastinum count ratio
LBD	Lewy body spectrum disorders
MCI	Mild cognitive impairment
MMSE	Mini-mental status examination
MP4A	*N*-[^{11}C]-methyl-4-piperidyl acetate
MRI	Magnetic resonance imaging
MSA	Multiple system atrophy
MTL	Medial temporal lobe
NAA	*N*-acetyl aspartate
NFTs	Neurofibrillary tangles
PCC	Posterior cingulate cortex
PD	Parkinson's disease
PDD	Parkinson's disease dementia
PET	Positron emission tomography
PFC	Prefrontal cortex
PSP	Progressive nuclear palsy
p-tau	Phosphorylated-tau
ROI	Region of interest
SPECT	Single-photon emission computed tomography
SPs	Senile plaques
T1	T1-weighted
T2	T2-weighted
t-tau	Total-tau
VaD	Vascular dementia
WM	White matter
WMH	White matter hyperintensities
αSyn	α-synuclein.

1. INTRODUCTION

Alzheimer's disease (AD) is the most common form of neurodegenerative dementia with momentous global health burden. AD is neuropathologically characterized by the presence of extracellular amyloid-beta (Aβ) plaques, intracellular neurofibrillary tangles (NFTs) composed of hyperphosphorylated tau protein, and cerebral amyloid angiopathy (CAA) at post-mortem examination **(Figure 1)** [1, 2]. These characteristic lesions, identified as the neuropathological hallmarks of AD, lead to neurotransmitter dysfunctions, of which cholinergic deficits are often the most profound. These abnormalities in neurotransmission are closely or contemporarily followed by neuronal loss in the medial temporal lobe (MTL) region of the brain early in the course of AD [2, 3]. This complex interplay of protein pathology, neuronal degeneration and synaptic dysfunction lead to the clinical symptoms of AD, of which memory loss is usually the most prominent and earliest symptom in the majority of AD patients. Although other cognitive domains, such as language and visuospatial functions, can be affected earlier in atypical AD presentations, such cases are less common [4].

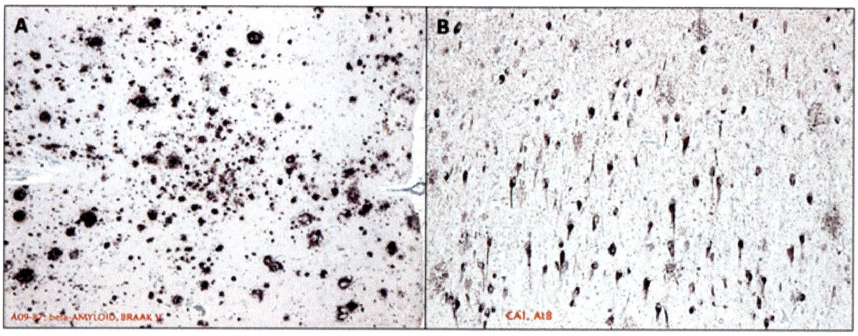

Figure 1. Histological staining of microscopic Alzheimer's disease pathology showing (A) astrocytic amyloid-beta plaques in frontal regions of the brain, and (B) neurofibrillary tangles in the CA1 region of the hippocampus.

Lewy body spectrum disorders (LBD) are the second most common group of heterogeneous neurodegenerative syndromes that share clinical features of parkinsonism, dementia, fluctuations in attention and alertness, as well as visual hallucinations [5-7]. LBD include dementia with Lewy bodies (DLB) and Parkinson's disease (PD) with and without dementia (PDD). LBD are neuropathologically characterized by the presence of intraneuronal inclusions (called Lewy bodies) containing abnormal aggregations of the α-synuclein (αSyn) protein **(Figure 2)** [5]. These Lewy bodies are preferentially distributed in the brain stem, limbic and/or neocortical structures [5, 6]. DLB and PDD are clinically differentiated from each other based on the time of onset of Parkinsonian symptoms relative to the development of dementia [5, 6]. The onset of dementia within 12 months of or contemporarily with motor symptoms qualifies as DLB; whereas in PDD, motor symptoms must precede the dementia by at least a year [5, 7]. Early diagnosis is important in LBD due to differential prognostic and disease management approaches [6]. For example, the avoidance of potentially life-threatening reactions to neuroleptic medications in DLB patients critically depends upon an accurate early diagnosis [8]. Although, AD and LBD are the most common causes of neurodegenerative dementias in the elderly, these and other cerebrovascular pathologies frequently co-occur and contribute to substantial heterogeneity in the disease presentation and progression [9]. To aid in the differential diagnosis of these dementias, a range of biomarkers are actively being explored.

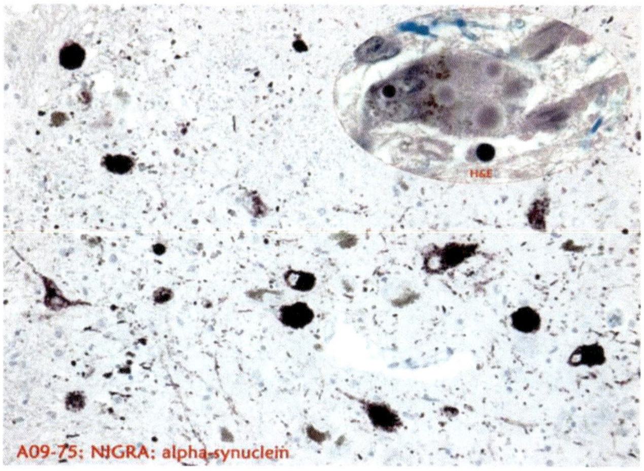

Figure 2. Histological staining of microscopic Lewy body pathology showing Lewy bodies, cytoplasmic stippling, neuropil grains and Lewy neurites immunostained by antibodies to α-synuclein.

A biomarker can be defined as a characteristic that is 'objectively measured and evaluated as an indicator of normal biology, pathological process or pharmacologic responses to a therapeutic intervention' [10]. In the context of neurodegenerative dementias, biomarkers can serve as sensitive and specific diagnostic tools in the early identification of the disease [11]. Biomarkers may assist in the treatment decision-making and show responsiveness to therapeutic interventions with measurable clinical outcomes [12]. In research settings, biomarkers may also aid in the screening of participants based on diagnostic or study-specific criteria. Biomarkers can be of different types: fluid-based measurements, such as phosphorylated-tau concentrations in the cerebrospinal fluid (CSF); or technically-derived neuroimaging correlates, such as reduced hippocampal volume as a surrogate for neuronal loss in structural magnetic resonance imaging (MRI) [11]. In this chapter, an overview of well-established and promising candidate biomarkers will be presented with emphasis on their distinguishing characteristics and patterns in AD and LBD.

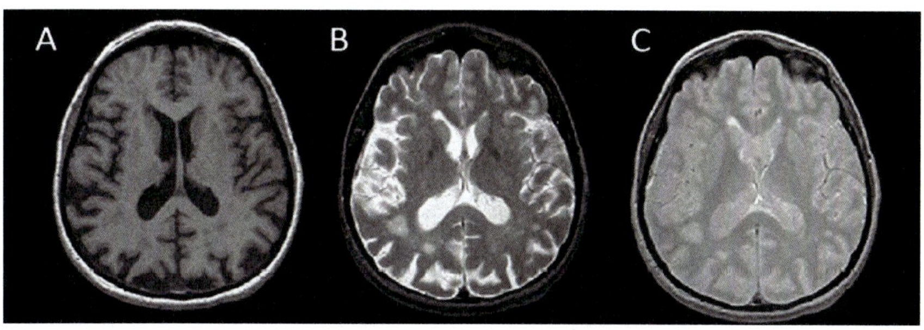

Figure 3. Axial views of the same slice as seen on a T1-weighted (A), T2-weighted (B), and proton density-weighted (C) magnetic resonance images.

2. Biomarkers Derived from Structural Magnetic Resonance Imaging (MRI) in AD and LBD

Conventional structural MRI uses T1-weighted (T1), T2-weighted (T2) and/or proton density-weighted sequences to derive regional or whole-brain volumetric changes **(Figure 3)**. The combination of these different sequences can provide a better contrast between the gray matter (GM), white matter (WM) and CSF, allowing for more precise tissue quantifications [13]. Several methods ranging from visual ratings to manual, automated and semi-automated segmentation techniques are routinely implemented to investigate whole-brain or *a priori* regions of interest (ROI) in terms of tissue volumetric or shape analyses. From an imaging biomarker prospective, quantification of structural changes, and patterns and rates of cerebral atrophy in cross-sectional and longitudinal designs have been of considerable interest.

2.1. Cross-sectional Profiles of Cerebral Atrophy

On structural MRI, AD is characterized by significant whole-brain and MTL atrophy compared with DLB, PDD, PD and normal controls [14-17]. MTL structures that include the hippocampus, parahippocampal gyrus, entorhinal cortex and amygdala, as well as the parietal lobe show significant thinning as compared to controls [11, 16]. DLB patients also show significant whole-brain atrophy, although to a lesser degree than in AD. Studies comparing atrophic patterns between AD and DLB found relatively focused atrophy of the midbrain, hypothalamus and substantia innominata in DLB with preservation of MTL, hippocampus and amygdala [18, 19]. Compared to normal controls, a diffuse pattern of cortical atrophy encompassing all four lobes was observed in PDD, which included temporal, occipital, right frontal and left parietal lobes; whereas, reduced GM volume involving the frontal lobes was prominent among PD patients [14]. When PDD and PD groups were directly compared, a greater GM atrophy in the occipital lobe was detected in PDD [14]. Therefore, based on this finding, partial volume effects due to neuronal loss may account for at least some of the occipital hypometabolism and hypoperfusion changes observed in LBD patients [20, 21]. Finally, pronounced cortical atrophy in temporal, parietal and occipital lobes was identified in DLB as compared to PDD groups, which is consistent with greater Aβ deposition as detected by positron emission tomography (PET) in DLB patients [15, 22, 23]. Interestingly, an association was also found between the duration of parkinsonism prior to dementia, and severity of cortical αSyn pathology and Aβ plaques. A more severe αSyn pathology along with plaque burden was associated with progressively shorter durations of PD prior to dementia onset, reinforcing a model with gradation of both αSyn and Aβ pathology across the LBD spectrum [24].

2.2. Longitudinal Rates of Cerebral Atrophy

Change in cerebral volume over a specific time period can be a powerful biomarker for monitoring disease progression and holds promise for tracking the therapeutic effects of disease-modifying therapies in clinical trials. Such MRI-based whole-brain or ROI atrophy rates can also serve as a surrogate for neuronal loss and may aid in diagnosis. Several longitudinal studies have assessed the rates of cerebral atrophy in AD and LBD. In AD, the annualized rate of brain atrophy is estimated at 2.4% versus 0.4% in normal controls [25]. A meta-analysis of nine studies estimated the annualized hippocampal atrophy rate at 4.7% in AD compared to 1.4% in normal controls [26]. A study by O'Brien et al. looked at the progressive brain atrophy on serial MRIs in DLB, AD and vascular dementia (VaD), and found the overall rates to be higher in dementia subjects than in controls [27]. In this study, although the differences between the three dementia subgroups were not statistically significant, the AD group had the highest rate (2%), followed by VaD (1.9%), DLB (1.4%) and then controls (0.5%) [27]. In a pathologically-proven AD sample, the rates of whole-brain atrophy (1.1%) and ventricular expansion (8.3%) were significantly greater compared with that of normal controls [28]. In a pure DLB group, these rates were not significantly different from normal controls; whereas in patients with mixed AD/DLB pathology, the rates were similar to those observed in the AD group (whole-brain atrophy rate of 1.3% and ventricular expansion of 7.2%) [28]. This suggests that αSyn pathology by itself may not result in significant global neuronal loss and that concomitant AD-type pathology is likely driving the loss of brain volume in these subjects, at least in earlier disease stages. In a comparison of annual brain atrophy rates in PD, PDD and controls, Burton et al. found rates to be elevated in PDD (1.1%) compared to PD (0.3%) and controls (0.3%) [29]. The whole-brain atrophy rate can be a robust longitudinal biomarker in AD subjects, and its utility in clinically-diagnosed DLB patients is limited by mixed pathologies. Further investigations with pathologically-proven samples are needed to precisely determine the cerebral atrophy rates in LBD.

2.3. Atrophy Patterns in Medial Temporal Lobe Structures

The medial temporal lobe (MTL) is an important MRI biomarker not only in AD, but also in LBD. The relative preservation of MTL is a consistent finding in DLB and PDD, and its atrophy is strongly suggestive of AD-type pathology. In fact, MTL atrophy on MRI was determined to be a highly accurate diagnostic marker of autopsy-confirmed AD (sensitivity 91% and specificity 94%) [30]. A review of atrophy patterns seen in AD and LBD across different MTL structures will now be presented.

2.3.1. Hippocampus

The hippocampus is a MTL structure with crucial roles in long-term memory storage and retrieval, and is one of the earliest sites of neuropathological involvement in AD [2]. The post-mortem examination of hippocampus in AD patients reveals patterns of Aβ deposition and progressive neurofibrillary changes across the different neuronal layers [2]. Structural MRI can be used to segment hippocampus as a specific ROI to investigate its volume and/or shape **(Figure 4)**. Such structural MRI studies have recognized smaller hippocampal volume as a robust imaging biomarker in AD patients [31, 32]. In contrast, the relative preservation of hippocampal volume in DLB compared to AD has been a consistent MRI finding, which has been incorporated into the revised DLB diagnostic criteria as a supportive feature [5, 19]. Other studies have examined sub-regional volumetric changes in the hippocampus. These studies have identified the cornu ammonis-1 (CA1) area of hippocampus to be smaller in AD, with relative preservation of CA1 in DLB and controls [33, 34]. The subiculum thickness was also found to be reduced in AD compared to controls and DLB [33]. Barber at al. investigated volumetric changes in MTL structures between AD and DLB groups, and identified hippocampal (and parahippocampal) volumes to be larger in DLB across the entire length of hippocampus [35]. Similarly, Camicioli et al. also found hippocampal volumes to be smaller in the patient groups, with a characteristic pattern: AD < PDD < PD < Controls [36]. In a recent cross-sectional study using ultra-high-field 7T MRI, the CA1 apical neuropil layer of the hippocampus was found to be thinner in mild AD subjects as compared to normal controls, with no change in the CA1 cell body layer or entire CA1 subfield [37]. At 7T field strength, the total hippocampal volumes did not differentiate between the mild AD and controls, but this higher resolution allowed for a sub-regional analysis of the CA1 neuropil layer, which was detected to be preferentially affected in mild AD patients versus controls [37]. Lastly, many studies have consistently associated the apolipoprotein-E ε4 allele (*APOE* ε4) with smaller hippocampal volumes in AD, which necessitates careful considerations in designing clinical trials [38, 39].

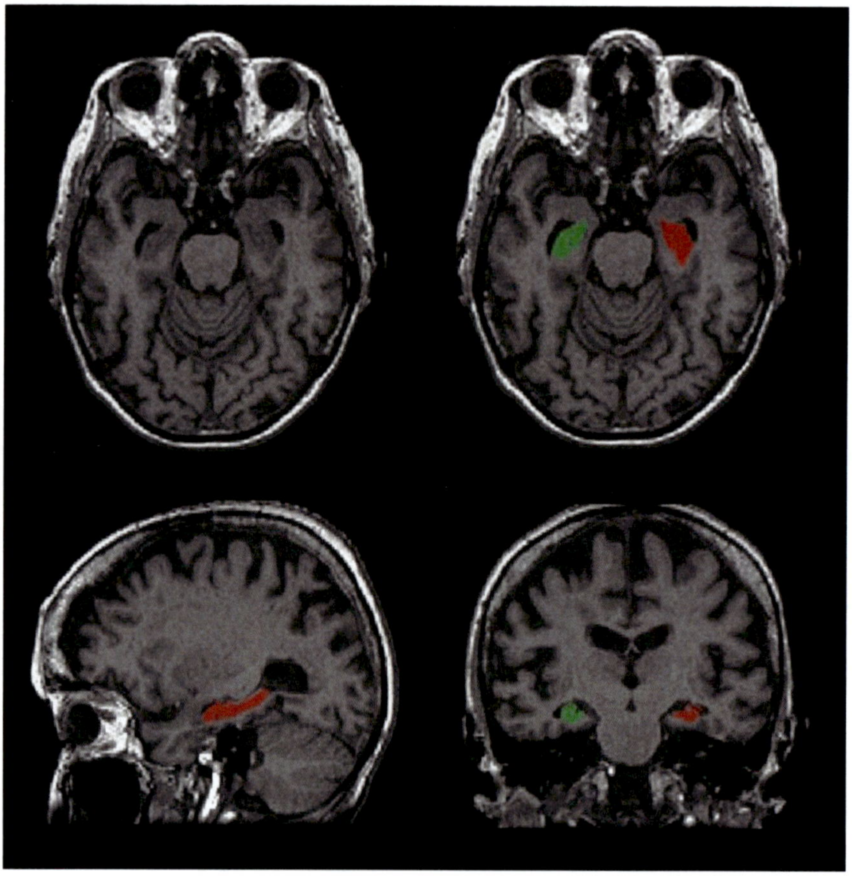

Figure 4. Hippocampal segmentation mask is overlayed on its T1-weighted image and displayed as a specific region of interest in axial (top-right), saggital (bottom-left) and coronal views (bottom-right) of the same patient.

Many studies examining the total or sub-regional hippocampal volumetric differences lack neuropathological confirmation, and differ in segmentation techniques and field strengths. Although 7T MRI may provide better resolution to detect early neurodegenerative changes, its clinical utility is currently limited as 7T MRIs are not used for clinical purposes and these high field strengths present greater susceptibility to motion artefacts. The CA1 hippocampal subfield may emerge as a sensitive biomarker; however, more research is needed to address the aforementioned limitations.

2.3.2. Entorhinal Cortex

The entorhinal cortex is regarded as the convergence point of highly complex multimodal and unimodal information, which is delivered and received from the hippocampal formation [40]. When compared with controls, the total entorhinal cortex volumes were found to be smaller in AD (21.9%), DLB (19.9%) and PDD (14.7%) subjects [41]. Goldman et al. compared entorhinal cortex volumes in PDD and PD patients and found substantially smaller volumes in PDD despite similar hippocampal volumes in the two groups [42]. It is suggested that MRI-based entorhinal cortex volume may better differentiate PDD from PD, especially when the hippocampal volumes do not account for the presenting cognitive impairments. Further research is needed in this area before any firm conclusions can be drawn.

2.3.3. Subcortical Structures

In LBD, dopamine transporter loss in the basal ganglia due to nigrostriatal degeneration is prominent [6]. A study performed volumetric quantifications of striatal structures that included caudate and putamen in PD patients, after controlling for the effects of age and gender. Caudate and putamen volumes were found to be significantly reduced in the PD group versus normal controls [43]. Similarly, Cousins et al. reported putamen volumes to be smaller in DLB patients compared with AD and controls, with no significant volumetric differences between AD and controls [44]. In the caudate nucleus, however, other studies failed to detect volumetric differences in PD or DLB subjects [45, 46]. Atrophy in the caudate was suggested to be non-specific, possibly representing part of the generalized brain volumetric loss and affliction of the fronto-subcortical circuits [46]. Future investigations are needed to reconcile these findings.

2.4. White Matter Hyperintensities

White matter hyperintensities (WMHs) are common and may be present in as many as 90-96% of individuals aged 60 and older [47, 48]. WMHs appear as focal, multifocal or confluent regions of hyperintensity on T2, proton density-weighted or fluid-attenuated inversion recovery (FLAIR) images, with slight hypointensity on T1 scans **(Figure 5 and 6)** [49, 50]. These WMHs can further be subclassified as involving the periventricular and deep white matter. Although the precise etiology and role of WMHs on dementia expression remain a matter of debate, several studies have associated WMHs with cognitive and executive functions, information processing speed and gait disturbances [51-54]. Burton et al. assessed the progression of WMHs in clinically-diagnosed dementias, and found significantly greater baseline WMHs in AD, but not in DLB or PDD [55]. The progression of WM lesions was found to be associated with the degree of baseline WMHs, rather than the diagnosis or severity of dementia [55]. A study by Barber et al. analyzed WM changes in AD, VaD and

LBD, and reported severe periventricular and deep WMHs in all dementia groups as compared to controls [56]. In this study, WMH scores were significantly greater in VaD in comparison with AD and LBD [56]. A significantly greater WMH load was also reported in PDD compared with PD [57]. In another study using a semi-quantitative scale, Barber at al. identified periventricular WMHs to be associated with atrophic processes, whereas deep WMHs were proposed to be the result of ischaemic risk factors [58]. In a large meta-analysis, WMHs strongly predicted an increased risk of dementia, stroke, as well as death [59].

WMHs can potentially serve as intermediate biomarkers of disease progression and treatment efficacy in clinical trials. Because WMH load is associated with increased cerebrovascular risks, its utility in stroke and dementia as clinical end-points can be valuable, both in research and clinical settings [59]. WMH volume can be quantified reliably and non-invasively, and its value as a continuous trait may provide adequate statistical power to detect changes in the disease progression and therapeutic responses [59]. Further studies are needed to clarify the role of progression of WMHs in AD and LBD.

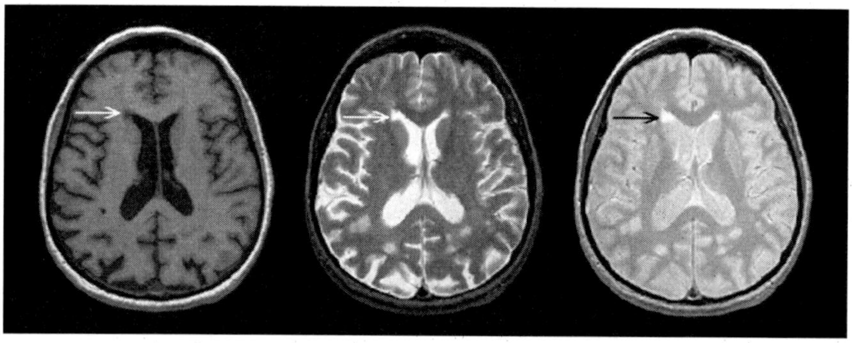

Figure 5. An example of periventricular white matter hyperintensities (arrow) as seen on the same axial slices on a T1-weighted (left), T2-weighted (middle), and proton density-weighted (right) magnetic resonance images. White matter hyperintensities appear as bright hyperintense regions on T2- and proton density-weighted images, with slight hypointensity on T1-weighted scans.

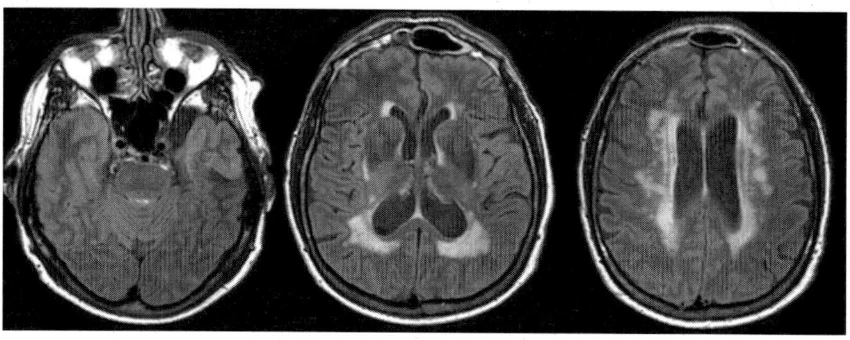

Figure 6. Fluid-attenuated inversion recovery (FLAIR) MRI of an elderly patient with vascular cognitive impairment due to cerebral small vessel disease [Adapted from Masellis et al. (2013)].

3. Biomarkers Derived from Diffusion Tensor Imaging (DTI) in AD and LBD

Diffusion tensor imaging (DTI) is an advanced neuroimaging technique that permits indirect measurements of brain microstructural integrity and enables elucidation of WM tracts in the brain circuitry [60, 61]. Using DTI, this tissue architectural information can be obtained by analyzing the overall displacement of water molecules in the brain (mean diffusivity), the degree of such displacement in space (anisotropy), as well as the direction of diffusivities [60]. Water tends to preferentially move along the underlying microstructural tracts and this physical property can be utilized in DTI to derive mean diffusivity ($\bar{D}$) and fractional anisotropy (FA) values, using whole-brain or ROI approaches. Several studies have reported the usefulness of DTI for examining tissue integrity, anatomical connectivity and pathophysiological mechanisms in DLB and AD.

Studies comparing AD with normal controls have reported higher $\bar{D}$ and lower FA in the corpus callosum and WM of temporal, frontal, parietal and occipital lobes of AD subjects [62-65]. Lower FA values in AD have also been consistently reported in the WM of MTL structures including the hippocampus, entorhinal cortex and parahippocampus, as well as in the temporal lobe and posterior cingulum [62, 63, 65, 66].

Firbank et al. compared DLB with AD showing decreased FA in the parietal lobe of DLB patients and increased apparent diffusion coefficient (ADC) in the left temporal lobe in AD [67]. In another study, Firbank et al. reported a bilateral region adjacent to the posterior cingulate cortex (PCC), where global atrophy correlated with FA in both AD and DLB [68]. This finding suggests that global atrophy may be associated with WM tract disruptions in PCC region. Bozzali et al. compared DLB with controls, and found WM abnormalities in the corpus callosum, frontal, parietal and occipital regions [69]. The selective involvement of these regions and less prominent temporal WM abnormalities align with the clinical and neuropsychological features of DLB. The same group also compared AD with controls, and found higher $\bar{D}$ and lower FA in the corpus callosum as well as in the WM of temporal, frontal and parietal lobes [62]. No difference in $\bar{D}$ and FA in occipital WM was detected between the two groups [62]. In DLB patients, Nedelska et al. showed reduced FA in parietooccipital WM compared to controls, and elevated FA in parahippocampal WM compared to AD – a finding that persisted after controlling for Aβ loads in the DLB group [70]. In terms of a biomarker viewpoint, DTI may have an important role as it may be employed to assess WM tract injury, integrity, early microarchitectural abnormalities, and to predict clinical outcomes. Further studies using standardized acquisition protocols and identical analytical methods are needed to further establish its validity, as well as to replicate and identify disease-specific signatures in AD and LBD.

4. Biomarkers Derived from Positron Emission Tomography (PET) in AD and LBD

Positron emission tomography (PET) is a functional neuroimaging technique that utilizes a variety of different radiotracers to visualize cerebral functions and pathological protein accumulation *in vivo* in neurodegenerative dementias. The brain Aβ burden has been widely assessed in AD and LBD using an ^{11}C-labelled thioflavin analogue, known as Pittsburgh compound-B (^{11}C-PIB), as well as other ^{18}F-labelled tracers that provide information independent from structural changes [71]. Cerebral glucose metabolism can be visualized using ^{18}F-labelled fluorodeoxyglucose radiotracer (^{18}F-FDG), where decreased local uptake is indicative of lower cerebral tissue metabolism. Their use in AD and LBD will now be discussed.

4.1. Role of FDG-PET

FDG-PET is a sensitive *in vivo* indicator of resting state metabolism and is reported to have a lower variability than standard neuropsychological measures across multiple centres [11, 72]. In AD, a consistent biparietotemporal hypometabolism is observed, including hypometabolism involving the precuneus and PCC [73, 74]. Using ^{18}F-FDG-PET, Gilman et al. compared local cerebral metabolism rates in AD and DLB, and found similar patterns of cerebral hypometabolism between the two groups except in the visual cortex, where the DLB group showed lower glucose metabolism in comparison with AD [20]. A multi-centered study replicated these findings in a larger sample and also indicated reduced ^{18}F-FDG uptake in hippocampus in AD [75]. The addition of hippocampal hypometabolism improved diagnostic specificity of AD from both DLB and frontotemporal dementia patients [75]. DLB and PDD patients both showed similar patterns of hypometabolism in the bilateral inferior, medial frontal and right parietal lobes, in comparison with PD patients [76]. These findings further highlight similar neurobiological mechanisms among DLB and PDD patients. When DLB and PDD groups were directly compared, hypometabolism in the anterior cingulate became prominent in DLB [76]. In a more recent investigation, Lim et al. compared the utility of ^{18}F-FDG-PET with ^{123}I-β-carbomethoxy-3ss-(4-iodophenyl) tropane SPECT (^{123}I-β-CIT-SPECT) imaging for the differentiation of DLB from AD [77]. Compared to AD, patients with DLB showed hypometabolism in the lateral occipital cortex on ^{18}F-FDG-PET with sensitivity of 88%, but relative preservation of the mid and posterior cingulate gyrus with 100% specificity – this finding was termed the 'Cingulate Island Sign' (CIS) [77]. Although ^{123}I-β-CIT-SPECT outperformed ^{18}F-FDG-PET, the incorporation of CIS was suggested to optimize the diagnostic specificity in ^{18}F-FDG-PET for DLB versus AD [77, 78]. This CIS on ^{18}F-FDG-PET was not associated with fibrillary Aβ deposits, but rather correlated with lower Braak NFT stages among DLB patients [79]. Finally, in a comparison with *N*-isopropyl-p-[^{123}I]iodoamphetamine (^{123}I-IMP) SPECT, the ^{18}F-FDG-PET was reported to be superior in detecting functional changes in DLB brains [80].

FDG-PET is considered a stable and valid biomarker, but its wider applicability is limited by costs and availability [11]. Nevertheless, few studies have utilized FDG-PET to detect treatment responses to cholinergic enhancers [81, 82].

4.2. Role of Amyloid PET

Cortical amyloid load as detected by ^{11}C-PIB-PET was found to be markedly elevated in AD as compared to DLB and controls, and these amyloidogenic changes tend to progress during the course of AD [83-85]. However, in another study, mean brain ^{11}C-PIB binding was found to be increased in 80% of DLB patients within the cingulum and striatal regions as compared to controls, while normal values were found in a PDD cohort [86]. The authors commented that the presence of amyloid pathology in DLB can contribute to the rapid progression of dementia in these patients [86]. Gomperts at al. also found the mean precuneus ^{11}C-PIB binding to be greater in DLB as compared to PD and PDD groups [87]. In general, studies find higher ^{11}C-PIB cortical binding in DLB than in PDD cohorts; whereas, other studies comparing DLB with PD/PDD do not find statistically significant differences [22, 23, 86, 88]. In these studies, similar trends in ^{11}C-PIB bindings were present: AD > DLB > PDD. The heterogeneity in results may be attributed to variability in the underlying pathological processes, such as the presence of mixed AD/LBD pathologies. Higher Aβ burden in DLB (versus low in PDD) may suggest an important role of Aβ in the timing of dementia onset relative to the motor symptoms and severity of cognitive impairments [88]. The occipital ^{11}C-PIB retention (relative to global cortical retention) was found to be lower in AD than in DLB, PDD or PD groups in a study [88]. Villemagne et al. utilized another amyloid tracer, ^{18}F-florbetaben, and found results comparable to ^{11}C-PIB demonstrating significantly greater neocortical binding in AD subjects compared to controls [23]. Most studies did not find ^{11}C-PIB binding to differ among PDD and PD subjects as compared to controls [89, 90]; however, when subjects were stratified into Aβ-positive and Aβ-negative scans based on a study-defined threshold, some studies showed higher proportions of Aβ-positive subjects in PDD groups [91, 92]. Post-mortem studies mirror these findings demonstrating greater Aβ deposition in DLB versus PDD or PD and in PDD versus PD [93, 94].

The presence of *APOE* ε4 was also associated with increased ^{11}C-PIB binding across AD, LBD and control groups and *APOE* ε4 prevalence was higher in Aβ-positive subjects as expected [84, 87, 92]. Using ^{11}C-PIB-PET, a study directly compared Aβ plaque loads in *APOE* ε4 carriers and non-carriers, and found more extensive ^{11}C-PIB binding bilaterally in temporoparietal and frontal cortices in *APOE* ε4 carriers [95]. It is suggested that *APOE* ε4 may independently influence the risk of dementia in PD, due to its association with the severity of cortical Lewy bodies and neurites [94]. In addition, several molecular and animal studies have supported the hypothesis of Aβ and αSyn synergism, suggesting increased propensity of αSyn to aggregate in the presence of Aβ, which further underscores *APOE* ε4 as a risk factor in synucleinopathies [96-99].

^{11}C-PIB-PET has a high sensitivity in detecting amyloid burden in AD, and may show promise as a therapeutic biomarker for drugs targeted at disrupting the cascade of amyloid aggregation. More studies are needed to assess its role in the onset and progression of cognitive symptoms in dementia [91]. An often-mentioned limitation of ^{11}C-PIB-PET is its non-specificity for neuritic plaques, as binding is also seen in those with diffuse plaques and CAA [91]. This may limit its replicability in neuropathological investigations that focus solely on neuritic plaques. Technical limitations include relatively lower resolution and less sensitivity in quantifying amyloid loads in *a priori* ROIs.

4.3. Role of Acetylcholine Esterase Activity on PET

A prominent cholinergic deficit is a feature of both AD and DLB, which is caused by neurodegeneration of cholinergic projections originating from the Nucleus Basalis of Meynert and the septal nuclei, as well as abnormalities in muscarinic and nicotinic receptors [100].

Cholinesterase inhibitors offer symptomatic improvements by inhibiting the breakdown of available acetylcholine into inactive choline and acetate metabolites [101]. Several radioligands have been developed to detect acetylcholine esterase and cholinergic receptor activity in AD and DLB; however, their efficacy as a biomarker is not yet proven [11]. A recent study using *N*-[^{11}C]-methyl-4-piperidyl acetate (MP4A) found significant reductions in acetylcholine esterase activity in DLB compared to AD in almost all volumes of interest [102]. Using the same radioligand, Bohnen at al. found donepezil induced reduction of 19.1% in acetylcholine esterase activity among mild AD patients, which correlated with improvement in neuropsychological performance [103]. These studies show potentially useful future applications, but further work is needed in this area to validate the biomarkers.

5. Biomarkers Derived from Single-Photon Emission Computed Tomography (SPECT) in AD and LBD

Single-photon emission computed tomography (SPECT) is an imaging technique that can be used to assess regional cerebral blood flow using gamma-emitting tracers, such as ^{99m}Tc-hexamethylpropyleneamineoxime (^{99m}Tc-HMPAO), ^{99m}Tc-ethyl cysteinate dimer (^{99m}Tc-ECD) (**Figure 7**) and ^{123}I-IMP [104]. These tracers are lipophilic and readily cross the blood brain barrier in a manner proportional to the cerebral flood flow allowing for both visual reads of tracer uptake and semi-quantification [104].

Using ^{99m}Tc-HMPAO as a tracer, Lobotesis et al. compared cerebral flood flow (CBF) among AD and DLB patients with SPECT [21]. Significant hypoperfusion was detected in frontal and medial temporal regions in AD, whereas the DLB group showed hypoperfusion in occipital areas compared to controls [21]. Upon direct comparisons, occipital hypoperfusion was the only differentiating radiographic feature between the AD and DLB groups [21]. Other studies also reported occipital hypoperfusion using ^{123}I-IMP [80], ^{99m}Tc-HMPAO [105, 106] and ^{99m}Tc-ECD [107] in DLB (**Figure 7**).

Nigrostriatal dopaminergic system integrity and degeneration can be assessed using ^{123}I-2β-carbometoxy-3β-(4-iodophenyl)-*N*-(3-fluoropropyl) nortropane (^{123}I-FP-CIT) as a SPECT tracer, which binds to dopamine transporters. Using ^{123}I-FP-CIT-SPECT, studies have found reduced striatal dopamine transporter uptake in DLB as compared to AD [108, 109]. Lower dopamine transporter functions were detected in the caudate and putamen in both DLB and PD patients versus AD and controls; whereas, uptake was similar among PD and DLB patients [108, 109]. The diagnostic accuracy of ^{123}I-FP-CIT-SPECT imaging in distinguishing probable DLB from other dementias was assessed in a multi-centered study, reporting a sensitivity of 78% and specificity of 90% at baseline [110]. In a 12-month follow-up of this sample, the clinical diagnosis of probable DLB and non-DLB remained relatively stable, while it changed for 44 subjects who were originally diagnosed as possible DLB at baseline [111]. Of these 44 subjects, the diagnoses of 19 cases were changed to probable DLB, 12 (63%) of whom had an abnormal ^{123}I-FP-CIT-SPECT at baseline [111]. Additionally, the clinical diagnosis of 7 patients diagnosed as possible DLB at baseline was revised to non-DLB at follow-up, all of which had normal ^{123}I-FP-CIT-SPECT at baseline [111]. It was concluded that abnormal uptake of ^{123}I-FP-CIT on SPECT in patients diagnosed as possible DLB is highly predictive of DLB, suggesting a useful role of this imaging technique in the differential diagnosis of uncertain DLB cases [111]. Another follow-up study of DLB and AD patients with neuropathological confirmation reported a sensitivity of 88% and specificity of 100% for the diagnosis of DLB with ^{123}I-FP-CIT-SPECT scans available [112]. In comparison, the sensitivity and specificity of clinical diagnosis alone was 75% and 42%, respectively [112].

SPECT scans to identify occipital hypoperfusion and striatal dopamine loss in DLB are clinically useful biomarkers and have been incorporated into the international consensus criteria of DLB [5]. It is worth noting that ^{123}I-FP-CIT-SPECT can be abnormal in other parkinsonian syndromes and will not differentiate DLB from other atypical parkinsonian syndromes and even PD itself [101, 113, 114].

6. Proton Magnetic Resonance Spectroscopy (^{1}H-MRS) as a Biomarker in AD and LBD

Proton magnetic resonance spectroscopy (^{1}H-MRS) provides biochemical information about compounds in brain tissues [115, 116]. MRS signals are less robust than structural MRI signals due to lower concentrations of metabolites in the brain tissue as compared to water. However, the compound N-acetyl aspartate (NAA) is found in the brain in high concentrations and is an indicator of neuronal health, number and integrity [117]. NAA levels drop upon neuronal loss or dysfunction, and are sometimes represented as a ratio of creatine (Cr) [116]. The concentration of Cr remains relatively constant in the healthy brain [116].

In AD, NAA and NAA/Cr levels are reduced [11, 118]. NAA levels in MTL along with other biomarkers may be helpful in identifying early AD pathology in at-risk individuals [119]. In a study of AD patients by Jessen et al., treatment with donepezil (a cholinergic enhancer) was associated with an increase in NAA and NAA/Cr values in the parietal lobe over a 3 month period [120]. Within the posterior cingulate gyrus as a voxel of interest, PDD subjects had lower NAA/Cr values as compared to PD and controls, which is in line with greater neurodegenerative changes in PDD [118, 121]. Another study found lower NAA/Cr ratios in the hippocampus of a DLB group as compared to controls [122]. Limitations of most studies are small sample sizes and differing voxels of interest. Although NAA concentrations using ^{1}H-MRS may not qualify as a biomarker at this time, future studies using this and other metabolites can enhance our understanding of the underlying pathological processes [115].

7. Biomarkers Derived from Functional Magnetic Resonance Imaging (fMRI) in AD and LBD

Functional magnetic resonance imaging (fMRI) is a blood oxygen level dependent (BOLD) non-invasive technique that measures neuronal activity, and relies upon the transient changes in blood flow, volume and oxyhemoglobin/deoxyhemoglobin ratios [123]. fMRI can be performed under experimental paradigms (task-based versus control conditions) or under resting-state conditions. Some studies measure functional connectivity (FC) patterns within the key brain circuits implicated in AD and LBD. One such network of regions that shows preferential activation at resting-state has been identified as the default mode network

(DMN), which includes medial prefrontal cortex (PFC), PCC, precuneus, and lateral parietal and medial temporal cortices [124]. Other regional brain networks have also been identified that show FC under task or resting-state conditions. Early detection of disturbances in the FC of these networks at preclinical stages may have potential roles as biomarkers of AD and LBD.

Some of the earliest works focused on MTL structures that used episodic memory tasks to compare BOLD responses in AD and MCI. In these studies, decreased hippocampal activity during encoding of new information was a consistent finding among the AD subjects [125, 126]. Wang et al. reported decreased resting-state FC of the hippocampus with key DMN regions including medial PFC, PCC, precuneus and ventral anterior cingulate cortex in mild AD subjects [127]. Other investigators have replicated these findings in AD [128-131]. These disruptions in the DMN circuitry were found to intensify with greater severity of AD [130]. While most resting-state fMRI studies report decreased FC in most DMN regions, some studies present evidence for increased FC in AD in certain regions [132]. These paradoxical increases in FC were observed between the left hippocampus and right lateral PFC, right insula, the inferior parietal regions [127, 133]; and between PCC and medial PFC [128]. Such hyperactivations were also found in MTL regions during episodic memory tasks among at-risk *APOE* ε4 carriers and MCI subjects [134, 135]. It is suggested that these hyperactivations represent the brain's compensatory response to early cognitive or neuronal damage [134, 136].

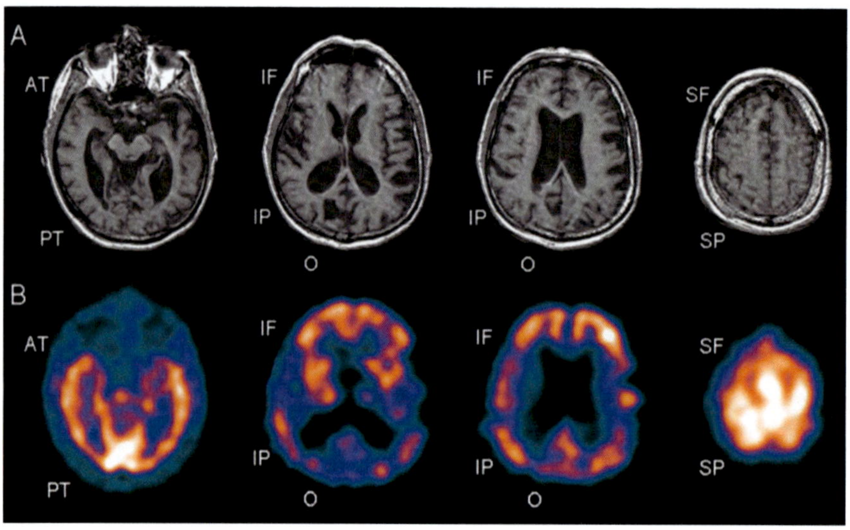

Figure 7. Corresponding **(A)** T1-weighted MRI, and **(B)** ^{99m}Tc-ethyl cysteinate dimer (^{99m}Tc-ECD) single photon emission computed tomography (SPECT) scans of a 79 year-old gentleman with a seven year history of Parkinson's disease (PD) who developed dementia, visual hallucinations and delusions five years after motor onset. MRI of the brain shows generalized atrophy slightly more prominent in the posterior and also involving the mesiotemporal regions bilaterally. The MRI findings may support a concomitant diagnosis of Alzheimer's disease. A brain SPECT revealed bilateral parieto-temporal hypoperfusion extending into the lateral occipital regions. These SPECT findings support a diagnosis of Parkinson's disease dementia. For the SPECT images, orange–yellow colors represent areas of high perfusion, while the blue–purple colors represent areas of low perfusion.

In PD patients, resting-state fMRI studies have reported increased FC between basal ganglia and motor regions, which have been identified as part of the basal ganglia-thalamocortical loop [137-141]. In these studies, reduced FC between putamen and parietal, and motor areas were also observed. Compared to controls, Peraza et al. showed altered resting-state FC within the fronto-parietal network in DLB, while disruptions in the supplementary motor area were apparent in PDD [142]. Generally, resting-state FC studies comparing AD and DLB groups have reported conflicting results with some studies showing greater, while others presenting reduced FC patterns compared to controls [132, 143]. Part of this variation may be attributed to variations in seed region selection and disease severity in these studies.

Other studies have investigated changes in DMN activity when switching from resting-state conditions to cognitively demanding tasks. In PD patients, van Eimeren et al. showed less deactivation of the PCC and precuneus regions during card-sorting task compared with simple sensory-motor task, suggesting failure in normal deactivation of DMN [144]. Schwindt et al. compared AD with normal controls during the resting-state and a simple visual task [131]. In this study, while the controls exhibited greater DMN connectivity during rest than task, the AD patients failed to show modulation of DMN activity between the two conditions. In addition, the degree of condition-dependent modulation in PCC and precuneus was predictive of mini-mental status examination (MMSE) scores [131].

These fMRI techniques have already been utilized to study responses to pharmacological treatments. A study linked enhanced cognition after rivastigmine treatment to altered BOLD activation patterns in the bilateral fusiform gyri and PFC in AD patients [145]. Saykin et al. assessed the therapeutic effects of donepezil in MCI patients using a working memory task, and found increased frontal activation relative to unmedicated controls [146].

fMRI using BOLD is a promising tool to assess early neurophysiological alterations in brain circuitry in dementia. It can also be applied to evaluate treatment effects of cognition-enhancing therapies and potentially serve as a secondary end-point in clinical trials. In light of its wider availability, non-invasiveness and relatively higher resolution, fMRI holds great potential to be a useful biomarker [147].

8. [^{123}I]Metaiodobenzylguanidine ([^{123}I]MIBG) Myocardial Scintigraphy to Assess Autonomic Dysfunction in AD and LBD

[^{123}I]Metaiodobenzylguanidine ([^{123}I]MIBG) is a radioiodinated structural analogue of norepinephrine, which is shown to compete and localize into postganglionic adrenergic neurons using identical cellular transport mechanisms [148, 149]. The uptake and localization of [^{123}I]MIBG can provide a useful measure of postganglionic sympathetic neuronal integrity and function [149]. Traditionally, the technique of [^{123}I]MIBG myocardial scintigraphy has been used to assess local myocardial sympathetic nerve damage in cardiovascular diseases. More recently, its use in the differential diagnosis of neurodegenerative diseases has been reported as autonomic dysfunction is frequent in LBD compared to AD [150, 151]. The uptake of [^{123}I]MIBG on myocardial scintigraphy is usually reported as a ratio of heart to mediastinum count densities (H/M ratio), which is a standard procedure employed in nuclear medicine. Several studies have demonstrated reduced [^{123}I]MIBG uptake in LBD as compared to AD and normal controls, with high discriminative accuracy between LBD and other dementias (sensitivity 95% and specificity 87%) [152-154]. Uptake ratios in AD and normal controls were not different in these studies. A study comparing the diagnostic value of myocardial [^{123}I]MIBG scintigraphy with occipital hypoperfusion on SPECT found [^{123}I]MIBG scintigraphy to be more sensitive in the differentiation of DLB from AD [155]. Similarly, another study found [^{123}I]MIBG myocardial scintigraphy to be superior to CSF markers in differentiating DLB from AD [156]. One advantage of this technique over FDG-PET is that it can distinguish DLB and PD from atypical parkinsonian syndromes, such as multiple system atrophy (MSA), corticobasal degeneration and progressive nuclear palsy (PSP). The [^{123}I]MIBG uptake ratios in these atypical parkinsonian syndromes were reported to be normal or only mildly reduced, as opposed to the significant reductions observed in DLB and PD versus normal controls [153, 157].

[^{123}I]MIBG myocardial scintigraphy appears to be a useful potential biomarker and may provide valuable adjunct evidence in the differential diagnosis of DLB from AD. However, there is a need for larger studies with pathologically-confirmed samples to tease out the confounding effects of vascular and mixed neuropathologies. Additionally, low myocardial [^{123}I]MIBG uptake is not specific to DLB and PD, and may also result due to cardiovascular morbidities, latent cardiac disorders and medications [101, 158].

9. Cerebrospinal Fluid (CSF) Biomarkers in AD and LBD

Biomarkers in AD can be represented by a dynamic clinicopathological model that reflects a temporal progression of the disease from preclinical phases to MCI and finally to dementia. According to this model proposed by Jack and collaborators, amyloid accumulation is an early preclinical event that leads to a cascade of successive neurodegenerative processes, including tau pathology, synaptic depletion and neuronal loss, eventually leading to a clinical diagnosis of dementia [159, 160]. The magnitude of the abnormality as proposed by this model may best be reflected in CSF due to its close contact with the brain tissue. The following four CSF biomarkers have been evaluated in many independent investigations: $A\beta_{40}$, $A\beta_{42}$, total tau and phosphorylated tau [11].

Amyloid precursor protein (APP) is an integral membrane protein, which can undergo differential cleavage via amyloidogenic or non-amyloidogenic pathways. The amyloidogenic pathway results in the formation of insoluble and hydrophobic $A\beta_{40}$ and $A\beta_{42}$ peptides that can aggregate forming an amyloid plaque [160, 161]. Soluble $A\beta_{42}$ neurotoxic aggregates, known as oligomers, may also form and lead to an increase in oligomer concentrations in CSF [162]. In AD, CSF levels of $A\beta_{42}$ or $A\beta_{42}/A\beta_{40}$ ratio progressively decline, whereas brain amyloidosis as detected by amyloid PET increases [163, 164]. This inverse relationship between CSF $A\beta_{42}$ concentrations and brain amyloidosis is thought to be the result of greater retention of Aβ-peptide moieties in the brain in the form of amyloid plaques.

Total-tau (t-tau) and phosphorylated-tau (p-tau) are the classic CSF biomarkers of neurodegeneration. Tau is a protein that is essential for proper assembly and stabilization of neuronal microtubules [165]. The functional expression of tau can be altered by abnormal hyperphosphorylation of serine and threonine residues that can aggregate to form NFTs – one of the hallmarks of AD [160]. Synaptic injury or cellular death results in the leakage of tau into the CSF and extracellular spaces. In AD and those MCI patients at the highest risk of developing AD, CSF levels of t-tau and p-tau are elevated compared to normal controls, which is in line with the neuropathological changes observed in AD [166].

The AD signature CSF profile: low $A\beta_{42}$ or $A\beta_{42}/A\beta_{40}$ ratio and high t-tau and p-tau, can be helpful as a biomarker to distinguish AD from normal controls and other non-AD forms of dementias, as well as to predict conversion from MCI to AD with good diagnostic accuracy (>80%) [166-168]. Compared to CSF, peripheral blood biomarkers are desirable due to easy accessibility; however, efforts have been hindered by their greater susceptibility to degradation and low concentrations in plasma.

In DLB, the CSF levels of $A\beta_{42}$ are lower than normal controls [169, 170]. Another study showed lower CSF levels of $A\beta_{42}$ in DLB patients with senile plaques (SPs), compared to DLB patients without SPs [171]. These studies reflect greater retention of $A\beta_{42}$ in brains with SPs and the corresponding decrease in CSF levels of $A\beta_{42}$ – an inverse relationship also seen in AD. The relative abundance of the oxidized version of $A\beta_{42}$ ($A\beta_{42}^{*}$) has also been reported to be elevated in DLB as compared to PDD and controls, and is proposed to be a specific marker of DLB pathophysiology [172]. It is noteworthy that $A\beta_{42}^{*}$ abundance was also found to be higher in AD [172]. Further studies are warranted to establish its precise role, replicability and potential usefulness as a biomarker in DLB. Other investigations have found that CSF levels of tau proteins are lower in DLB than in AD, but higher in DLB compared to PD and PDD groups [170, 173, 174]. This fits our general understanding of greater whole-brain neuronal loss in AD, followed by DLB and PD/PDD with lesser neurodegenerative changes at least in the earlier stages of the disease process.

As DLB is characterized by αSyn proteinopathy, some studies have aimed to measure the total αSyn levels in CSF and found them to be lower in αSyn-associated disorders of PD, DLB and MSA [175, 176]. This finding was suggested to be due to greater cerebral accumulation of αSyn aggregates in the form of Lewy bodies [175]. However, contradictory results were also reported where αSyn levels were shown to be elevated in DLB compared to AD and normal controls [177]. A recent meta-analysis of 17 studies found reduced CSF αSyn concentrations in PD patients compared to AD and controls, with no significant differences between PD and DLB or MSA [178]. Another meta-analysis looked at the CSF αSyn levels between synucleinopathies and PSP in 9 studies and found lower CSF concentrations in synucleinopathies versus PSP [179]. Although these meta-analyses show favourable results, further investigations are needed to reconcile negative findings. The CSF levels of αSyn may not be sufficient as a single 'stand-alone' diagnostic biomarker, but its role as an adjunct source of information in synucleinopathies seems promising.

CONCLUSION

In summary, a combination of different biomarkers can improve the differential diagnosis and it is hoped that future investigations will eventually facilitate a personalized medicine approach to the management of neurodegenerative diseases [180]. These biomarkers may eventually be able to provide powerful ways of measuring disease progression and therapeutic responses to drugs. The diagnostic and prognostic value of these biomarkers are dependent as much on the type as their methods of measurement [181]. Imaging, fluid and other candidate biomarkers have their own strengths and limitations. Despite great advances in neurodegenerative research in the past decade, more work is needed to refine measurement techniques, standardize research protocols and better understand the underlying pathological mechanisms.

ACKNOWLEDGMENTS

The authors would like to gratefully acknowledge Dr. Juan Bilbao for providing the neuropathology images. MM and SEB are supported by the Department of Medicine at Sunnybrook Health Sciences Centre and the University of Toronto. SEB is supported by the Brill Chair in Neurology and the Hurvitz Brain Sciences Program. US is supported by an Ontario Graduate Scholarship, Margaret and Howard Gamble Research Grant, Scace Graduate Fellowship in Alzheimer's Research, and an Institute of Medical Sciences Entrance Award.

REFERENCES

[1] Bird T. Genetic aspects of Alzheimer disease. *Genet Med*, 2008, 10(4), 231-239.

[2] Braak, H; Braak, E. Neuropathological stageing of Alzheimer-related changes. *Acta Neuropathol.*, 1991, 82(4), 239-259.

[3] Dubois, B; Feldman, HH; Jacova, C; Dekosky, ST; Barberger-Gateau, P; Cummings, J; Delacourte, A; Galasko, D; Gauthier, S; Jicha, G; Meguro, K; O'brien, J; Pasquier, F; Robert, P; Rossor, M; Salloway, S; Stern, Y; Visser, PJ; Scheltens, P. Research criteria for the diagnosis of Alzheimer's disease: revising the NINCDS-ADRDA criteria. *Lancet Neurol.*, 2007 Aug, 6(8), 734-746.

[4] Lam, B; Masellis, M; Freedman, M; Stuss, DT; Black, SE. Clinical, imaging, and pathological heterogeneity of the Alzheimer's disease syndrome. *Alzheimers Res Ther.*, 2013 Jan 9, 5(1), 1.

[5] McKeith, IG; Dickson, DW; Lowe, J; Emre, M; O'Brien, JT; Feldman, H; Cummings, J; Duda, JE; Lippa, C; Perry, EK; Aarsland, D; Arai, H; Ballard, CG; Boeve, B; Burn, DJ; Costa, D; Del Ser, T; Dubois, B; Galasko, D; Gauthier, S; Goetz, CG; Gomez-Tortosa, E; Halliday, G; Hansen, LA; Hardy, J; Iwatsubo, T; Kalaria, RN; Kaufer, D; Kenny, RA; Korczyn, A; Kosaka,, K; Lee, VM; Lees, A; Litvan, I; Londos, E; Lopez, OL; Minoshima, S; Mizuno, Y; Molina, JA; Mukaetova-Ladinska, EB; Pasquier, F; Perry, RH; Schulz, JB; Trojanowski, JQ; Yamada, M. Consortium on DLB. Diagnosis and management of dementia with Lewy bodies: third report of the DLB Consortium. *Neurology*, 2005 Dec 27, 65(12), 1863-1872.

[6] McKeith, I; Mintzer, J; Aarsland, D; Burn, D; Chiu, H; Cohen-Mansfield, J; Dickson, D; Dubois, B; Duda, JE; Feldman, H; Gauthier, S; Halliday, G; Lawlor, B; Lippa, C; Lopez, OL; Carlos Machado, J; O'Brien, J; Playfer, J; Reid, W. International Psychogeriatric Association Expert Meeting on DLB. Dementia with Lewy bodies. *Lancet Neurol.*, 2004 Jan, 3(1), 19-28.

[7] Dubois, B; Burn, D; Goetz, C; Aarsland, D; Brown, RG; Broe, GA; Dickson, D; Duyckaerts, C; Cummings, J; Gauthier, S; Korczyn, A; Lees, A; Levy, R; Litvan, I; Mizuno, Y; McKeith, IG; Olanow, CW; Poewe, W; Sampaio, C; Tolosa, E; Emre, M. Diagnostic procedures for Parkinson's disease dementia: recommendations from the movement disorder society task force. *Mov Disord.*, 2007 Dec, 22(16), 2314-2324.

[8] Aarsland, D; Perry, R; Larsen, JP; McKeith, IG; O'Brien, JT; Perry, EK; Burn, D; Ballard, CG. Neuroleptic sensitivity in Parkinson's disease and parkinsonian dementias. *J Clin Psychiatry.*, 2005 May, 66(5), 633-637.

[9] Rahimi, J; Kovacs, GG. Prevalence of mixed pathologies in the aging brain. *Alzheimers Res Ther.*, 2014 Nov 21, 6(9), 82.

[10] Biomarkers Definitions Working Group. Biomarkers and surrogate endpoints: preferred definitions and conceptual framework. *Clin Pharmacol Ther.*, 2001 Mar, 69(3), 89-95.

[11] Hampel, H; Frank, R; Broich, K; Teipel, SJ; Katz, RG; Hardy, J; Herholz, K; Bokde, AL; Jessen, F; Hoessler, YC; Sanhai, WR; Zetterberg, H; Woodcock, J; Blennow, K. Biomarkers for Alzheimer's disease: academic; industry and regulatory perspectives. *Nat Rev Drug Discov.*, 2010 Jul, 9(7), 560-574.

[12] Frank, R; Hargreaves, R. Clinical biomarkers in drug discovery and development. *Nat Rev Drug Discov.*, 2003 Jul, 2(7), 566-580.

[13] Kovacevic, N; Lobaugh, NJ; Bronskill, MJ; Levine, B; Feinstein, A; Black, SE. A robust method for extraction and automatic segmentation of brain images. *Neuroimage.*, 2002 Nov, 17(3), 1087-1100.

[14] Burton, EJ; McKeith, IG; Burn, DJ; Williams, ED; O'Brien, JT. Cerebral atrophy in Parkinson's disease with and without dementia: a comparison with Alzheimer's disease, dementia with Lewy bodies and controls. *Brain.*, 2004 Apr, 127(Pt 4), 791-800.

[15] Beyer, MK; Larsen, JP; Aarsland, D. Gray matter atrophy in Parkinson disease with dementia and dementia with Lewy bodies. *Neurology.*, 2007 Aug 21, 69(8), 747-754.

[16] Blanc, F; Colloby, SJ; Philippi, N; de Pétigny, X; Jung, B; Demuynck, C; Phillipps, C; Anthony, P; Thomas, A; Bing, F; Lamy, J; Martin-Hunyadi, C; O'Brien, JT; Cretin, B; McKeith, I; Armspach, JP; Taylor, JP. Cortical Thickness in Dementia with Lewy Bodies and Alzheimer's Disease: A Comparison of Prodromal and Dementia Stages. *PLoS One.*, 2015 Jun 10, 10(6), e0127396.

[17] McKhann, GM; Knopman, DS; Chertkow, H; Hyman, BT; Jack, CR; Jr; Kawas, CH; Klunk, WE; Koroshetz, WJ; Manly, JJ; Mayeux, R; Mohs, RC; Morris, JC; Rossor, MN; Scheltens, P; Carrillo, MC; Thies, B; Weintraub, S; Phelps, CH. The diagnosis of dementia due to Alzheimer's disease: recommendations from the National Institute on Aging-Alzheimer's Association workgroups on diagnostic guidelines for Alzheimer's disease. *Alzheimers Dement.*, 2011 May, 7(3), 263-269.

[18] Whitwell, JL; Weigand, SD; Shiung, MM; Boeve, BF; Ferman, TJ; Smith, GE; Knopman, DS; Petersen, RC; Benarroch, EE; Josephs, KA; Jack, CR. Jr. Focal atrophy in dementia with Lewy bodies on MRI: a distinct pattern from Alzheimer's disease. *Brain.*, 2007 Mar, 130(Pt 3), 708-719.

[19] Burton, EJ; Karas, G; Paling, SM; Barber, R; Williams, ED; Ballard, CG; McKeith, IG; Scheltens, P; Barkhof, F; O'Brien, JT. Patterns of cerebral atrophy in dementia with Lewy bodies using voxel-based morphometry. *Neuroimage.*, 2002 Oct, 17(2), 618-630.

[20] Gilman, S; Koeppe, RA; Little, R; An, H; Junck, L; Giordani, B; Persad, C; Heumann, M; Wernette, K. Differentiation of Alzheimer's disease from dementia with Lewy

bodies utilizing positron emission tomography with [18F]fluorodeoxyglucose and neuropsychological testing. *Exp Neurol.*, 2005 Feb, 191 Suppl 1, S95-S103.

[21] Lobotesis, K; Fenwick, JD; Phipps, A; Ryman, A; Swann, A; Ballard, C; McKeith, IG; O'Brien, JT. Occipital hypoperfusion on SPECT in dementia with Lewy bodies but not AD. *Neurology.*, 2001 Mar 13, 56(5), 643-649.

[22] Foster, ER; Campbell, MC; Burack, MA; Hartlein, J; Flores, HP; Cairns, NJ; Hershey, T; Perlmutter, JS. Amyloid imaging of Lewy body-associated disorders. *Mov Disord.*, 2010 Nov 15, 25(15), 2516-2523.

[23] Villemagne, VL; Ong, K; Mulligan, RS; Holl, G; Pejoska, S; Jones, G; O'Keefe, G; Ackerman, U; Tochon-Danguy, H; Chan, JG; Reininger, CB; Fels, L; Putz, B; Rohde, B; Masters, CL; Rowe, CC. Amyloid imaging with (18)F-florbetaben in Alzheimer disease and other dementias. *J Nucl Med.*, 2011 Aug, 52(8), 1210-1217.

[24] Ballard, C; Ziabreva, I; Perry, R; Larsen, JP; O'Brien, J; McKeith, I; Perry, E; Aarsland, D. Differences in neuropathologic characteristics across the Lewy body dementia spectrum. *Neurology.*, 2006 Dec 12, 67(11), 1931-1934.

[25] Fox, NC; Cousens, S; Scahill, R; Harvey, RJ; Rossor, MN. Using serial registered brain magnetic resonance imaging to measure disease progression in Alzheimer disease: power calculations and estimates of sample size to detect treatment effects. *Arch Neurol.*, 2000 Mar, 57(3), 339-344.

[26] Barnes, J; Bartlett, JW; van de Pol, LA; Loy, CT; Scahill, RI; Frost, C; Thompson, P; Fox, NC. A meta-analysis of hippocampal atrophy rates in Alzheimer's disease. *Neurobiol Aging.*, 2009 Nov, 30(11), 1711-1723.

[27] O'Brien, JT; Paling, S; Barber, R; Williams, ED; Ballard, C; McKeith, IG; Gholkar, A; Crum, WR; Rossor, MN; Fox, NC. Progressive brain atrophy on serial MRI in dementia with Lewy bodies, AD, and vascular dementia. *Neurology.*, 2001 May 22, 56(10), 1386-1388.

[28] Whitwell, JL; Jack, CR; Jr; Parisi, JE; Knopman, DS; Boeve, BF; Petersen, RC; Ferman, TJ; Dickson, DW; Josephs, KA. Rates of cerebral atrophy differ in different degenerative pathologies. *Brain.*, 2007 Apr, 130(Pt 4), 1148-1158.

[29] Burton, EJ; McKeith, IG; Burn, DJ; O'Brien, JT. Brain atrophy rates in Parkinson's disease with and without dementia using serial magnetic resonance imaging. *Mov Disord.* 2005 Dec, 20(12), 1571-1576.

[30] Burton, EJ; Barber, R; Mukaetova-Ladinska, EB; Robson, J; Perry, RH; Jaros, E; Kalaria, RN; O'Brien, JT. Medial temporal lobe atrophy on MRI differentiates Alzheimer's disease from dementia with Lewy bodies and vascular cognitive impairment: a prospective study with pathological verification of diagnosis. *Brain.*, 2009 Jan, 132(Pt 1), 195-203.

[31] Dubois, B; Feldman, HH; Jacova, C; Hampel, H; Molinuevo, JL; Blennow, K; DeKosky, ST; Gauthier, S; Selkoe, D; Bateman, R; Cappa, S; Crutch, S; Engelborghs, S; Frisoni, GB; Fox, NC; Galasko, D; Habert, MO; Jicha, GA; Nordberg, A; Pasquier, F; Rabinovici, G; Robert, P; Rowe, C; Salloway, S; Sarazin, M; Epelbaum, S; de Souza, LC; Vellas, B; Visser, PJ; Schneider, L; Stern, Y; Scheltens, P; Cummings, JL. Advancing research diagnostic criteria for Alzheimer's disease: the IWG-2 criteria. *Lancet Neurol.*, 2014 Jun, 13(6), 614-629.

[32] Laakso, MP; Soininen, H; Partanen, K; Helkala, EL; Hartikainen, P; Vainio, P; Hallikainen, M; Hänninen, T; Riekkinen, PJ Sr. Volumes of hippocampus, amygdala

and frontal lobes in the MRI-based diagnosis of early Alzheimer's disease: correlation with memory functions. *J Neural Transm Park Dis Dement Sect.* 1995, 9(1), 73-86.

[33] Firbank, MJ; Blamire, AM; Teodorczuk, A; Teper, E; Burton, EJ; Mitra, D; O'Brien, JT. High resolution imaging of the medial temporal lobe in Alzheimer's disease and dementia with Lewy bodies. *J Alzheimers Dis.*, 2010, 21(4), 1129-1140.

[34] Mak, E; Li, S; Williams, GB; Watson, R; Firbank, M; Blamire, A; O'Brien, J. Differential Atrophy of Hippocampal Subfields: A Comparative Study of Dementia with Lewy Bodies and Alzheimer Disease. *Am J Geriatr Psychiatry.*, 2015 Jun 25.

[35] Barber, R; McKeith, IG; Ballard, C; Gholkar, A; O'Brien, JT. A comparison of medial and lateral temporal lobe atrophy in dementia with Lewy bodies and Alzheimer's disease: magnetic resonance imaging volumetric study. *Dement Geriatr Cogn Disord.*, 2001 May-Jun, 12(3), 198-205.

[36] Camicioli, R; Moore, MM; Kinney, A; Corbridge, E; Glassberg, K; Kaye, JA. Parkinson's disease is associated with hippocampal atrophy. *Mov Disord.*, 2003 Jul, 18(7), 784-790.

[37] Kerchner, GA; Hess, CP; Hammond-Rosenbluth, KE; Xu, D; Rabinovici, GD; Kelley, DA; Vigneron, DB; Nelson, SJ; Miller, BL. Hippocampal CA1 apical neuropil atrophy in mild Alzheimer disease visualized with 7-T MRI. *Neurology.*, 2010 Oct 12, 75(15), 1381-1387.

[38] Hashimoto, M; Yasuda, M; Tanimukai, S; Matsui, M; Hirono, N; Kazui, H; Mori, E. Apolipoprotein E epsilon 4 and the pattern of regional brain atrophy in Alzheimer's disease. *Neurology.*, 2001 Oct 23, 57(8), 1461-1466.

[39] Pievani, M; Galluzzi, S; Thompson, PM; Rasser, PE; Bonetti, M; Frisoni, GB. APOE4 is associated with greater atrophy of the hippocampal formation in Alzheimer's disease. *Neuroimage.*, 2011 Apr 1, 55(3), 909-919.

[40] Canto, CB; Wouterlood, FG; Witter, MP. What does the anatomical organization of the entorhinal cortex tell us? *Neural Plast.* 2008, 2008, 381243.

[41] Kenny, ER; Burton, EJ; O'Brien, JT. A volumetric magnetic resonance imaging study of entorhinal cortex volume in dementia with lewy bodies. A comparison with Alzheimer's disease and Parkinson's disease with and without dementia. *Dement Geriatr Cogn Disord.*, 2008, 26(3), 218-225.

[42] Goldman, JG; Stebbins, GT; Bernard, B; Stoub, TR; Goetz, CG; deToledo-Morrell, L. Entorhinal cortex atrophy differentiates Parkinson's disease patients with and without dementia. *Mov Disord.*, 2012 May, 27(6), 727-734.

[43] Pitcher, TL; Melzer, TR; Macaskill, MR; Graham, CF; Livingston, L; Keenan, RJ; Watts, R; Dalrymple-Alford, JC; Anderson, TJ. Reduced striatal volumes in Parkinson's disease: a magnetic resonance imaging study. *Transl Neurodegener.*, 2012 Aug 21, 1(1), 17.

[44] Cousins, DA; Burton, EJ; Burn, D; Gholkar, A; McKeith, IG; O'Brien, JT. Atrophy of the putamen in dementia with Lewy bodies but not Alzheimer's disease: an MRI study. *Neurology.*, 2003 Nov 11, 61(9), 1191-1195.

[45] Barber, R; McKeith, I; Ballard, C; O'Brien, J. Volumetric MRI study of the caudate nucleus in patients with dementia with Lewy bodies, Alzheimer's disease, and vascular dementia. *J Neurol Neurosurg Psychiatry.*, 2002 Mar, 72(3), 406-407.

[46] Almeida, OP; Burton, EJ; McKeith, I; Gholkar, A; Burn, D; O'Brien, JT. MRI study of caudate nucleus volume in Parkinson's disease with and without dementia with Lewy bodies and Alzheimer's disease. *Dement Geriatr Cogn Disord.*, 2003, 16(2), 57-63.
[47] Longstreth, WT; Jr; Manolio, TA; Arnold, A; Burke, GL; Bryan, N; Jungreis, CA; Enright, PL; O'Leary, D; Fried, L. Clinical correlates of white matter findings on cranial magnetic resonance imaging of 3301 elderly people. The Cardiovascular Health Study. *Stroke.*, 1996 Aug, 27(8), 1274-1282.
[48] de Leeuw, FE; de Groot, JC; Achten, E; Oudkerk, M; Ramos, LM; Heijboer, R; Hofman, A; Jolles, J; van Gijn, J; Breteler, MM. Prevalence of cerebral white matter lesions in elderly people: a population based magnetic resonance imaging study. The Rotterdam Scan Study. *J Neurol Neurosurg Psychiatry.* 2001 Jan, 70(1), 9-14.
[49] Black, S; Gao, F; Bilbao, J. Understanding white matter disease: imaging-pathological correlations in vascular cognitive impairment. *Stroke.*, 2009 Mar, 40(3 Suppl), S48-52.
[50] Wardlaw, JM; Smith, C; Dichgans, M. Mechanisms of sporadic cerebral small vessel disease: insights from neuroimaging. *Lancet Neurol.*, 2013 May, 12(5), 483-497.
[51] Garde, E; Lykke Mortensen, E; Rostrup, E; Paulson, OB. Decline in intelligence is associated with progression in white matter hyperintensity volume. *J Neurol Neurosurg Psychiatry.*, 2005 Sep, 76(9), 1289-1291.
[52] Prins, ND; van Dijk, EJ; den Heijer, T; Vermeer, SE; Jolles, J; Koudstaal, PJ; Hofman, A; Breteler, MM. Cerebral small-vessel disease and decline in information processing speed, executive function and memory. *Brain.*, 2005 Sep, 128(Pt 9), 2034-2041.
[53] Ramirez, J; McNeely, AA; Scott, CJ; Stuss, DT; Black, SE. Subcortical hyperintensity volumetrics in Alzheimer's disease and normal elderly in the Sunnybrook Dementia Study: correlations with atrophy, executive function, mental processing speed, and verbal memory. *Alzheimers Res Ther.*, 2014 Aug 11, 6(4), 49.
[54] Kramer, JH; Reed, BR; Mungas, D; Weiner, MW; Chui, HC. Executive dysfunction in subcortical ischaemic vascular disease. *J Neurol Neurosurg Psychiatry.*, 2002 Feb, 72(2), 217-220.
[55] Burton, EJ; McKeith, IG; Burn, DJ; Firbank, MJ; O'Brien, JT. Progression of white matter hyperintensities in Alzheimer disease, dementia with lewy bodies, and Parkinson disease dementia: a comparison with normal aging. *Am J Geriatr Psychiatry.*, 2006 Oct, 14(10), 842-849.
[56] Barber, R; Scheltens, P; Gholkar, A; Ballard, C; McKeith, I; Ince, P; Perry, R; O'Brien, J. White matter lesions on magnetic resonance imaging in dementia with Lewy bodies, Alzheimer's disease, vascular dementia, and normal aging. *J Neurol Neurosurg Psychiatry.* 1999 Jul, 67(1), 66-72.
[57] Beyer, MK; Aarsland, D; Greve, OJ; Larsen, JP. Visual rating of white matter hyperintensities in Parkinson's disease. *Mov Disord.*, 2006 Feb, 21(2), 223-229.
[58] Barber, R; Gholkar, A; Scheltens, P; Ballard, C; McKeith, IG; O'Brien, JT. MRI volumetric correlates of white matter lesions in dementia with Lewy bodies and Alzheimer's disease. *Int J Geriatr Psychiatry.*, 2000 Oct, 15(10), 911-916.
[59] Debette, S; Markus, HS. The clinical importance of white matter hyperintensities on brain magnetic resonance imaging: systematic review and meta-analysis. *BMJ.*, 2010 Jul 26, 341, c3666.
[60] Le Bihan, D. Looking into the functional architecture of the brain with diffusion MRI. *Nat Rev Neurosci.*, 2003, 4, 469–480.

[61] Bozzali, M; Cherubini, A. Diffusion tensor MRI to investigate dementias: a brief review. *Magn Reson Imaging.*, 2007, 25, 969–977.
[62] Bozzali, M; Falini, A; Franceschi, M; Cercignani, M; Zuffi, M; Scotti, G; Comi, G; Filippi, M. White matter damage in Alzheimer's disease assessed *in vivo* using diffusion tensor magnetic resonance imaging. *J Neurol Neurosurg Psychiatry.*, 2002, 72, 742–746.
[63] Fellgiebel, A; Wille, P; Müller, MJ; Winterer, G; Scheurich, A; Vucurevic, G; Schmidt, LG; Stoeter, P. Ultrastructural hippocampal and white matter alterations in mild cognitive impairment: a diffusion tensor imaging study. *Dement Geriatr Cogn Disord.*, 2004, 18(1), 101-108.
[64] Head, D; Buckner, RL; Shimony, JS; Williams, LE; Akbudak, E; Conturo, TE; McAvoy, M; Morris, JC; Snyder, AZ. Differential vulnerability of anterior white matter in nondemented aging with minimal acceleration in dementia of the Alzheimer type: evidence from diffusion tensor imaging. *Cereb Cortex.*, 2004 Apr, 14(4), 410-423.
[65] Stebbins, GT; Murphy, CM. Diffusion tensor imaging in Alzheimer's disease and mild cognitive impairment. *Behav Neurol.*, 2009, 21(1), 39-49.
[66] Choo, IH; Lee, DY; Oh, JS; Lee, JS; Lee, DS; Song, IC; Youn, JC; Kim, SG; Kim, KW; Jhoo, JH; Woo, JI. Posterior cingulate cortex atrophy and regional cingulum disruption in mild cognitive impairment and Alzheimer's disease. *Neurobiol Aging.*, 2010 May, 31(5), 772-779.
[67] Firbank, MJ; Blamire, AM; Krishnan, MS; Teodorczuk, A; English, P; Gholkar, A; Harrison, RM; O'Brien, JT. Diffusion tensor imaging in dementia with Lewy bodies and Alzheimer's disease. *Psychiatry Res.*, 2007, 155, 135–145.
[68] Firbank, MJ; Blamire, AM; Krishnan, MS; Teodorczuk, A; English, P; Gholkar, A; Harrison, R; O'Brien, JT. Atrophy is associated with posterior cingulate white matter disruption in dementia with Lewy bodies and Alzheimer's disease. *Neuroimage.*, 2007, 36, 1–7.
[69] Bozzali, M; Falini, A; Cercignani, M; Baglio, F; Farina, E; Alberoni, M; Vezzulli, P; Olivotto, F; Mantovani, F; Shallice, T; Scotti, G; Canal, N; Nemni, R. Brain tissue damage in dementia with Lewy bodies: an *in vivo* diffusion tensor MRI study. *Brain.*, 2005; 128(Pt 7), 1595–1604.
[70] Nedelska, Z; Schwarz, CG; Boeve, BF; Lowe, VJ; Reid, RI; Przybelski, SA; Lesnick, TG; Gunter, JL; Senjem, ML; Ferman, TJ; Smith, GE; Geda, YE; Knopman, DS; Petersen, RC; Jack, CR; Jr; Kantarci, K. White matter integrity in dementia with Lewy bodies: a voxel-based analysis of diffusion tensor imaging. *Neurobiol Aging.*, 2015 Jun, 36(6), 2010-2017.
[71] Rowe, CC; Villemagne, VL. Brain amyloid imaging. *J Nucl Med.*, 2011 Nov, 52(11), 1733-1740.
[72] Herholz, K; Perani, D; Salmon, E; Franck, G; Fazio, F; Heiss, WD; Comar, D. Comparability of FDG PET studies in probable Alzheimer's disease. *J Nucl Med.*, 1993 Sep, 34(9), 1460-1466.
[73] Alexander, GE; Chen, K; Pietrini, P; Rapoport, SI; Reiman, EM. Longitudinal PET Evaluation of Cerebral Metabolic Decline in Dementia: A Potential Outcome Measure in Alzheimer's Disease Treatment Studies. *Am J Psychiatry.*, 2002 May, 159(5), 738-745.

[74] Duara, R; Grady, C; Haxby, J; Sundaram, M; Cutler, NR; Heston, L; Moore, A; Schlageter, N; Larson, S; Rapoport, SI. Positron emission tomography in Alzheimer's disease. *Neurology.*, 1986 Jul, 36(7), 879-887.

[75] Mosconi, L; Tsui, WH; Herholz, K; Pupi, A; Drzezga, A; Lucignani, G; Reiman, EM; Holthoff, V; Kalbe, E; Sorbi, S; Diehl-Schmid, J; Perneczky, R; Clerici, F; Caselli, R; Beuthien-Baumann, B; Kurz, A; Minoshima, S; de Leon, MJ. Multicenter standardized 18F-FDG PET diagnosis of mild cognitive impairment, Alzheimer's disease, and other dementias. *J Nucl Med.*, 2008 Mar, 49(3), 390-398.

[76] Yong, SW; Yoon, JK; An, YS; Lee, PH. A comparison of cerebral glucose metabolism in Parkinson's disease, Parkinson's disease dementia and dementia with Lewy bodies. *Eur J Neurol.*, 2007 Dec, 14(12), 1357-1362.

[77] Lim, SM; Katsifis, A; Villemagne, VL; Best, R; Jones, G; Saling, M; Bradshaw, J; Merory, J; Woodward, M; Hopwood, M; Rowe, CC. The 18F-FDG PET cingulate island sign and comparison to 123I-beta-CIT SPECT for diagnosis of dementia with Lewy bodies. *J Nucl Med.*, 2009 Oct, 50(10), 1638-1645.

[78] Imamura, T; Ishii, K; Sasaki, M; Kitagaki, H; Yamaji, S; Hirono, N; Shimomura, T; Hashimoto, M; Tanimukai, S; Kazui, H; Mori, E. Regional cerebral glucose metabolism in dementia with Lewy bodies and Alzheimer's disease: a comparative study using positron emission tomography. *Neurosci Lett.*, 1997 Oct 10, 235(1-2), 49-52.

[79] Graff-Radford, J; Murray, ME; Lowe, VJ; Boeve, BF; Ferman, TJ; Przybelski, SA; Lesnick, TG; Senjem, ML; Gunter, JL; Smith, GE; Knopman, DS; Jack, CR; Jr; Dickson, DW; Petersen, RC; Kantarci, K. Dementia with Lewy bodies, basis of cingulate island sign. *Neurology.*, 2014 Aug 26, 83(9), 801-809.

[80] Ishii, K; Hosaka, K; Mori, T; Mori, E. Comparison of FDG-PET and IMP-SPECT in patients with dementia with Lewy bodies. *Ann Nucl Med.*, 2004 Jul, 18(5), 447-451.

[81] Teipel, SJ; Drzezga, A; Bartenstein, P; Möller, HJ; Schwaiger, M; Hampel, H. Effects of donepezil on cortical metabolic response to activation during (18)FDG-PET in Alzheimer's disease; a double-blind cross-over trial. *Psychopharmacology (Berl).*, 2006 Jul, 187(1), 86-94.

[82] Heiss, WD; Hebold, I; Klinkhammer, P; Ziffling, P; Szelies, B; Pawlik, G; Herholz, K. Effect of piracetam on cerebral glucose metabolism in Alzheimer's disease as measured by positron emission tomography. *J Cereb Blood Flow Metab.* 1988 Aug, 8(4), 613-617.

[83] Kantarci, K; Lowe, VJ; Boeve, BF; Weigand, SD; Senjem, ML; Przybelski, SA; Dickson, DW; Parisi, JE; Knopman, DS; Smith, GE; Ferman, TJ; Petersen, RC; Jack, CR. Jr. Multimodality imaging characteristics of dementia with Lewy bodies. *Neurobiol Aging.*, 2012 Sep, 33(9), 2091-2105.

[84] Rowe, CC; Ng, S; Ackermann, U; Gong, SJ; Pike, K; Savage, G; Cowie, TF; Dickinson, KL; Maruff, P; Darby, D; Smith, C; Woodward, M; Merory, J; Tochon-Danguy, H; O'Keefe, G; Klunk, WE; Mathis, CA; Price, JC; Masters, CL; Villemagne, VL. Imaging beta-amyloid burden in aging and dementia. *Neurology.*, 2007 May 15, 68(20), 1718-1725.

[85] Engler, H; Forsberg, A; Almkvist, O; Blomquist, G; Larsson, E; Savitcheva, I; Wall, A; Ringheim, A; Långström, B; Nordberg, A. Two-year follow-up of amyloid deposition in patients with Alzheimer's disease. *Brain.*, 2006 Nov, 129(Pt 11), 2856-2866.

[86] Edison, P; Rowe, CC; Rinne, JO; Ng, S; Ahmed, I; Kemppainen, N; Villemagne, VL; O'Keefe, G; Någren, K; Chaudhury, KR; Masters, CL; Brooks, DJ. Amyloid load in Parkinson's disease dementia and Lewy body dementia measured with [11C]PIB positron emission tomography. *J Neurol Neurosurg Psychiatry.*, 2008 Dec, 79(12), 1331-1338.

[87] Gomperts, SN; Locascio, JJ; Marquie, M; Santarlasci, AL; Rentz, DM; Maye, J; Johnson, KA; Growdon, JH. Brain amyloid and cognition in Lewy body diseases. *Mov Disord.*, 2012 Jul, 27(8), 965-973.

[88] Gomperts, SN; Rentz, DM; Moran, E; Becker, JA; Locascio, JJ; Klunk, WE; Mathis, CA; Elmaleh, DR; Shoup, T; Fischman, AJ; Hyman, BT; Growdon, JH; Johnson, KA. Imaging amyloid deposition in Lewy body diseases. *Neurology.*, 2008 Sep 16, 71(12), 903-910.

[89] Maetzler, W; Reimold, M; Liepelt, I; Solbach, C; Leyhe, T; Schweitzer, K; Eschweiler, GW; Mittelbronn, M; Gaenslen, A; Uebele, M; Reischl, G; Gasser, T; Machulla, HJ; Bares, R; Berg, D. [11C]PIB binding in Parkinson's disease dementia. *Neuroimage.*, 2008 Feb 1, 39(3), 1027-1033.

[90] Jokinen, P; Scheinin, N; Aalto, S; Någren, K; Savisto, N; Parkkola, R; Rokka, J; Haaparanta, M; Röyttä, M; Rinne, JO. [(11)C]PIB-, [(18)F]FDG-PET and MRI imaging in patients with Parkinson's disease with and without dementia. *Parkinsonism Relat Disord.*, 2010 Dec, 16(10), 666-670.

[91] Donaghy, P; Thomas, AJ; O'Brien, JT. Amyloid PET Imaging in Lewy body disorders. *Am J Geriatr Psychiatry.*, 2015 Jan, 23(1), 23-37.

[92] Maetzler, W; Liepelt, I; Reimold, M; Reischl, G; Solbach, C; Becker, C; Schulte, C; Leyhe, T; Keller, S; Melms, A; Gasser, T; Berg, D. Cortical PIB binding in Lewy body disease is associated with Alzheimer-like characteristics. *Neurobiol Dis.*, 2009 Apr, 34(1), 107-112.

[93] Harding, AJ; Halliday, GM. Cortical Lewy body pathology in the diagnosis of dementia. *Acta Neuropathol.*, 2001 Oct, 102(4), 355-363.

[94] Irwin, DJ; White, MT; Toledo, JB; Xie, SX; Robinson, JL; Van Deerlin, V; Lee, VM; Leverenz, JB; Montine, TJ; Duda, JE; Hurtig, HI; Trojanowski, JQ. Neuropathologic substrates of Parkinson disease dementia. *Ann Neurol.*, 2012 Oct, 72(4), 587-598.

[95] Drzezga, A; Grimmer, T; Henriksen, G; Mühlau, M; Perneczky, R; Miederer, I; Praus, C; Sorg, C; Wohlschläger, A; Riemenschneider, M; Wester, HJ; Foerstl, H; Schwaiger, M; Kurz, A. Effect of APOE genotype on amyloid plaque load and gray matter volume in Alzheimer disease. *Neurology.*, 2009 Apr 28, 72(17), 1487-1494.

[96] Pletnikova, O; West, N; Lee, MK; Rudow, GL; Skolasky, RL; Dawson, TM; Marsh, L; Troncoso, JC. Abeta deposition is associated with enhanced cortical alpha-synuclein lesions in Lewy body diseases. *Neurobiol Aging.*, 2005 Aug-Sep, 26(8), 1183-1192.

[97] Masliah, E; Rockenstein, E; Veinbergs, I; Sagara, Y; Mallory, M; Hashimoto, M; Mucke, L. beta-amyloid peptides enhance alpha-synuclein accumulation and neuronal deficits in a transgenic mouse model linking Alzheimer's disease and Parkinson's disease. *Proc Natl Acad Sci U S A.* 2001 Oct 9, 98(21), 12245-12250.

[98] Clinton, LK; Blurton-Jones, M; Myczek, K; Trojanowski, JQ; LaFerla FM. Synergistic Interactions between Abeta, tau, and alpha-synuclein, acceleration of neuropathology and cognitive decline. *J Neurosci.*, 2010 May 26, 30(21), 7281-7289.

[99] Tsuang, D; Leverenz, JB; Lopez, OL; Hamilton, RL; Bennett, DA; Schneider, JA; Buchman, AS; Larson, EB; Crane, PK; Kaye, JA; Kramer, P; Woltjer, R; Trojanowski, JQ; Weintraub, D; Chen-Plotkin, AS; Irwin, DJ; Rick, J; Schellenberg, GD; Watson, GS; Kukull, W; Nelson, PT; Jicha, GA; Neltner, JH; Galasko, D; Masliah, E; Quinn, JF; Chung, KA; Yearout, D; Mata, IF; Wan, JY; Edwards, KL; Montine, TJ; Zabetian, CP. APOE ε4 increases risk for dementia in pure synucleinopathies. *JAMA Neurol.*, 2013 Feb, 70(2), 223-228.

[100] Duda, JE. Pathology and neurotransmitter abnormalities of dementia with Lewy bodies. *Dement Geriatr Cogn Disord.*, 2004, 17 Suppl 1, 3-14.

[101] Sinha, N; Firbank, M; O'Brien, JT. Biomarkers in dementia with Lewy bodies, a review. *Int J Geriatr Psychiatry.*, 2012 May, 27(5), 443-453.

[102] Shimada, H; Hirano, S; Sinotoh, H; Ota, T; Tanaka, N; Sato, K; Yamada, M; Fukushi, K; Irie, T; Zhang, MR; Higuchi, M; Kuwabara, S; Suhara, T. Dementia with Lewy bodies can be well-differentiated from Alzheimer's disease by measurement of brain acetylcholinesterase activity-a [(11)C]MP4A PET study. *Int J Geriatr Psychiatry.*, 2015 Nov, 30(11), 1105-1113.

[103] Bohnen, NI; Kaufer, DI; Hendrickson, R; Ivanco, LS; Lopresti, BJ; Koeppe, RA; Meltzer, CC; Constantine, G; Davis, JG; Mathis, CA; Dekosky, ST; Moore, RY. Degree of inhibition of cortical acetylcholinesterase activity and cognitive effects by donepezil treatment in Alzheimer's disease. *J Neurol Neurosurg Psychiatry.* 2005 Mar, 76(3), 315-319.

[104] Saha, GB; MacIntyre, WJ; Go, RT. Radiopharmaceuticals for brain imaging. *Semin Nucl Med.*, 1994 Oct, 24(4), 324-349.

[105] Shimizu, S; Hanyu, H; Kanetaka, H; Iwamoto, T; Koizumi, K; Abe, K. Differentiation of dementia with Lewy bodies from Alzheimer's disease using brain SPECT. *Dement Geriatr Cogn Disord.*, 2005, 20(1), 25-30.

[106] Colloby, SJ; Fenwick, JD; Williams, ED; Paling, SM; Lobotesis, K; Ballard, C; McKeith, I; O'Brien, JT. A comparison of (99m) Tc-HMPAO SPET changes in dementia with Lewy bodies and Alzheimer's disease using statistical parametric mapping. *Eur J Nucl Med Mol Imaging.*, 2002 May, 29(5), 615-622.

[107] Ceravolo, R; Volterrani, D; Gambaccini, G; Rossi, C; Logi, C; Manca, G; Berti, C; Mariani, G; Murri, L; Bonuccelli, U. Dopaminergic degeneration and perfusional impairment in Lewy body dementia and Alzheimer's disease. *Neurol Sci.*, 2003 Oct, 24(3), 162-163.

[108] O'Brien, JT; Colloby, S; Fenwick, J; Williams, ED; Firbank, M; Burn, D; Aarsland, D; McKeith, IG. Dopamine transporter loss visualized with FP-CIT SPECT in the differential diagnosis of dementia with Lewy bodies. *Arch Neurol.*, 2004 Jun, 61(6), 919-925.

[109] Walker, Z; Costa, DC; Walker, RW; Shaw, K; Gacinovic, S; Stevens, T; Livingston, G; Ince, P; McKeith, IG; Katona, CL. Differentiation of dementia with Lewy bodies from Alzheimer's disease using a dopaminergic presynaptic ligand. *J Neurol Neurosurg Psychiatry.*, 2002 Aug, 73(2), 134-140.

[110] McKeith, I; O'Brien, J; Walker, Z; Tatsch, K; Booij, J; Darcourt, J; Padovani, A; Giubbini, R; Bonuccelli, U; Volterrani, D; Holmes, C; Kemp, P; Tabet, N; Meyer, I; Reininger, C. DLB Study Group. Sensitivity and specificity of dopamine transporter

imaging with 123I-FP-CIT SPECT in dementia with Lewy bodies: a phase III, multicentre study. *Lancet Neurol.*, 2007 Apr, 6(4), 305-313.

[111] O'Brien, JT; McKeith, IG; Walker, Z; Tatsch, K; Booij, J; Darcourt, J; Marquardt, M; Reininger, C. DLB Study Group. Diagnostic accuracy of 123I-FP-CIT SPECT in possible dementia with Lewy bodies. *Br J Psychiatry.*, 2009 Jan, 194(1), 34-39.

[112] Walker, Z; Jaros, E; Walker, RW; Lee, L; Costa, DC; Livingston, G; Ince, PG; Perry, R; McKeith, I; Katona, CL. Dementia with Lewy bodies: a comparison of clinical diagnosis, FP-CIT single photon emission computed tomography imaging and autopsy. *J Neurol Neurosurg Psychiatry.*, 2007 Nov, 78(11), 1176-1181.

[113] Jauković, L; Ilić, TV; Dopudja, M; Ajdinović, B. 123I-FP-CIT brain SPECT (DaTSCAN) imaging in the diagnosis of patients with movement disorders--first results. *Vojnosanit Pregl.* 2012 Feb, 69(2), 157-162.

[114] Kemp, PM; Hoffmann, SA; Tossici-Bolt, L; Fleming, JS; Holmes, C. Limitations of the HMPAO SPECT appearances of occipital lobe perfusion in the differential diagnosis of dementia with Lewy bodies. *Nucl Med Commun.*, 2007 Jun, 28(6), 451-456.

[115] Watson, R; Blamire, AM; O'Brien, JT. Magnetic resonance imaging in lewy body dementias. *Dement Geriatr Cogn Disord.*, 2009, 28(6), 493-506.

[116] Soares, DP; Law, M. Magnetic resonance spectroscopy of the brain: review of metabolites and clinical applications. *Clin Radiol.*, 2009 Jan, 64(1), 12-21.

[117] Moffett, JR; Ross, B; Arun, P; Madhavarao, CN; Namboodiri, AM. N-Acetylaspartate in the CNS: from neurodiagnostics to neurobiology. *Prog Neurobiol.*, 2007 Feb, 81(2), 89-131.

[118] Griffith, HR; den Hollander, JA; Okonkwo, OC; O'Brien, T; Watts, RL; Marson, DC. Brain metabolism differs in Alzheimer's disease and Parkinson's disease dementia. *Alzheimers Dement.*, 2008 Nov, 4(6), 421-427.

[119] Chao, LL; Schuff, N; Kramer, JH; Du, AT; Capizzano, AA; O'Neill, J; Wolkowitz, OM; Jagust, WJ; Chui, HC; Miller, BL; Yaffe, K; Weiner, MW. Reduced medial temporal lobe N-acetylaspartate in cognitively impaired but nondemented patients. *Neurology.*, 2005 Jan 25, 64(2), 282-289.

[120] Jessen, F; Traeber, F; Freymann, K; Maier, W; Schild, HH; Block, W. Treatment monitoring and response prediction with proton MR spectroscopy in AD. *Neurology.*, 2006 Aug 8, 67(3), 528-530.

[121] Griffith, HR; den Hollander, JA; Okonkwo, OC; O'Brien, T; Watts, RL; Marson, DC. Brain N-acetylaspartate is reduced in Parkinson disease with dementia. *Alzheimer Dis Assoc Disord.*, 2008 Jan-Mar, 22(1), 54-60.

[122] Xuan, X; Ding, M; Gong, X. Proton magnetic resonance spectroscopy detects a relative decrease of N-acetylaspartate in the hippocampus of patients with dementia with Lewy bodies. *J Neuroimaging.*, 2008 Apr, 18(2), 137-141.

[123] Logothetis, NK; Pauls, J; Augath, M; Trinath, T; Oeltermann, A. 2001. Neurophysiological investigation of the basis of the fMRI signal. *Nature*, 412, 150–157.

[124] Buckner, RL; Andrews-Hanna, JR; Schacter, DL. The brain's default network: anatomy, function, and relevance to disease. *Ann N Y Acad Sci.*, 2008 Mar, 1124, 1-38.

[125] Small, SA; Perera, GM; DeLaPaz, R; Mayeux, R; Stern, Y. Differential regional dysfunction of the hippocampal formation among elderly with memory decline and Alzheimer's disease. *Ann Neurol.*, 1999 Apr, 45(4), 466-472.

[126] Rombouts, SA; Barkhof, F; Veltman, DJ; Machielsen, WC; Witter, MP; Bierlaagh, MA; Lazeron, RH; Valk, J; Scheltens, P. 2000. Functional MR imaging in Alzheimer's disease during memory encoding. *Am J Neuroradiol*, 21, 1869–1875.

[127] Wang, L; Zang, Y; He, Y; Liang, M; Zhang, X; Tian, L; Wu, T; Jiang, T; Li, K. Changes in hippocampal connectivity in the early stages of Alzheimer's disease: evidence from resting state fMRI. *Neuroimage.*, 2006 Jun, 31(2), 496-504.

[128] Zhang, HY; Wang, SJ; Xing, J; Liu, B; Ma, ZL; Yang, M; Zhang, ZJ; Teng, GJ. Detection of PCC functional connectivity characteristics in resting-state fMRI in mild Alzheimer's disease. *Behav Brain Res.*, 2009 Jan 30, 197(1), 103-108.

[129] Wu, X; Li, R; Fleisher, AS; Reiman, EM; Guan, X; Zhang, Y; Chen, K; Yao, L. Altered default mode network connectivity in Alzheimer's disease--a resting functional MRI and Bayesian network study. *Hum Brain Mapp.*, 2011 Nov, 32(11), 1868-1881.

[130] Zhang, HY; Wang, SJ; Liu, B; Ma, ZL; Yang, M; Zhang, ZJ; Teng, GJ. Resting brain connectivity: changes during the progress of Alzheimer disease. *Radiology.*, 2010 Aug, 256(2), 598-606.

[131] Schwindt, GC; Chaudhary, S; Crane, D; Ganda, A; Masellis, M; Grady, CL; Stefanovic, B; Black, SE. Modulation of the default-mode network between rest and task in Alzheimer's Disease. *Cereb Cortex.*, 2013 Jul, 23(7), 1685-1694.

[132] Hafkemeijer, A; van der Grond, J; Rombouts, SA. (2012) Imaging the default mode network in aging and dementia. *Biochim Biophys Acta*, 1822, 431-441.

[133] Kenny ER; Blamire AM; Firbank MJ; O'Brien JT. Functional connectivity in cortical regions in dementia with Lewy bodies and Alzheimer's disease. *Brain.*, 2012 Feb, 135(Pt 2), 569-581.

[134] Dickerson, BC; Salat, DH; Bates, JF; Atiya, M; Killiany, RJ; Greve, DN; Dale, AM; Stern, CE; Blacker, D; Albert, MS; et al. 2004. Medial temporal lobe function and structure in mild cognitive impairment. *Ann Neurol*, 56, 27–35.

[135] Celone, KA; Calhoun, VD; Dickerson, BC; Atri, A; Chua, EF; Miller, SL; DePeau, K; Rentz, DM; Selkoe, DJ; Blacker, D; Albert, MS; Sperling, RA. Alterations in memory networks in mild cognitive impairment and Alzheimer's disease: an independent component analysis. *J Neurosci.*, 2006 Oct 4, 26(40), 10222-10231.

[136] Johnson, KA; Fox, NC; Sperling, RA; Klunk, WE. Brain imaging in Alzheimer disease. *Cold Spring Harb Perspect Med.*, 2012 Apr,. 2(4), a006213.

[137] Wu, T; Long, X; Wang, L; Hallett, M; Zang, Y; Li, K; Chan, P. Functional connectivity of cortical motor areas in the resting state in Parkinson's disease. *Hum Brain Mapp.*, 2011 Sep, 32(9), 1443-1457.

[138] Helmich, RC; Derikx, LC; Bakker, M; Scheeringa, R; Bloem, BR; Toni, I. Spatial remapping of cortico-striatal connectivity in Parkinson's disease. *Cereb Cortex.*, 2010, 20, 1175–1186.

[139] Baudrexel, S; Witte, T; Seifried, C; et al. Resting state fMRI reveals increased subthalamic nucleus-motor cortex connectivity in Parkinson's disease. *Neuroimage.*, 2011, 55, 1728–1738.

[140] Kwak, Y; Peltier, S; Bohnen, NI; Müller, ML; Dayalu, P; Seidler, RD. Altered resting state cortico-striatal connectivity in mild to moderate stage Parkinson's disease. *Front Syst Neurosci.*, 2010, 4, 143.

[141] Pievani, M; de Haan, W; Wu, T; Seeley, WW; Frisoni, GB. Functional network disruption in the degenerative dementias. *Lancet Neurol.*, 2011 Sep, 10(9), 829-843.
[142] Peraza, LR; Colloby, SJ; Firbank, MJ; Greasy, GS; McKeith, IG; Kaiser, M; O'Brien, J; Taylor, JP. Resting state in Parkinson's disease dementia and dementia with Lewy bodies: commonalities and differences. *Int J Geriatr Psychiatry.*, 2015 Nov, 30(11), 1135-1146.
[143] Franciotti, R; Falasca, NW; Bonanni, L; Anzellotti, F; Maruotti, V; Comani, S; Thomas, A; Tartaro, A; Taylor, JP; Onofrj, M. Default network is not hypoactive in dementia with fluctuating cognition: an Alzheimer disease/dementia with Lewy bodies comparison. *Neurobiol Aging.*, 2013 Apr, 34(4), 1148-1158.
[144] van Eimeren, T; Monchi, O; Ballanger, B; Strafella, AP. Dysfunction of the default mode network in Parkinson disease: a functional magnetic resonance imaging study. *Arch Neurol.*, 2009 Jul, 66(7), 877-883.
[145] Rombouts, SA; Barkhof, F; Van Meel, CS; Scheltens, P. Alterations in brain activation during cholinergic enhancement with rivastigmine in Alzheimer's disease. *J Neurol Neurosurg Psychiatry.*, 2002 Dec, 73(6), 665-671.
[146] Saykin, AJ; Wishart, HA; Rabin, LA; Flashman, LA; McHugh, TL; Mamourian, AC; Santulli, RB. Cholinergic enhancement of frontal lobe activity in mild cognitive impairment. *Brain.*, 2004 Jul, 127(Pt 7), 1574-1583.
[147] Sperling, R. Potential of functional MRI as a biomarker in early Alzheimer's disease. *Neurobiol Aging.*, 2011 Dec, 32 Suppl 1, S37-43.
[148] Gasnier, B; Roisin, MP; Scherman, D; Coornaert, S; Desplanches, G; Henry, JP. Uptake of meta-iodobenzylguanidine by bovine chromaffin granule membranes. *Mol Pharmacol.*, 1986 Mar, 29(3), 275-280.
[149] Braune, S; Reinhardt, M; Schnitzer, R; Riedel, A; Lücking, CH. Cardiac uptake of [123I]MIBG separates Parkinson's disease from multiple system atrophy. *Neurology.*, 1999 Sep 22, 53(5), 1020-1025.
[150] Goldstein, DS; Holmes, CS; Dendi, R; Bruce, SR; Li, ST. Orthostatic hypotension from sympathetic denervation in Parkinson's disease. *Neurology.*, 2002 Apr 23, 58(8), 1247-1255.
[151] Allan, LM; Ballard, CG; Allen, J; Murray, A; Davidson, AW; McKeith, IG; Kenny, RA. Autonomic dysfunction in dementia. *J Neurol Neurosurg Psychiatry.*, 2007 Jul, 78(7), 671-677.
[152] Hanyu, H; Shimizu, S; Hirao, K; Sakurai, H; Iwamoto, T; Chikamori, T; Hida, S; Yamashina, A; Koizumi, K; Abe, K. The role of 123I-metaiodobenzylguanidine myocardial scintigraphy in the diagnosis of Lewy body disease in patients with dementia in a memory clinic. *Dement Geriatr Cogn Disord.*, 2006, 22(5-6), 379-384.
[153] Taki, J; Yoshita, M; Yamada, M; Tonami, N. Significance of 123I-MIBG scintigraphy as a pathophysiological indicator in the assessment of Parkinson's disease and related disorders: it can be a specific marker for Lewy body disease. *Ann Nucl Med.*, 2004 Sep, 18(6), 453-461.
[154] Yoshita, M; Taki, J; Yamada, M. A clinical role for [(123)I]MIBG myocardial scintigraphy in the distinction between dementia of the Alzheimer's-type and dementia with Lewy bodies. *J Neurol Neurosurg Psychiatry.*, 2001 Nov, 71(5), 583-588.

[155] Hanyu, H; Shimizu, S; Hirao, K; Kanetaka, H; Iwamoto, T; Chikamori, T; Usui, Y; Yamashina, A; Koizumi, K; Abe, K. Comparative value of brain perfusion SPECT and [(123)I]MIBG myocardial scintigraphy in distinguishing between dementia with Lewy bodies and Alzheimer's disease. *Eur J Nucl Med Mol Imaging.*, 2006 Mar, 33(3), 248-253.

[156] Wada-Isoe, K; Kitayama, M; Nakaso, K; Nakashima, K. Diagnostic markers for diagnosing dementia with Lewy bodies: CSF and MIBG cardiac scintigraphy study. *J Neurol Sci.*, 2007 Sep 15, 260(1-2), 33-37.

[157] Braune, S; Reinhardt, M; Schnitzer, R; Riedel, A; Lücking, CH. Cardiac uptake of [123I]MIBG separates Parkinson's disease from multiple system atrophy. *Neurology.*, 1999 Sep 22, 53(5), 1020-1025.

[158] Nagayama, H; Hamamoto, M; Ueda, M; Nagashima, J; Katayama, Y. Reliability of MIBG myocardial scintigraphy in the diagnosis of Parkinson's disease. *J Neurol Neurosurg Psychiatry.*, 2005 Feb, 76(2), 249-251.

[159] Jack, CR; Jr; Knopman, DS; Jagust, WJ; Shaw, LM; Aisen, PS; Weiner, MW; Petersen, RC; Trojanowski, JQ. Hypothetical model of dynamic biomarkers of the Alzheimer's pathological cascade. *Lancet Neurol.*, 2010 Jan, 9(1), 119-128.

[160] Rosa-Neto, P; Hsiung, GY; Masellis, M. CCDTD4 participants. Fluid biomarkers for diagnosing dementia: rationale and the Canadian Consensus on Diagnosis and Treatment of Dementia recommendations for Canadian physicians. *Alzheimers Res Ther.*, 2013 Nov 25, 5(Suppl 1), S8.

[161] Seeman, P; Seeman, N. Alzheimer's disease: β-amyloid plaque formation in human brain. *Synapse.*, 2011 Dec, 65(12), 1289-1297.

[162] Gao, CM; Yam, AY; Wang, X; Magdangal, E; Salisbury, C; Peretz, D; Zuckermann, RN; Connolly, MD; Hansson, O; Minthon, L; Zetterberg, H; Blennow, K; Fedynyshyn, JP; Allauzen, S. Aβ40 oligomers identified as a potential biomarker for the diagnosis of Alzheimer's disease. *PLoS One.*, 2010 Dec 30, 5(12), e15725.

[163] Tolboom, N; van der Flier, WM; Yaqub, M; Boellaard, R; Verwey, NA; Blankenstein, MA; Windhorst, AD; Scheltens, P; Lammertsma, AA; van Berckel, BN. Relationship of cerebrospinal fluid markers to 11C-PiB and 18F-FDDNP binding. *J Nucl Med.*, 2009 Sep, 50(9), 1464-1470.

[164] Weigand, SD; Vemuri, P; Wiste, HJ; Senjem, ML; Pankratz, VS; Aisen, PS; Weiner, MW; Petersen, RC; Shaw, LM; Trojanowski, JQ; Knopman, DS; Jack, CR; Jr; Alzheimer's Disease Neuroimaging Initiative. Transforming cerebrospinal fluid Aβ42 measures into calculated Pittsburgh Compound B units of brain Aβ amyloid. *Alzheimers Dement.*, 2011 Mar, 7(2), 133-141.

[165] Kolarova, M; García-Sierra, F; Bartos, A; Ricny, J; Ripova, D. Structure and pathology of tau protein in Alzheimer disease. *Int J Alzheimers Dis.*, 2012, 2012, 731526.

[166] lennow, K; Hampel, H. CSF markers for incipient Alzheimer's disease. *Lancet Neurol.*, 2003 Oct, 2(10), 605-613.

[167] Andreasen, N; Minthon, L; Davidsson, P; Vanmechelen, E; Vanderstichele, H; Winblad, B; Blennow, K. Evaluation of CSF-tau and CSF-Abeta42 as diagnostic markers for Alzheimer disease in clinical practice. *Arch Neurol.*, 2001 Mar, 58(3), 373-379.

[168] Hansson, O; Zetterberg, H; Buchhave, P; Londos, E; Blennow, K; Minthon, L. Association between CSF biomarkers and incipient Alzheimer's disease in patients with mild cognitive impairment: a follow-up study. *Lancet Neurol.*, 2006 Mar, 5(3), 228-234.

[169] Kanemaru, K; Kameda, N; Yamanouchi, H. Decreased CSF amyloid beta42 and normal tau levels in dementia with Lewy bodies. *Neurology.*, 2000 May 9, 54(9), 1875-1876.

[170] Mollenhauer, B; Cepek, L; Bibl, M; Wiltfang, J; Schulz-Schaeffer, WJ; Ciesielczyk, B; Neumann, M; Steinacker, P; Kretzschmar, HA; Poser, S; Trenkwalder, C; Otto, M. Tau protein, Abeta42 and S-100B protein in cerebrospinal fluid of patients with dementia with Lewy bodies. *Dement Geriatr Cogn Disord.*, 2005, 19(2-3), 164-170.

[171] Slaets, S; Le Bastard, N; Theuns, J; Sleegers, K; Verstraeten, A; De Leenheir, E; Luyckx, J; Martin, JJ; Van Broeckhoven, C; Engelborghs, S. Amyloid pathology influences aβ1-42 cerebrospinal fluid levels in dementia with lewy bodies. *J Alzheimers Dis.*, 2013, 35(1), 137-146.

[172] Mollenhauer, B; Esselmann, H; Trenkwalder, C; Schulz-Schaeffer, W; Kretzschmar, H; Otto, M; Wiltfang, J; Bibl, M. CSF amyloid-β peptides in neuropathologically diagnosed dementia with Lewy bodies and Alzheimer's disease. *J Alzheimers Dis.*, 2011, 24(2), 383-391.

[173] Parnetti, L; Lanari, A; Amici, S; Gallai, V; Vanmechelen, E; Hulstaert, F. Phospho-Tau International Study Group. CSF phosphorylated tau is a possible marker for discriminating Alzheimer's disease from dementia with Lewy bodies. Phospho-Tau International Study Group. *Neurol Sci.*, 2001 Feb, 22(1), 77-78.

[174] Andersson, M; Zetterberg, H; Minthon, L; Blennow, K; Londos, E. The cognitive profile and CSF biomarkers in dementia with Lewy bodies and Parkinson's disease dementia. *Int J Geriatr Psychiatry.*, 2011 Jan, 26(1), 100-105.

[175] Kasuga, K; Tokutake, T; Ishikawa, A; Uchiyama, T; Tokuda, T; Onodera, O; Nishizawa, M; Ikeuchi, T. Differential levels of alpha-synuclein, beta-amyloid42 and tau in CSF between patients with dementia with Lewy bodies and Alzheimer's disease. *J Neurol Neurosurg Psychiatry.*, 2010 Jun, 81(6), 608-610.

[176] Wennström, M; Surova, Y; Hall, S; Nilsson, C; Minthon, L; Boström, F; Hansson, O; Nielsen, HM. Low CSF levels of both α-synuclein and the α-synuclein cleaving enzyme neurosin in patients with synucleinopathy. *PLoS One.*, 2013, 8(1), e53250.

[177] Kapaki, E; Paraskevas, GP; Emmanouilidou, E; Vekrellis, K. The diagnostic value of CSF α-synuclein in the differential diagnosis of dementia with Lewy bodies vs. normal subjects and patients with Alzheimer's disease. *PLoS One.*, 2013 Nov 25, 8(11), e81654.

[178] Gao, L; Tang, H; Nie, K; Wang, L; Zhao, J; Gan, R; Huang, J; Zhu, R; Feng, S; Duan, Z; Zhang, Y; Wang, L. Cerebrospinal fluid alpha-synuclein as a biomarker for Parkinson's disease diagnosis: a systematic review and meta-analysis. *Int J Neurosci.*, 2015, 125(9), 645-654.

[179] Sako, W; Murakami, N; Izumi, Y; Kaji, R. Reduced alpha-synuclein in cerebrospinal fluid in synucleinopathies: evidence from a meta-analysis. *Mov Disord.*, 2014 Nov, 29(13), 1599-1605.

[180] Masellis, M; Sherborn, K; Neto, P; Sadovnick, DA; Hsiung, GY; Black, SE; Prasad, S; Williams, M; Gauthier, S. Early-onset dementias: diagnostic and etiological considerations. *Alzheimers Res Ther.*, 2013 Jul 31, 5(Suppl 1), S7.

[181] Frisoni, GB; Bocchetta, M; Chételat, G; Rabinovici, GD; de Leon, MJ; Kaye, J; Reiman, EM; Scheltens, P; Barkhof, F; Black, SE; Brooks, DJ; Carrillo, MC; Fox, NC; Herholz, K; Nordberg, A; Jack, CR; Jr; Jagust, WJ; Johnson, KA; Rowe, CC; Sperling, RA; Thies, W; Wahlund, LO; Weiner, MW; Pasqualetti, P; Decarli, C. ISTAART's NeuroImaging Professional Interest Area. Imaging markers for Alzheimer disease: which vs how. *Neurology.*, 2013 Jul 30, 81(5), 487-500.

In: Progressive Cognitive Impairment …
Editor: Gediminas Peter Gliebus
ISBN: 978-1-63485-221-0

Chapter 3

FUNCTION AND DYSFUNCTION OF THE PREFRONTAL LOBES IN NEURODEGENERATIVE DISEASES

Alexandre Henri-Bhargava[1,2,*]
Donald T. Stuss[3,4,5] ***and Morris Freedman***[4,6,7]
[1]University of British Columbia (Island Medical Program), Victoria, B.C., Canada
[2]Division of Medical Sciences, University of Victoria, Victoria, B.C., Canada
[3]University of Toronto, Toronto, Ontario, Canada
[4]Rotman Research Institute, Baycrest, Toronto, Ontario, Canada
[5]Sunnybrook Health Sciences Centre, Toronto, Ontario, Canada
[6]Department of Medicine, Division of Neurology, Baycrest, Mt Sinai Hospital, and University of Toronto, Canada
[7]Sam and Ida Ross Memory Clinic, Baycrest, Toronto, Ontario, Canada

ABSTRACT

Clinical assessment of the functions of the prefrontal cortex in physiological and pathological states is dependent on one's model of prefrontal function. There is no overarching "frontal lobe syndrome"; rather, the prefrontal cortices are involved in a number of distinct cognitive and social-behavioural processes. Stuss, Shallice, Alexander and Picton studied patients with focal lesions. They found that damage to anterior cingulate and other superior medial prefrontal regions caused deficits in *energization*, which manifests clinically as a spectrum of disorders characterized by difficulty initiating and sustaining a response on cognitive testing and in daily behaviour. Damage to right dorsolateral prefrontal cortex (DLPFC) caused deficits in *monitoring*, and damage to left DLPFC caused deficits in *task setting*. Injury to ventromedial prefrontal cortex caused deficits in *emotional or behavioural self-regulation*; this may not be easily detected

* Correspondence to: alexhb@uvic.ca.

through bedside tests and requires careful history taking and observation for accurate diagnosis. Finally, damage to the frontal poles caused deficits in *metacognitive functions*. These different prefrontal areas participate in distinct cortico-striato-pallido-thalamo-cortical loops, but also form parts of larger scale frontal connectivity networks. Prefrontal dysfunction can be a symptom of the subcortical dementias, which include Parkinson's disease and vascular dementia among many others. Prefrontal dysfunction is also found in the frontotemporal dementias, and can also be present in the behavioural/dysexecutive variant of Alzheimer's disease. Bedside clinical tests and methods of observation are described that are sensitive to dysfunction of the prefrontal lobes.

Terminology

Descriptions of prefrontal lobe functions have been associated with confusing terminology. In this chapter, terms are defined in a manner that will be useful for clinicians without sacrificing specificity. Strictly speaking, "frontal functions" include the functions of the primary and secondary motor cortices, as well as other areas such as the frontal eye fields. These will not be discussed. Instead the focus will be on higher order cognitive and social-emotional functions that rely heavily upon more anterior structures within the frontal lobes, and which are termed "prefrontal functions." It should be noted that many often use the term "frontal function" synonymously with "prefrontal function," even though these are technically not equivalent.

The term "executive function" is even more problematic; there are myriad definitions for this term. In this chapter executive functions are defined as a set of interrelated cognitive processes required for complex goal-directed activity, including processes such as planning, monitoring, goal-setting, etc. Disruption of these functions are most often observed after damage to the frontal lobes [1]. The terms "executive function" and "frontal or prefrontal lobe function" have often been used synonymously. However, the prefrontal lobes are involved in more than those cognitive functions usually considered to be "executive." Furthermore, regions outside the frontal lobes are involved in many executive functions [2]. In addition, executive functions refer to cognitive processes whereas the prefrontal lobes define an anatomical structure [3]. For these reasons, "executive functions" are not equivalent to "prefrontal functions," even though many executive functions are highly dependent upon the prefrontal cortices (Figure 1).

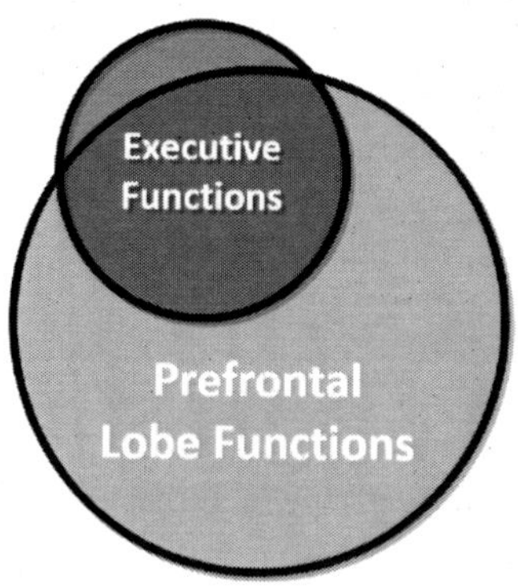

Figure 1. Relationship between prefrontal lobe functions and executive functions.

NEUROANATOMY OF PREFRONTAL FUNCTIONS

Stuss' Model of Prefrontal Function

There are different models of prefrontal function. Stuss, Shallice, Alexander and Picton, based on review of literature and a theoretical hypothesis, proposed that prefrontal lobe abilities consist of different functional categories interacting to achieve complex human behaviours [4]. To prove this, they examined patients with focal damage to specific frontal areas on theoretically derived experimental tests. The results indicated four anatomically segregated functions of the prefrontal lobes: energization, executive, behavioural/emotional self-regulation, and metacognition [3]. This model is an elaboration of the processes involved in the influential Supervisory System model of Norman and Shallice [5].

Deficits in *energization,* defined as "the process of initiating and sustaining any response," were secondary to damage to anterior cingulate and other superior medial prefrontal regions (SMPFC). Only two functions fit the classical definition of *executive functions*, and these were related to lateral frontal regions: right dorsolateral prefrontal cortex (DLPFC) - monitoring; left DLPFC - task setting, or planning. Monitoring is the process of checking a task over time and adjusting behaviour as needed for successful completion. Task Setting refers to putting in place a plan in response to a stimulus or demand, e.g., learning to drive a car, organizing the plan, and coordinating processes required to carry out the task such as putting the foot on the brake, as opposed to the gas pedal, when stopping the car [6].

Deficits in processes involving *emotional or behavioural self-regulation* occurred in patients with injuries to ventromedial prefrontal cortex. Finally, patients with damage to the frontal poles (FPs) may have deficits in *metacognitive functions* such as self-awareness and ability to take the perspective of others, i.e., theory of mind (ToM) [3, 7].

Cortico-Striato-Pallido-Thalamo-Cortical Loops

The frontal lobes do not function as a single neuroanatomical unit. Early on, researchers identified neural projections from the frontal lobes to corpus striatum, from corpus striatum to globus pallidus, from globus pallidus to thalamus, and from thalamus back to the frontal lobes. These have been called cortico-striatal-pallidal-thalamic loops (also shortened to frontal-subcortical circuits). Research in the 1970's and 1980's, particularly through axonal tracer studies in primates, culminated in a model of these loops proposed by Alexander, Delong and Strick, and which continues to form the basis of our understanding of frontal lobe function and connectivity [8]. This model proposes distinct, parallel cortico-striato-pallido-thalamo-cortical loops, subserving distinct functions. Refinements to this model have revealed loops involved in motor function, cognitive function, and social-emotional processing [9]. These loops originate from primary motor cortex and supplementary motor area, frontal and supplementary eye fields, DLPFC, lateral prefrontal cortex (LatPFC), medial OFC, and anterior cingulate cortex (ACC) and frontal insular (FI) regions. They are illustrated in Figure 2.

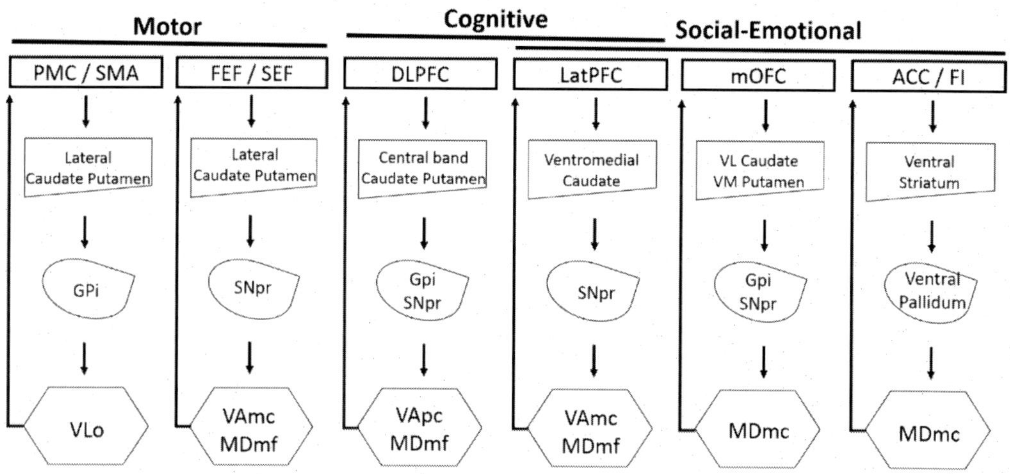

Figure 2. Frontal-Subcortical Circuits, based on Seeley's update of Alexander, Delong and Strick's model. Note that these loops are simplified; additional areas project to the striatum including areas outside of the frontal lobes. There are also myriad cortico-cortical and cortico-limbic connections that interconnect these loops. ACC = anterior cingulate cortex; DLPFC = dorsolateral prefrontal cortex; FEF = frontal eye fields; FI = frontal insula; GPi = globus pallidus pars compacta; LatPFC = lateral prefrontal cortex; MDmc = medialis dorsalis, pars magnocellularis; MDmf = medialis dorsalis, pars multiformis; mOFC = medial orbitofrontal cortex; SEF = supplementary eye fields; SMA = supplemental motor area; SNpr = subtantia nigra pars reticularis; VAmc = ventralis anterior, pars magnocellularis; VApc = ventralis anterior, pars parvocellularis; VL = ventrolateral; VLo = ventralis lateralis, pars oralis; VM = ventromedial.

Integration of the Two Models

Stuss' model has been mapped onto the cortico-striatal loop model [3]. The DLPFC loop is involved in cognitive functions including task setting and monitoring, lateralized to the left and right hemispheres, respectively [6]. However, there is an additional LatPFC loop that is not accounted for in Stuss' model. It has been argued that this prefrontal region is mainly involved in stopping, shifting, and inhibition of undesired responses, and is therefore at a crossroads between cognitive and social-emotional processes [9, 10]. In contrast, Stuss and colleagues did not find experimental evidence of an independent inhibitory function in lesion studies. Instead, based on parsimony they argued that inhibition was a psychological construct, the functions of which could be accounted for by more fundamental frontal lobe processes, either singularly or combination of energization, task setting and monitoring [6].

The OFC loop is involved in emotional and behavioural self-regulation [11]. This regulation, however, may occur through more basic cognitive processes in which the OFC plays a role. Some have argued for the division of the OFC into a ventral and medial portion, based on distinct connectivity patterns [12]. Ventral OFC receives multimodal sensory input, particularly from sensory modalities related to appetitive drives (e.g., taste and visceral afferents), whereas the medial OFC provides output to visceromotor structures in the brainstem and hypothalamus, in addition to its projections to ventral striatum [12]. The OFC is therefore well suited to its role in dynamically updating the value of available rewards or options in the context of the current internal state of the individual. Indeed, imaging studies have demonstrated a role for the medial OFC in determining and updating the value of sensory stimuli and future outcomes. In keeping with this notion, patients with damage to orbitofrontal cortex are inconsistent when making basic preference choices [13].

The ACC circuit (SMPFC) is involved in *energization* in Stuss' model [3]. Functional neuroimaging studies suggest a role for error monitoring subserved by this circuit [14]. Some such studies have postulated a role for this area in determining and updating the value of future actions, although this observation may be biased by task specificity as differing experimental tasks require different levels of energization [15, 16].

The metacognitive processes putatively located in the FPs are not part of any of these loops. It is thought that the FPs integrate information from diverse prefrontal cortical regions, without themselves having direct subcortical connections. Because the frontal pole is connected to both OFC and SMPFC, it has been suggested that this region can integrate information about the value of future outcomes and of future actions [15, 17]. However, the precise mechanisms whereby this leads to metacognitive processes are unclear.

Larger-Scale Frontal Networks

Further insights into prefrontal function have been gained in the past decade by studying brain regions that are functionally connected. Using resting state functional MRI, Seeley and colleagues identified an executive control network (ECN), and a salience network (SN) [18]. The ECN demonstrates that the DLPFC is functionally connected with the dorsal caudate nucleus and anterior thalamus (confirming functional linkage of the anatomically linked frontal-subcortical loops), and also with parietal areas and other frontal areas. The SN consists of a functional linkage between the ACC and FI, as well as subcortical structures, limbic structures, and importantly the OFC. This demonstrates cross-connectivity between different frontal-subcortical loops at a functionally connected network level, even though their distinctness was highlighted earlier.

Zhou and Seeley postulated that the "frontoinsula represents the major afferent SN hub, representing subjective "feeling states" by integrating inputs from the interoceptive stream with those arriving from other networks, whereas the ACC serves as an efferent SN hub for mobilizing visceroautonomic, emotional, cognitive, and behavioral responses to the salience detected in the frontoinsula" [19]. Thus, whereas the ventral/medial OFC system is involved in the valuation of outcome or reward options, the SN mobilizes visceral/emotional responses to salience and weighs these outcome values to guide behavior.

Clinical Assessment of Prefrontal Functions

This chapter will focus mainly on so-called "bedside" tests of prefrontal function, meaning tests that can be easily administered in routine clinical settings without use of special equipment or test materials. There are many tests used to probe prefrontal lobe function that are more typically used by neuropsychologists than physicians, and these will only be briefly touched upon. However, the principles regarding testing prefrontal functions remain the same, whether one uses bedside tests or formal neuropsychological tests.

Interpreting performance on tests of prefrontal lobe function requires experience and skill. Failure is relative, not absolute, and performance may be inconsistent. Furthermore, inconsistent performance on cognitive tasks, in and of itself, is a symptom of prefrontal lobe dysfunction [20].

An important point to highlight is that, although tests may be sensitive to lesions in selective prefrontal brain regions, patients may be impaired on these measures for reasons unrelated to prefrontal functions. For example, even though tests of verbal fluency are sensitive to prefrontal lesions, patients with language deficits due to temporal or parietal lesions may also have reduced verbal fluency. Therefore, since patients may be impaired on a given cognitive test for different reasons, interpretation of the findings will depend upon the context in which the deficits occur, the nature of the errors, and the comparison of the performance on one test in relation to others.

Thus, there are no "true" tests of prefrontal functions. Instead, there are tests that tap into one or more of the processes related to specific frontal regions. The same applies to executive function. Deficits in executive function detected by cognitive tasks are identified by the nature of the errors, and not simply by poor overall performance on a given test. For example, on a test of list learning, false positive errors suggest a task setting deficit with failure of setting a criterion to respond by only producing words on the list. In contrast, recalling the same word twice suggests poor monitoring of previously recalled words. Thus, it is not the list learning task itself that is a measure of executive function but the component processes of task setting and monitoring involved in completing the task. It should also be noted that there are not many validity studies of many of these tests in patients with focal lesions, and there are still questions of sensitivity and specificity.

Dorsolateral Prefrontal Functions

Clinical tests of prefrontal function have been developed over the last half-century, beginning with the work of Alexandre Luria, whose tests are still often used in routine clinical practice [21]. The vast majority of these tests tap into DLPFC functions. They examine distinct components of cognitive functions, and often are not all impaired in the same patient. This gives further support to the concept that functions of the frontal lobes are subserved by distinct sub-component processes.

A number of tests of DLPFC function require special materials for administration that are often not readily available in a physician's office or at the bedside. These tests are typically administered by neuropsychologists. Only one such popular test will be discussed, i.e., the Wisconsin Card Sorting Test (WCST). In contrast, many other tests can be readily administered in an office or "bedside" setting using only pencil and paper. An exhaustive description of all available tests is beyond the scope of this chapter, but some of the more commonly used tests will be discussed.

The *Wisconsin Card Sorting Test* (WCST) is used widely in experimental psychology and for clinical neuropsychological assessment, and is sensitive to deficits in executive function. A standard approach involves presenting patients with cards that can be sorted according to different criteria (colour, form, number). Patients are required to discover the sorting rules based upon feedback from the examiner. The first rule is to sort the cards by "colour." After 10 correct sorts, the criteria are changed to "form" without warning. After 10 correct sorts to "form," the criteria are then changed to "number," and then back to "colour" with the sequence being repeated until 6 sorts have been completed or 128 cards have been used up. Thus patients must discover the rule of sorting to colour, maintain this set, and then shift set after the sorting rule changes [22]. The WCST measures executive functions of task setting (discovering the sorting rule) and monitoring (maintaining the rule until it changes). A deficit in the process of task setting suggests a left DLPFC lesion whereas a deficit in monitoring suggests right DLPFC damage. This is most apparent by analyzing an individual's reaction to instructions: The first administration of the test will stress more an individual's ability to analyze and plan response, being more sensitive to left DLPFC damage; if errors are made after instructions are given, the problems are most likely sensitive to monitoring [23]. It is important to determine which version of the card sorting test has been used, since a version commonly used in the U.S. provides more details about the rules in an attempt to eliminate confusion, and in so doing potentially stresses more the process of monitoring rather than task setting or planning [24]. The requirement for a deck of stimulus cards precludes its widespread use as a standard bedside test.

Digit span backwards is commonly used as a bedside test of working memory due to DLPFC function [25]. It is generally administered after digit span forwards, a test of working memory that simply consists of determining the longest string of digits that a patient can repeat back. The backwards digit span test requires the patient to repeat the string in reverse order. This involves working memory as well as the executive functions of task setting, i.e., repeating the digits in reverse order as opposed to forwards, and monitoring, i.e., repeating the digits only once. Scoring options include noting the longest string of numbers that can be successfully repeated backward, and a discrepancy score between the forward and reverse digit span. This test is easy to administer at the bedside, but lacks specificity.

Due to impaired monitoring and task setting, patients with DLPFC damage may have difficulty performing tasks requiring sequencing of successive motor actions. Such tasks were initially developed by Luria and are easy to administer at the bedside [21]. These include a motor task known as the *Luria hand sequences*, in which patients are required to repetitively place their hand on the table in a "fist – edge – palm" sequence. A written equivalent of this task involves asking a patient to copy and continue drawing a sequence of alternating square-like and triangular figures. A related task that is more sensitive to deficiencies of monitoring is the multiple loops task in which patients are required to repetitively draw three loops without perseverating by drawing more than three loops [26]. Task setting is required for acquiring the set necessary to carry out the task. Monitoring is required to determine when to shift from one aspect of the task to another, such as stopping after drawing three loops and shifting to draw another figure with three loops. Patients who had undergone prefrontal leucotomies, which spares the DLPFC, are not impaired on these tests [27].

Various versions of the *go/no-go* task are popularly used to test DLPFC function, although patients may be impaired on these measures following medial frontal lesions [25]. Luria's original task involves raising one finger in response to one tap ("go") but making no movement in response to two taps ("no-go"). A modification of this task involves instructions to raise one finger in response to two taps and two fingers in response to one tap. This test involves executive functions of task setting, i.e., learning the target responses, and monitoring the stimuli to determine which response to make.

Tests of abstract thinking have long been used as tests of executive function. Popular among these is the *similarities test* wherein subjects are presented with two stimuli (words or objects) and asked in what way they are alike. Correct answers require mentally placing both stimuli into the same superordinate taxonomic categorization (task setting). This "consists of grouping objects or words according to their common features at a high level of generality" and has been shown to activate left peri-Sylvian prefrontal regions on PET scanning [28, 29]. Interpretation of proverbs has been proposed as an equivalent test of abstract thinking. However, the correct interpretation of a proverb may have more to do with having access to previously-learned semantic knowledge of the proverb's meaning, and therefore may be more a test of semantic memory [30]. Thus testing similarities may be preferable to proverbs, but even here familiarity may affect performance.

Lexical (phonemic) word-list generation is another common measure of executive function [31]. Patients are asked to name as many words beginning with a certain letter as possible in one minute, excluding proper names. A popular version of this test is the *FAS test*, where patients are asked to perform the task three times using each of the letters "F," "A," and "S." Normative values for performance on this task are available [32]. This task has been shown to be most impaired in patients with left DLPFC damage, although patients with medial frontal lesions can also be impaired due to deficits in energization [6, 33]. This test taps into multiple component sub-processes of the brain including retrieval, updating, shifting, inhibition, and energization [6, 34]. Task setting is required to generate as many different words as possible without false positive errors such as listing proper names. Monitoring is required to avoid repeating the same word.

Design fluency is the non-verbal homologue of lexical word-list generation. There are various versions of this task. At its most simple level, patients can be asked to draw as many unique figures as possible in a limited amount of time. This task was shown to be most impaired in patients with right DLPFC lesions [35]. In a more standardized version, patients are shown a matrix of five dots and asked to make as many unique figures as possible by joining the dots using straight lines, in one minute [36]. Various more complex versions of this task are available but become more cumbersome to use at the bedside and may be best used in the context of neuropsychological assessment [37].

Whereas word and design fluency tap into multiple components of DLPFC function, other tasks may tap into more basic components. The *Trail-making Test* (TMT) is employed as a popular test of DLPFC function [38]. Patients are presented with a sheet of paper with 25 circles. In *Part A*, the circles contain the numbers 1 to 25, and patients must connect the circles in ascending order by number as quickly as possible without making errors; thus testing basic visuomotor attention and scanning, as well as motor and visual search speed. In *Part B*, the circles contain the letters A to L and the numbers 1 to 13. Patients must alternate from number to letter in increasing order as quickly as possible without making errors. TMT Part B relies more heavily on task setting and monitoring, as compared to Part A. The TMT is easily administered at the bedside [39]. It should be noted that dysfunction outside of the DLPFC can cause impairment on the TMT, thus making it sensitive for prefrontal dysfunction but not always specific for DLPFC dysfunction [40].

The *clock drawing* test is easy and quick to administer at the bedside. Several processes are involved in *clock drawing* and include planning, monitoring, visuospatial function, and abstraction. Choosing the time setting is important for sensitivity of clock drawing as a cognitive assessment tool. Setting the time at 10 after 11 is one of the more sensitive times and illustrates the role of abstraction on the clock drawing task. For this time setting, the "10" must be mentally recoded so that the minute hand is set on the number "2." Patients with frontal lobe lesions who are impaired in abstract thinking tend to make stimulus-bound errors and process the "10" in a perceptual fashion rather than at a semantic level. Consequently they tend to place the minute hand on the "10' rather than the "2." [41] Executive functions required for clock drawing include task setting to plan the layout of the clock including the size and shape of the contour, placement of the numbers, and setting the time. Monitoring is required to avoid duplicating numbers and drawing extra hands, as well as self-correcting errors such as poor number placement.

Test batteries exist that incorporate several of the above tests. The *Executive Interview (EXIT-25)* is a widely-available 25-item assessment battery that incorporates a wide array of bedside tests, including many of those discussed above. It takes 15 minutes or more to administer and requires a freely-obtainable stimulus booklet [42]. Another popular battery is the *Frontal Assessment Battery (FAB),* which incorporates lexical word fluency, similarities, conflicting instructions, go/no-go, Luria hand sequences, and a measure of environmental dependency [43]. Scores less than 14/18 are considered suggestive of "frontal impairment," although strictly speaking, this battery mainly tests DLPFC functions. Of particular interest to clinicians, this battery was initially validated as a method for distinguishing non-Alzheimer dementias with primarily prefrontal dysfunction from the more typical amnestic syndrome of Alzheimer's disease (AD). The EXIT-25 and the FAB have been found to correlate quite closely, with the FAB being shorter and easier to administer [44].

Medial Prefrontal Functions

As discussed above, the SMPFC, and in particular the ACC, is involved in monitoring the value of future actions in response to internal states [15]. Therefore, dysfunction of this area leads to difficulties in initiating internally-driven actions. At the moderate and severe ends of the spectrum, this type of dysfunction is usually apparent from the patient history and behavioural observations. Deficits can range from apathy, a mild quantitative reduction in internally-generated behaviour, to a more significant reduction, termed abulia, or at the most severe extreme, akinetic mutism, in which there is a severe loss of all internally-generated behaviour [45, 46]. Different forms of apathy can be described which probably have differing neural bases [47]. Only some types of apathy can be considered amotivational. Furthermore, the terms apathy and abulia are at times used interchangeably in clinical settings [48].

Apart from careful clinical observation, bedside tests are rarely used to determine the presence or severity of an apathy syndrome. However, there are several rating scales that can be used to supplement clinical observation. The *Apathy Evaluation Scale* (AES) is a validated 18-item scale that is freely accessible, easy to administer, and comes in self-administered, informant-administered, and clinician-administered versions [49].

Some of the bedside tests of DLPFC function described earlier likely also tap into SMPFC function. Lexical word fluency was described above as a test of DLPFC function. However, in their experiments with patients who had lesions to SMPFC, Stuss and colleagues found deficiencies on this task as well [33]. More specifically, patients with SMPFC lesions named fewer words in the latter portion of the naming task, indicating that they had difficulty sustaining their effort due to poor energization. Patients with SMPFC damage also perform poorly on tasks requiring speeded responses [3]. Thus it should be expected that general psychomotor speed will be reduced in patients with superior medial damage. Psychomotor speed is not typically measured at the bedside, but usually commented upon in behavioural observations. Another cognitive task that is sensitive to medial frontal lesions is the *object alternation test* [50, 51, 52]. This test is also sensitive to orbitofrontal lesions and is described in the next section below.

Although apathy and amotivational syndromes are classically described as the hallmark of damage to the SMPFC, as well as the associated circuitry involving the ventral striatum (in particular the nucleus accumbens) and ventral pallidum (see Figure 2), such syndromes can develop with frontal and subcortical damage outside these areas. In fact, the driving mechanism producing some of these syndromes may often hinge on reduced output from the basal ganglia to any of the frontal-subcortical loops [53]. Amotivational syndromes, apathy, or other forms of reduced response to internal stimuli may therefore also be seen with dysfunction of the SMPFC or the basal ganglia.

In summary, behavioural observations for reduced psychomotor speed, apathy, abulia, or in extreme cases akinetic mutism, form the cornerstone of "testing" for SMPFC. Clinical rating scales can be used to bolster these observations. Reduced performance on speeded cognitive tasks or failure to maintain performance may also provide clues to the presence of SMPFC or basal ganglia dysfunction.

Orbitofrontal Functions

Dysfunction of the orbitofrontal areas produces changes in behaviour, emotion, appetite regulation, and social cognition. Seemingly unrelated behavioural disturbances may arise from a central problem in the evaluation of outcomes (including rewards) and options for action. These can include hyperphagia or altered food preferences, sexually inappropriate behaviour, loss of social decorum, jocularity, argumentativeness, capriciousness, narrowed or inappropriate preoccupations, and even criminal behaviour. When dysfunction is restricted to the orbitofrontal area of the brain, performance on tests of DLPFC function described above may be normal. The only clinical signs of OFC dysfunction may be evident from careful history taking or clinical observation of aberrant behaviour. However, formal clinical assessment scales may be helpful. For example, the *Frontal Behavioral Inventory* (FBI) is a clinician-administered assessment scale given to caregivers to aid in the diagnosis of behavioural variant frontotemporal dementia (bvFTD), and captures many of the abnormal behaviours that can be seen with OFC dysfunction. The FBI has also been used to demonstrate OFC dysfunction in neurological diseases other than bvFTD, and in traumatic brain injury [54, 55].

It can be difficult to distinguish aberrant behaviour in a neurologically intact individual with an unusual personality from early or mild signs of OFC dysfunction. Because standard bedside cognitive tests and clinical neuropsychological measures are relatively insensitive to OFC dysfunction, there is a need for development of cognitive tests of OFC function. One candidate is the *object alternation test*, a task adopted from the non-human animal literature to study cognitive function in humans and which has been shown by Freedman and colleagues to be sensitive to ventrolateral-orbitofrontal and medial frontal dysfunction in humans [50, 51]. During this task, a penny is placed under one of two objects. Subjects are required to learn that the object under which a penny is located is being alternated after each correct response. Freedman et al. showed the object alternation test is a highly sensitive measure of medial frontal function in bvFTD [52]. A limitation of the object alternation test for bedside use is that a test apparatus or computer program is required.

A battery of tests termed the *Executive and Social Cognition Battery* (ESCB) has been proposed as a sensitive measure of OFC dysfunction in bvFTD [56]. The components of the ESCB are derived from the experimental psychology literature and are thought to be tests of day-to-day activities in a "real-life" environment. These tests require specific stimuli including card decks, which restrict the utility of the ESCB as a bedside test; however, this battery may find utility within a more lengthy neuropsychological assessment.

Frontal Polar Functions

The FPs appear to be involved in metacognitive tasks such as perceiving one's own emotional state, perceiving emotional states of others, and understanding what another person may be thinking. The abilities to impute the mental states of oneself and others are referred to as theory of mind (ToM) [57]. ToM can be assessed using experimental tests such as the *false belief tasks* [58, 59, 60]. For example, on first order false belief tasks, stories are presented to a subject in which someone (Person A) puts an object away in the presence of another individual (Person B) and then leaves the room. Person B then moves the object to a different location while Person A is away. Person A returns and the subject is asked a belief question, i.e., "Where does Person A think that the object is?" Correctly answering this question requires the subject to take the mental perspective of Person A. Other ToM tasks involve recognition of humour from cartoons and stories which require the reader to understand a mind state [61]. ToM deficits have been demonstrated in patients with focal frontal lobe lesions, Parkinson's disease, AD, and bvFTD [59, 60, 62]. However, ToM is not routinely tested in clinical practice, although it certainly could be. Usually, deficits in ToM are imputed from the patient's history, for example when deficits in empathy are reported. The application of experimental ToM tasks to routine clinical practice is an untapped area of research.

Disorders of Prefrontal Functions in Neurodegenerative Diseases

There is a vast and interesting literature pertaining to disordered frontal lobe function in psychiatric disease and acquired neurological brain injury. However, this chapter will focus on disorders of the prefrontal lobes in neurodegenerative diseases. When dealing with neurodegenerative diseases affecting the prefrontal lobes, a useful heuristic has been to divide disorders between so-called "subcortical" and "cortical" dementias. The characteristic features of each are discussed below.

Subcortical Dementias

The term subcortical dementia was first used to describe cognitive deficits associated with progressive supranuclear palsy and Huntington's disease [63, 64]. It is now used to describe a syndrome associated with dysfunction of the frontal-subcortical loops and often involves damage to both cortical and subcortical structures pathologically [65]. A preferable term may be fronto-subcortical dementia since the neuropsychological deficits associated with subcortical dementia are often related to frontal system dysfunction [66]. In fact, these terms are often used interchangeably. In contrast to the subcortical dementias, the cortical dementias are syndromes in which disorders of memory, language, perception and praxis are prominent [67].

Clinically, patients with subcortical dementia tend to demonstrate features of SMPFC and DLPFC dysfunction. The classical profile of patients with subcortical dementia is characterized by forgetfulness, impaired manipulation of acquired knowledge (e.g., calculating and abstracting ability), personality changes marked by apathy or depression with occasional episodes of irritability, and slowed thought processes [63]. Patients usually demonstrate deficits in energization, performing poorly on speeded tasks. Memory encoding, a medial temporal function, is largely intact. However, retrieval, which relies on frontal-subcortical systems, may be impaired. Working memory may also be impaired. For example, patients may perform poorly on the reverse digit span task [68]. Patients may also be impaired on experimental measures of DLPFC functions, as well as clinical measures such as the TMT [69]. In addition, word list generation may be impaired. Aphasia is uncommon, although patients often have slow speech and dysarthria.

Subcortical dementias are caused by disorders affecting the subcortical grey matter structures, such as Parkinson's disease, Huntington's disease, progressive supranuclear palsy, thalamic degeneration, and AIDS dementia complex, or by disorders of the white matter connections between the prefrontal lobes and the subcortical grey matter structures, such as subcortical vascular cognitive impairment, idiopathic normal pressure hydrocephalus, or multiple sclerosis. In addition, frontal cortex may be affected [65]. It is likely that the specific characteristic of a subcortical dementia may relate to the specific frontal-subcortical pathway involved.

Behavioural Variant Frontotemporal Dementia (bvFTD)

Arnold Pick first described forms of dementia with focal atrophy, particularly in the frontal and temporal lobes [70]. These are now considered part of the spectrum of frontotemporal lobar degeneration (FTLD), which is a group of related but pathologically diverse neurodegenerative diseases that preferentially affect the frontal and temporal lobes. FTLD presents with a number of phenotypes determined by the anatomical sites of maximal involvement. The most common phenotype of FTLD is bvFTD [71].

Distinct histopathological forms of FTLD exist, involving different patterns of accumulations of one of two major proteins in most cases, Tau and TDP-43. In inherited forms, there may be mutations in one of several genes. However, the most common mutations involve the C9orf72, tau (MAPT) and progranulin (GRN) genes [71]. Yet almost every one of these histopathologic and genetic variants can lead to the clinical bvFTD phenotype. For the most part, the phenotype is dictated by the brain regions affected rather than the pathology itself. In most cases of bvFTD, neurodegeneration affects the VMPFC, ACC, and FI preferentially [72]. These are the major nodes of the SN, and it has therefore been argued that bvFTD is a disease of the SN [73]. These nodes of the SN are also brain regions that contain a distinct type of neuron called von Economo neurons (VENs), which are only found in highly-evolved primates (including humans), certain cetaecans, and African elephants. VENs appear to be the early victims of neurodegeneration in bvFTD [74]. It appears that VENs are particularly sensitive to the pathogenic processes occurring in FTLD, although the mechanisms are unknown. This results in degeneration of the VEN-rich brain areas that form the SN. The degeneration and subsequent dysfunction of the SN leads to signs of bvFTD.

As would be predicted from degeneration of the SN, the clinical features of bvFTD are those of OFC and SMPFC dysfunction [75]. Patients present with early apathy and inertia (SMPFC signs), as well as socially inappropriate behaviour (OFC signs) [76]. Usually there is also a significant loss of empathy and lack of insight, which may reflect involvement of the FI in the SN.

As the disease progresses, degeneration in bvFTD affects other parts of the prefrontal cortex. In more moderate stages of the illness, symptoms of EN dysfunction may emerge, concurrent with atrophy of the DLPFC. It is at this point that patients with bvFTD may become impaired on tests of DLPFC function that were mentioned above; although early on in the disease they may perform such tasks normally.

Behavioural/Dysexecutive Variant of Alzheimer's Disease

Alzheimer's disease (AD) is the prototypical example of cortical dementia and usually presents as an amnestic syndrome. However, there may be an atypical presentation with primarily prefrontal features. Johnson and colleagues identified a subset of patients with pathologically-proven AD, whose early predominant clinical presentation reflected a disturbance of executive function [77]. They termed this the "frontal variant of Alzheimer's" and demonstrated an aberrant pattern of neurofibrillary tangle deposition, more concentrated in the prefrontal cortices. In contrast, these are more concentrated in mesial temporal structures in typical AD. Subsequent studies have refined this concept and identified patients with AD and predominant executive dysfunction, such as that described by Johnson and colleagues, as well as patients with prominent bvFTD-like behavioural disturbances [77, 78]. The term behavioural/dysexecutive variant of AD has been proposed for this presentation. Interestingly, on neuroimaging, patients with the behavioural/dysexecutive variant of AD demonstrate more prominent atrophy in the parietotemporal areas bilaterally, similar to typical AD patients, and much less atrophy of the frontal regions than is seen in patients with bvFTD [78]. Therefore, disease preferentially affecting the prefrontal cortices may not necessarily account for the symptoms of the behavioural/dysexecutive variant, and additional mechanisms may be in play whereby a minority of patients with AD show symptoms of DLPFC or of SMPFC/OFC dysfunction.

Conclusion

This chapter has discussed the cognitive and social-behavioural functions of the prefrontal regions of the brain. It is no longer thought that there is a single overarching "frontal lobe syndrome." Rather, the prefrontal cortices are involved in a number of distinct cognitive and social-behavioural processes. As a useful heuristic, three main syndromes can be discussed, which appear to have distinct anatomical substrates. DLPFC dysfunction causes mainly executive function difficulties that can be identified using bedside tests. OFC dysfunction causes impairments of interpersonal conduct that cannot easily be detected using bedside cognitive tests and that require careful history taking and behavioural observations to identify. SMPFC dysfunction causes difficulty with energization which may manifest clinically as a spectrum of disorders characterized by difficulty initiating and sustaining a response on cognitive testing and in daily behaviour. The FPs are involved in metacognitive processes.

The discovery of functionally connected networks of brain activity, such as the EN and SN provide an alternate way of viewing prefrontal function, and in particular illustrate how function of the OFC and SMPFC are connected. Early on in bvFTD, the SN is preferentially affected, giving rise to aberrant interpersonal conduct, loss of empathy, and poor insight with spared cognitive functions. Later on in the course of bvFTD, the EN is affected and patients demonstrate executive function difficulties.

Neurodegenerative diseases affecting the frontal lobes can generally be divided into subcortical and cortical dementias. Subcortical dementias manifest with deficiencies of energization, amotivational syndromes, and executive function difficulties. AD is the prototypical cortical dementia and usually presents as an amnestic syndrome associated with prominent parietotemporal pathology. However, a behavioural/dysexecutive variant of AD may represent an additional prefrontal dementia, although in this condition the neurodegeneration is more widespread, and the reasons why primarily prefrontal functions are affected remains to be elucidated.

Acknowledgments

M. Freedman receives support from the Saul A. Silverman Family Foundation as a Canada International Scientific Exchange Program and the Morris Kerzner Memorial Fund.

References

[1] Lezak MD. *Neuropsychological Assessment.* 3rd ed. New York, NY: Oxford University Press; 1995.

[2] Nowrangi MA, Lyketsos C, Rao V, Munro CA. Systematic Review of Neuroimaging Correlates of Executive Functioning: Converging Evidence From Different Clinical Populations. *J Neuropsychiatry Clin Neurosci.* 2014 Apr 1;26(2):114–25.

[3] Stuss DT. Functions of the Frontal Lobes: Relation to Executive Functions. *J Int Neuropsychol Soc.* 2011 Sep;17(05):759–65.

[4] Stuss DT, Shallice T, Alexander MP, Picton TW. A Multidisciplinary Approach to Anterior Attentional Functions. *Ann N Y Acad Sci.* 1995 Dec 1;769(1):191–212.

[5] Norman D, Shallice T. Attention to Action: Willed and Automatic Control of Behavior. In: Davidson R, Schwartz R, Shapiro D, editors. *Consciousness and Self-Regulation: Advances in Research and Theory IV.* Plenum Press; 1986.

[6] Stuss DT, Alexander MP. Is There a Dysexecutive Syndrome? *Philos Trans R Soc B Biol Sci.* 2007 May 29;362(1481):901–15.
[7] Cicerone K, Levin H, Malec J, Stuss D, Whyte J. Cognitive Rehabilitation Interventions for Executive Function: Moving From Bench to Bedside in Patients with Traumatic Brain Injury. *J Cogn Neurosci.* 2006 Jul;18(7):1212–22.
[8] Alexander GE, DeLong MR, Strick PL. Parallel Organization of Functionally Segregated Circuits Linking Basal Ganglia and Cortex. *Annu Rev Neurosci.* 1986;9(1):357–81.
[9] Seeley WW. An Overview of Brain Networks Emphasizing Frontal Systems. In: *67th Annual Meeting of the American Academy of Neurology.* Washington, DC; 2015.
[10] Robbins TW. Shifting and Stopping: Fronto-striatal Substrates, Neurochemical Modulation and Clinical Implications. *Philos Trans R Soc Lond B Biol Sci.* 2007 May 29;362(1481):917–32.
[11] Kringelbach ML, Rolls ET. The Functional Neuroanatomy of the Human Orbitofrontal Cortex: Evidence from Neuroimaging and Neuropsychology. *Prog Neurobiol.* 2004 Apr;72(5):341–72.
[12] Öngür D, Price JL. The Organization of Networks within the Orbital and Medial Prefrontal Cortex of Rats, Monkeys and Humans. *Cereb Cortex.* 2000 Mar 1;10(3):206–19.
[13] Henri-Bhargava A, Simioni A, Fellows LK. Ventromedial Frontal Lobe Damage Disrupts the Accuracy, but not the Speed, of Value-Based Preference Judgments. *Neuropsychologia.* 2012 Jun;50(7):1536–42.
[14] Bush G, Luu P, Posner MI. Cognitive and Emotional Influences in Anterior Cingulate Cortex. *Trends Cogn Sci.* 2000 Jun 1;4(6):215–22.
[15] Amodio DM, Frith CD. Meeting of Minds: the Medial Frontal Cortex and Social Cognition. *Nat Rev Neurosci.* 2006 Apr;7(4):268–77.
[16] Floden D, Vallesi A, Stuss DT. Task Context and Frontal Lobe Activation in the Stroop Task. *J Cogn Neurosci.* 2011 Apr;23(4):867–79.
[17] Ramnani N, Owen AM. Anterior Prefrontal Cortex: Insights into Function from Anatomy and Neuroimaging. *Nat Rev Neurosci.* 2004 Mar;5(3):184–94.
[18] Seeley WW, Menon V, Schatzberg AF, Keller J, Glover GH, Kenna H, et al. Dissociable Intrinsic Connectivity Networks for Salience Processing and Executive Control. *J Neurosci.* 2007 Feb 28; 27(9):2349–56.
[19] Zhou J, Seeley WW. Network Dysfunction in Alzheimer's Disease and Frontotemporal Dementia: Implications for Psychiatry. *Biol Psychiatry.* 2014 Apr 1;75(7):565–73.
[20] Stuss DT, Murphy KJ, Binns MA, Alexander MP. Staying on the Job: the Frontal Lobes Control Individual Performance Variability. *Brain.* 2003 Nov 1;126(11):2363–80.
[21] Luria AR. *Human Brain and Psychological Processes. New* York, NY: Harper and Row; 1966.
[22] Milner B. Effects of Different Brain Lesions on Card Sorting: The Role of the Frontal Lobes. *Arch Neurol.* 1963 Jul 1;9(1):90–100.
[23] Stuss DT, Levine B, Alexander MP, Hong J, Palumbo C, Hamer L, et al. Wisconsin Card Sorting Test Performance in Patients with Focal Frontal and Posterior Brain Damage: Effects of Lesion Location and Test Structure on Separable Cognitive Processes. *Neuropsychologia.* 2000 Apr;38(4):388–402.
[24] Nelson HE. A modified card sorting test sensitive to frontal lobe defects. *Cortex J Devoted Study Nerv Syst Behav.* 1976 Dec;12(4):313–24.

[25]MacPherson SE, Sala SD, Cox SR, Girardi A, Iveson MH. *Handbook of Frontal Lobe Assessment.* Oxford, UK: Oxford University Press; 2015. 449 p.

[26]Strub RL, Black FW. *The Mental Status Examination in Neurology.* F.A. Davis Company; 2000. 208 p.

[27]Benson DF, Stuss DT. Motor abilities after frontal leukotomy. *Neurology.* 1982 Dec;32(12):1353–7.

[28]Rozencwajg P, Bertoux ML. Categorization and Aging as Measured by an Adapted Version of Wechsler's Similarities Test. *Curr Psychol Lett Behav Brain Cogn.* 2008;24(2).

[29]Chase TN, Fedio P, Foster NL, Brooks R, Di Chiro G, Mansi L. Wechsler Adult Intelligence Scale Performance. Cortical Localization by Fluorodeoxyglucose F 18-Positron Emission Tomography. *Arch Neurol.* 1984 Dec;41(12):1244–7.

[30]Kaiser NC, Lee GJ, Lu PH, Mather MJ, Shapira J, Jimenez E, et al. What Dementia Reveals About Proverb Interpretation and its Neuroanatomical Correlates. *Neuropsychologia.* 2013 Aug;51(9):1726–33.

[31]Borkowski JG, Benton AL, Spreen O. Word fluency and brain damage. *Neuropsychologia.* 1967 May;5(2):135–40.

[32]Tombaugh TN, Kozak J, Rees L. Normative Data Stratified by Age and Education for Two Measures of Verbal Fluency: FAS and Animal Naming. *Arch Clin Neuropsychol.* 1999 Feb;14(2):167–77.

[33]Stuss DT, Alexander MP, Hamer L, Palumbo C, Dempster R, Binns M, et al. The effects of focal anterior and posterior brain lesions on verbal fluency. *J Int Neuropsychol Soc.* 1998 May;4(03):265–78.

[34]Fisk JE, Sharp CA. Age-Related Impairment in Executive Functioning: Updating, Inhibition, Shifting, and Access. *J Clin Exp Neuropsychol.* 2004 Oct 1;26(7):874–90.

[35]Jones-Gotman M, Milner B. Design fluency: the invention of nonsense drawings after focal cortical lesions. *Neuropsychologia.* 1977;15(4-5):653–74.

[36]Regard M, Strauss E, Knapp P. Children's production on verbal and non-verbal fluency tasks. *Percept Mot Skills.* 1982 Dec;55(3 Pt 1):839–44.

[37]Suchy Y, Kraybill ML, Gidley Larson JC. Understanding design fluency: motor and executive contributions. *J Int Neuropsychol Soc JINS.* 2010 Jan;16(1):26–37.

[38]Reitan RM. The relation of the Trail Making Test to organic brain damage. *J Consult Psychol.* 19(5):393–4.

[39]Tombaugh TN. Trail Making Test A and B: normative data stratified by age and education. *Arch Clin Neuropsychol Off J Natl Acad Neuropsychol.* 2004;19(2):203–14.

[40]Stuss DT, Bisschop SM, Alexander MP, Levine B, Katz D, Izukawa D. The Trail Making Test: a study in focal lesion patients. *Psychol Assess.* 2001 Jun;13(2):230–9.

[41]Freedman M, Leach L, Kaplan E, Winocur G, Shulman KI, Delis DC. *Clock drawing: a neuropsychological analysis.* New York: Oxford University Press; 1994. 182 p.

[42]Royall DR. Executive cognitive impairment: a novel perspective on dementia. *Neuroepidemiology.* 2000 Dec;19(6):293–9.

[43]Dubois B, Slachevsky A, Litvan I, Pillon B. The FAB A frontal assessment battery at bedside. *Neurology.* 2000 Dec 12;55(11):1621–6.

[44]Moorhouse P, Gorman M, Rockwood K. Comparison of EXIT-25 and the Frontal Assessment Battery for evaluation of executive dysfunction in patients attending a memory clinic. *Dement Geriatr Cogn Disord.* 2009;27(5):424–8.

[45]Brown RG, Pluck G. Negative symptoms: the "pathology" of motivation and goal-directed behaviour. *Trends Neurosci.* 2000 Sep;23(9):412–7.

[46]Marin RS, Wilkosz PA. Disorders of Diminished Motivation. *J Head Trauma Rehabil Disord Self-Aware.* 2005 Aug;20(4):377–88.

[47]Stuss DT, van Reekum R, Murphy KJ. Differentiation of States and Causes of Apathy. In: Borod J, editor. *The Neuropsychology of Emotion.* New York, NY: Oxford University Press; 2012. p. 340–63.

[48]D'Souza G, Kakoullis A, Hegde N, Tadros G. Recognition and management of abulia in the elderly. *Prog Neurol Psychiatry.* 2010 Nov 1;14(6):24–8.

[49]Marin RS, Biedrzycki RC, Firinciogullari S. Reliability and validity of the apathy evaluation scale. *Psychiatry Res.* 1991 Aug;38(2):143–62.

[50]Freedman M. Object alternation and orbitofrontal system dysfunction in Alzheimer's and Parkinson's disease. *Brain Cogn.* 1990 Nov;14(2):134–43.

[51]Freedman M, Black S, Ebert P, Binns M. Orbitofrontal function, object alternation and perseveration. *Cereb Cortex.* 1998;8(1):18–27.

[52]Freedman M, Binns MA, Black SE, Levine B, Miller BL, Ramirez J, et al. Object Alternation: A Novel Probe of Medial Frontal Function in Frontotemporal Dementia. *Alzheimer Dis Assoc Disord.* 2013;27(4):316–23.

[53]Levy R, Dubois B. Apathy and the Functional Anatomy of the Prefrontal Cortex–Basal Ganglia Circuits. *Cereb Cortex.* 2006 Jul 1;16(7):916–28.

[54]Gündüz T, Emir Ö, Kürtüncü M, Mutlu M, Tumaç A, Akca S, et al. Cognitive impairment in neuro-Behcet's disease and multiple sclerosis: a comparative study. *Int J Neurosci.* 2012 Nov;122(11):650–6.

[55]Pachalska M, Talar J, Kurzbauer H, Frańczuk B, Grochmal-Bach B, Macqueen BD. Differential diagnosis of frontal syndrome in patients with closed-head injuries. *Ortop Traumatol Rehabil.* 2002 Jan 31;4(1):81–7.

[56]Torralva T, Roca M, Gleichgerrcht E, Bekinschtein T, Manes F. A neuropsychological battery to detect specific executive and social cognitive impairments in early frontotemporal dementia. *Brain.* 2009;132(Pt 5):1299–309.

[57]Premack D, Woodruff G. Does the chimpanzee have a theory of mind? *Behav Brain Sci.* 1978 Dec;1(04):515–26.

[58]Stone VE, Baron-Cohen S, Knight RT. Frontal Lobe Contributions to Theory of Mind. *J Cogn Neurosci. 1998* Sep 1;10(5):640–56.

[59]Stuss DT, Gallup GG, Alexander MP. The frontal lobes are necessary for "theory of mind." *Brain.* 2001 Feb;124(Pt 2):279–86.

[60]Freedman M, Stuss DT. Theory of Mind in Parkinson's disease. *J Neurol Sci.* 2011 Nov 15;310(1–2):225–7.

[61]Gallagher HL, Happé F, Brunswick N, Fletcher PC, Frith U, Frith CD. Reading the mind in cartoons and stories: an fMRI study of "theory of mind" in verbal and nonverbal tasks. *Neuropsychologia.* 2000;38(1):11–21.

[62]Freedman MM, Binns MA, Black SEM, Murphy CB, Stuss DT. Theory of Mind and Recognition of Facial Emotion in Dementia: Challenge to Current Concepts. *Alzheimer Dis Assoc Disord.* 2013 Mar;27(1):56–61.

[63]Albert ML, Feldman RG, Willis AL. The "subcortical dementia" of progressive supranuclear palsy. *J Neurol Neurosurg Psychiatry.* 1974;37(2):121–30.

[64]McHugh P, Folstein MF. Psychiatric syndromes of Huntington's chorea: a clinical and phenomenologic study. In: Benson DF, Blumer D, editors. *Psychiatric Aspects of Neurological Disease.* New York, NY: Grune and Stratton; 1975. p. 267–86.

[65]Bonelli RM, Cummings JL. Frontal-subcortical dementias. *The Neurologist.* 2008 Mar;14(2):100–7.

[66]Freedman M, Albert M. Subcortical Dementia. In: Vinken P, Bruyn G, Klawans H, editors. *Handbook of Clinical Neurology.* New York, NY: Elsevier; 1985. p. 311–6.

[67]Albert ML. Subcortical dementia: historical review and personal view. *Neurocase.* 2005 Aug;11(4):243–5.

[68]Lamar M, Price CC, Libon DJ, Penney DL, Kaplan E, Grossman M, et al. Alterations in working memory as a function of leukoaraiosis in dementia. *Neuropsychologia.* 2007 Jan 28;45(2):245–54.

[69]Freedman M, Oscar-Berman M. Selective delayed response deficits in parkinson's and alzheimer's disease. *Arch Neurol.* 1986 Sep 1;43(9):886–90.

[70]Pick A. Über primäre progressive Demenz bei Erwachsenen. *Prag Med Wochenschr.* 1904;29:417–20.

[71]Miller BL. *Frontotemporal Dementia.* New York, NY: Oxford University Press; 2014. 200 p.

[72]Karageorgiou E, Miller BL. Frontotemporal lobar degeneration: a clinical approach. *Semin Neurol.* 2014 Apr;34(2):189–201.

[73]Seeley WW, Crawford RK, Zhou J, Miller BL, Greicius MD. Neurodegenerative diseases target large-scale human brain networks. *Neuron.* 2009 Apr 16;62(1):42–52.

[74]Santillo AF, Englund E. Greater loss of von Economo neurons than loss of layer II and III neurons in behavioral variant frontotemporal dementia. *Am J Neurodegener Dis.* 2014 Sep 6;3(2):64–71.

[75]Rascovsky K, Hodges JR, Kipps CM, Johnson JK, Seeley WW, Mendez MF, et al. Diagnostic criteria for the behavioral variant of frontotemporal dementia (bvFTD): current limitations and future directions. *Alzheimer Assoc Disord.* 2007;21(4):S14–8.

[76]Viskontas IV, Possin KL, Miller BL. Symptoms of Frontotemporal Dementia Provide Insights into Orbitofrontal Cortex Function and Social Behavior. *Ann N Y Acad Sci.* 2007;1121(Linking affect to Action: Critical Contributions of the Orbitofrontal Cortex):528–45.

[77]Johnson JK, Head E, Kim R, Starr A, Cotman CW. Clinical and pathological evidence for a frontal variant of Alzheimer disease. *Arch Neurol.* 1999 Oct;56(10):1233–9.

[78]Ossenkoppele R, Pijnenburg YAL, Perry DC, Cohn-Sheehy BI, Scheltens NME, Vogel JW, et al. The behavioural/dysexecutive variant of Alzheimer's disease: clinical, neuroimaging and pathological features. *Brain.* 2015;138(9):2732–49.

In: Progressive Cognitive Impairment …
Editor: Gediminas Peter Gliebus
ISBN: 978-1-63485-221-0

Chapter 4

Action-Intentional Disorders in Neurodegenerative Diseases

Kenneth M. Heilman*[*], *MD, Arash Salardini, MD, and Adam D. Falchook, MD
Department of Neurology, and Center of Neuropsychological Studies at the University of Florida and the Malcom Randall Veterans Affairs Hospital, Gainesville, FL, US

Abstract

The action-intentional disorders are often associated with many progressive degenerative and vascular cerebral disorders as well as endocrine, metabolic and psychiatric disorders. While clinicians rarely test for disorder of this system, they are often responsible for serious disabilities, dependency and a reduction of quality of life. This chapter reviews the four major forms of action-intentional disorders including impairments of action initiation, impersistence, defective response inhibition, and perseveration, as well as the subtypes of each of these disorders. The symptoms, signs and means of testing patients for each of these action-intentional disorders will be described. In addition, the pathophysiology of these disorders as well as some of the diseases that can induce these disorders will also be discussed. In regard to treatment, when possible the underlying disease must be treated and while some possible treatments will be discussed much further research is needed to increase our understanding of the pathophysiology of these disorders as well as their treatment.

Movement-Action Programming: "How" and "When"

Humans are almost always either altering their environment or themselves. Our bone-joint structure, the muscles that move these joints and the nerves that activate these muscles permit us to make almost an infinite number of different movements, at different speeds with different forces. In order to successfully alter our environment or ourselves we need to have

[*] Correspondence to: Heilman@neurology.ufl.edu.

movement programs that will allow us to be successfully at making these changes and there are two major types of programs that govern our actions and allow us to achieve our goals.

The praxis system contains the programs that allow a person to know 'how' to position their hand and arm when interacting with objects or holding a tool or implement that will alter objects. In addition, these praxis programs allow a person to know 'how' to move their joints, including those joints that need to perform the correct movement and those that need to be stabilized. Many purposeful actions require the movements of several joints and these programs allow us to know 'how' several joints should be moved in relation to each other. Praxic programs also allow us to control the speed of various portions of our limb, as well as 'how' much force is needed [1].

In order to successfully interact in our environment in addition to knowing 'how' to act we also need to know 'when" to act. The brains network that regulates-control 'when' programs we call the action-intentional system (AIS). The AIS or 'when' system is a brain network that determines; 1) action initiation or when a goal oriented motor action or series of actions should be started; 2) action inhibition-when not to initiate a motor action; 3) perseverance-when to continue a motor action or series of actions; 4) termination-when to discontinue or finish an action or a motor task [2].

Relationships between Components of Sensory-Attention and Action-Intention

Awareness and Initiation: The human brain has limited processing capacity and just as the sensory systems receive more information than the brain can fully process, humans have a limit on the number of actions they can simultaneously perform. Thus, humans must triage incoming stimuli as well as actions they will perform and selective sensory-attention as well as selective action-intention are triaging tools used by the our brains to allocate the limited processing resources to successfully interact with our environment and achieve our goals. For example, now when you are reading this chapter, before I mentioned your right foot you were probably unaware of the sensation coming from that foot even though it was being stimulated. In addition, you are probably not moving this foot. However, even if I did not mention your foot and a bug crawled on your foot you would become aware of the sensation coming from your foot and would stop reading this chapter. You also would probably rapidly move this foot.

A person's brain has to decide which, if any incoming stimuli to process and which not to process, a decision that may be based on past, present, and/or future goals. Initiation of actions is necessary for a person to achieve a relevant goal. If the action is not relevant to achieve a goal, this action often should be inhibited to preserve limited intentional resources for those actions that are necessary or desired.

Vigilance and Persistence: After the brain initiates attention to a stimulus or a set of stimuli, in order to fully process these stimuli, the brain may need to continue to attend to these stimuli until they are no longer relevant. Thus, after you get this bug off your foot you may again attend to this chapter and continue to attend until you complete reading this entire chapter. This process is called vigilance. In a similar fashion some interactions with the environment or one's self require continuous action, repeated actions or series of actions, and this ability to continue a needed action or actions is called motor persistence. So for example, if you are reading this chapter in the book and you are holding this book you would need to continue holding this book.

Sensory Extinction/Habituation and Action Termination: The computer on this chapter is being written makes a very low buzzing noise. When this computer is first turned on we hear this noise but then as we continue to write we no longer are aware of this noise. Thus, when a stimulus is novel, or meaningful, a person will most often attend to this stimulus because its significance is unknown. However, if the person's brain determines that this stimulus is insignificant (like the noise coming from computer), awareness of this stimulus will end. In a similar fashion, when an action is completed, a person should discontinue this action, and if the action is not achieving the relevant goal it should also be terminated. For example, after I complete writing this chapter I will stop pressing the letter keys.

ACTION-INTENTIONAL DISORDERS

Action-intentional disorders can be categorized into four broad categories which include: disorders of action initiation, defective response inhibition, impersistence, failure of termination.

Impaired Initiation

Akinesia

Akinesia is defined as the inability to initiate a goal oriented movement. There are many reasons why a patient may be impaired at initiating a goal oriented movement and these include weakness, inattention, impaired comprehension or understanding the need to initiate a movement. Akinesia is the failure to initiate an action that is not caused by these other factors.

There are several different forms of akinesia and akinesia can be classified by: the part of the body that is impaired, the direction or spatial location of the movement that should be initiated, and whether thc movement is initiated in response to an internal drive or motivated by the perception of an external stimulus.

Global Akinesia: In regard to body part, akinesia can be global and patients with global akinesia fail to initiate any action with any part of their body, in any part of space, both spontaneously and even to external stimuli such as commands [3, 4].

Akinesia Paradoxica*:* Some patients with global akinesia, are impaired at self-initiation of actions, but can initiate an action in response to an external stimuli, and other can spontaneously initiate actions but fail to initiated an action in response to certain stimuli and their failure to initiate an action is not related to inattention.

Abulia: Whereas akinesia is a failure to initiate a goal directed action, abulia is a decrease in the frequency of self-initiated goal directed activities. Movement monitors can be used in an attempt to quantify abulia, but these monitors cannot record whether a person's action and activities are self-initiated, versus initiated in response to environmental stimuli, and cannot determine if these actions are goal oriented. Another method of assessing for abulia is to have a family member keep records of the patient's goal oriented behaviors. The term "apathy" has been defined as a lack of passion or emotional indifference; however, now many people use this term to also describe abulia. Questionnaires have been developed to assess apathy and abulia. Whereas questionnaires, such as the Lille Apathy Rating Scale, were primarily developed to assess apathy and abulia in patients with Parkinson's disease, and the Apathy Evaluation Scale (AES) was developed by Marin for assessing patients with traumatic brain injury, these scales do have several questions that assess for a reduction of goal oriented behaviors (e.g., Getting things started on his/her own is important to her/him.), but these scales are subjective [5, 6].

Limb Akinesia: Patients with unilateral neglect can be unaware of or inattentive to stimuli presented to one side of space or even on one side of their body [7]. Similarly, in some patients akinesia can be observed in the limbs on one side of the body [8-10]. Sometimes clinically, limb akinesia or motor neglect can be confused with a hemiparesis or hemiplegia; however, when patients with a hemiplegia are asked to move an arm they will often make some shoulder and trunk movements, and even show by their facial expressions that they are making an effort, but the patients with limb akinesia often will not demonstrated evidence they are attempting to make the requested movement [8, 11]. In addition, studies such as motor evoked potentials can reveal in these patients that the corticospinal system is intact [12].

Spatial Akinesia: This form of akinesia takes place in one side of peripersonal space, a disorder also called hemispatial akinesia. For example, a patient with a hemispatial akinesia may fail to use his or her arm when it is in contralesional space, but be able to move it when it is in ipsilesional space [9]. In addition, some patients with primarily unilateral right hemisphere lesions, when asked to close their eyes and to first point to their middle of their chest and then to point straight out in front of them (midsagittal plane) will deviate to the side of their hemispheric lesion [13].

Directional Akinesia: An akinesia can also occur for actions that take place in a certain direction, such as leftward or rightward. This directional akinesia can occur with attempted movements of the arms, the head and the eyes [14]. For example, if coins are distributed over a table and a patient with a right hemispheric lesions, who is blindfolded, is asked to pick up all the coins on the table, he or she will often start picking up coins on the ipsilateral side and then may pick up only those coins on the side ipsilateral to their hemispheric injury, because they fail to move their hand toward the contralesional side and thus fail to explore this part of the table to learn if coins are present. De Renzi et al. first showed this using a maze, and posited that the patients who fail to explore one part of space, may not have a representation of this part of space; [15] however, this disorder cannot be explained by spatial inattention since the patient can only sense or detect the presence of the coin after they have moved. A somewhat similar phenomenon can occur with the eyes. Clinicians often call this a gaze palsy, but this disorder is not caused by weakness, and can even be reversed by putting cold water in the patient's ear and thus gaze palsy is often a form a directional akinesia [16].

Hypokinesia: Patients with milder forms of akinesia may be slower to initiate responses than normal people, and this is called hypokinesia [2]. Hypokinesia, like akinesia can be observed for the entire body or different part of the body (e.g., limbs), on one side of the body, or a portion of egocentric (body centered) space. Hypokinesia can even be directional. One of the best means of testing for hypokinesia is reaction times; however, when using reaction times, attentional disorders may also be responsible for slowed reaction times.

Motor Extinction: Some patients with action-intentional disorders demonstrate a phenomenon called motor extinction [17]. Patient with sensory extinction can detect a single stimulus presented to one or the other side of the body, or visual field; however, when both sides are simultaneously stimulated a person may only detect the stimulus on one side. When testing for motor extinction a patient can be asked to close their eyes and to report if they were touched on the left, right or both hands. If they have sensory extinction it may be difficult to test them for motor extinction, but if they do not show sensory extinction, the examiner can then ask the patient to lift the hand or hands touched by the examiner. The patient with motor extinction will lift each hand when it is the only hand that is touched, but when both hands are touched the patient with motor extinction will only lift the hand ipsilateral to the injured hemisphere. However, there are also some patients who will lift the contralesional hand after a delay. This type of inability to perform simultaneous movements is called motor extinction.

Defective Response Inhibition

Defective response inhibition is characterized by performing actions in response to stimuli when these responses are not relevant for achieving specific goals. Patients with defective response inhibition have a decreased ability to inhibit incorrect actions that are directed to these stimuli. Whereas defective response inhibition is almost always evoked by a stimulus, there are many means by which this abnormal behavior can be elicited and there are several forms of defective response that are similar to the subdivisions of akinesia. For example, defective response inhibition may be seen in a specific part of the body such as the eyes or upper limbs. Defective response inhibition may be on one side of space or in one direction. In general defective response inhibition can be considered a form of an adherence disorders.

Tactile Adherence Disorders

Grasp Reflex: The adherence disorder most often assessed by neurologists is the grasp reflex, where patients close their hands around any object that touches their palm even when told by the examiner to keep their hand relaxed.

Tactile Mitgehen: Some patients when asked to keep their hands and arms relaxed on their lap and they are touched on their finger by the examiner who then moves his hand slowly upward, and that patient will move their hand off their lap so that it stays in contact with the examiner's hand. This phenomenon has been called "tactile mitgehen." [18]

Tactile Defective Response Inhibition: In this task the patient, who is sitting, is asked to put their hands (palm down) on their lap. They are then asked to close their eyes and if the examiner touches the back of their left hand they are, as rapidly as possible, to lift their right hand and if the examiner touches their back of their right hand they are to lift their left hand. Any lifting of the hand that is touched is considered an error. In our clinic we touch our patients' hands 10 times (5 to each hand in a random order). If a patient lifts the touched hand more than two times it is probably abnormal [19].

Visual Adherence Disorders

Magnetic Apraxia: Some patients with adherence disorders do not even need to be touched in their palm or finger but when they see the examiner move his or her hand they will reach out to grab the examiner's hand. This visual adherence disorder was called "magnetic apraxia" by Denny-Brown and Chambers [20].

Visual and Facial Grasp: A "visual grasp "is a disorder where again the patient magnetically follows an object they see, even when told to keep the eyes fixated on another object in the room. For example, when patients are asked to fixate on a cross on a wall and an examiner attempts to view their fundi they will look right into the light of the ophthalmoscope. When examining ocular pursuit by asking a patient to fixate on a moving finger, some patients will fail to move their eyes along with the finger and instead fixate on the examiner's face. This adherence behavior is called a "facial grasp." [21]

Visual-Ocular Response Inhibition: In this task the examiner stands directly in front of the patient and the patient is asked to look at the examiner's eyes. The examiner raises his arms so that they are parallel to the patient's eyes with one hand in each visual field. They are then told if the examiner moves her or his left hand they should look to the examiner opposite (right hand) and vice versa. In our clinic we do this 10 times (5 with each hand in a random order).

Echopraxia: Some patients will mirror the examiner's movements, and this behavioral disorder is called "echopraxia." AR Luria developed an excellent test for echopraxia [22]. The patient is asked to make a fist with one hand and the examiner also makes a fist. The patients is then told when the examiner lifts one finger the patient is to hold up two fingers and when the examiner holds up two fingers the patient is to hold up one finger. The examiner then randomly holds up one or two fingers for a total of 10 trials. If a patient holds up the same number of fingers as the examiner, this patient has a form of echopraxia.

Finger Response Inhibition; *Go No-Go*: To examine defective response inhibition of the fingers, Luria used a 'go no-go paradigm.' In this test the patient is asked to make a fist with either hand. The examiner explains to the patient that if the examiner puts up one finger the patient is to put up two fingers, and if the examiner puts up two fingers the patient is not to put up any fingers [22]. In this test the patient can make two types of errors, defective response inhibition (putting up any fingers when the examiner put up two fingers and echopraxia (putting up one finger when the examiner puts up one finger). In research settings, response inhibition is often assessed with go no-go computerized reaction time paradigms.

Utilization Behavior: Lhermitte describe patients who demonstrated what he called "utilization behavior." [23] When objects are place before these patients, like a pen and piece of paper, without any request by the examiner, they would pick up and manipulate or use these objects, such as writing on this paper.

Motor (Action) Impersistence

In order to successful interact with environment not only does a person have to initiate goal oriented activities and avoid performing activities that do not lead to this goal, but often achieving a goal requires either a continuous action or the continuation of a series of actions. When a person discontinues a goal oriented activity before it is completed this deficit is call motor impersistence. Motor impersistence, like akinesia can be observed for a body part, such as the eyes, mouth, tongue, limbs, or whole body, as well as be directional or even hemispatial.

This disorder of motor persistence was described by Fisher who examined patients by requesting that they keep their eyes closed and tongue protruded [24]. Subsequently, Kertesz et al. suggested that that the addition of mouth opening even makes Fisher's test more sensitive [25]. Directional impersistence may be assess by have participant maintain gaze directed to one side and then the other side. In our clinic we usually have our patients maintain this posture for 20 seconds. Limb-hand impersistence can be tested by using a force dynamometer and having subjects maintain a force [26].

Motor Perseveration

The continuation of an action or a series of actions after the task is completed is called motor perseveration. Another form of motor perseveration is when an action or series of actions is continued when it appears that this activity is not allowing or not helping a person to achieve their goal. We call the former type 'terminal motor perseveration' and the other type "flawed perseveration." Sandson and Albert described two major forms of terminal motor perseveration [27]. Patients who show 'recurrent perseveration' repeats a prior action after the task requirements have changed, and patients who demonstrated 'continuous perseveration' continues the same action even after the task is completed and this repetition of this action is counter-productive.

There are several means of testing for recurrent and continuous perseveration. One means is by asking the patient to copy the examiner's actions. The examiner performs three series of hand actions described by Luria, where the seated examiner softly hits own lap with his fist, then the ulnar edge of his open hand and then with the palm of his open hand. Patients with recurrent perseveration may use their fist followed by the open hand and then again the fist, which would be recurrent perseveration; however, these errors may be related to an impaired action working memory deficit. Alternatively, the examiner may ask patients draw a series of alternating triangles and squares or write the alternating letters of "n" and "m."

Luria assessed patients for continuous perseveration by having them draw a triple loop [22]. Patients with the continuous form of motor perseveration may continue to draw loops even after they completed drawing the triple loops. We have found that Dubois et al's clapping test is often a more sensitive test for detecting continuous perseveration [28]. We ask the patient to copy what we are doing. Then we clap our hands, about one clap per second and after 3 claps we stop. If a patient claps more than 3 times they have perseveration.

Perseveration like other form of action intentional disorders can be seen in one upper limb, or on one side of space [29, 30]. Patients with spatial neglect from right hemisphere lesions often show perseveration on the cancellation task [30, 31]. There appears to be three types of perseveration on the cancellation task, one where the patient continues to cancel the same target (continuous), another where the patient returns to a previously cancelled target and cancels it again (recurrent), and one were the patient makes a cancellation mark where there is no target. Gandola et al., call this last type "'flying marks" and suggests that they are a form a defective response inhibition.

THE ANATOMY OF THE ACTION-INTENTIONAL NETWORK

Almost all action intentional disorders are associated with frontal dysfunction. Just like the executive of a corporation who must get input from all divisions of a business before he or she can productively manage the corporation, the frontal lobes receive input from many different areas of the brain. The frontal lobes receives input from areas of the limbic system important in mediating emotions, the hypothalamus important in mediating homeostasis of the internal organs, input from the sensory association areas that contain the percepts of incoming stimuli and from posterior regions of multimodal and polymodal cortex which store declarative information and knowledge. Based on this input the frontal lobe can determine whether an action is needed and when needed, the type of action that is required. The frontal lobe also has basal ganglia and thalamic connections and receives neurotransmitter-neuromodulator input from the midbrain and these inputs from these subcortical structures are critical for normal frontal lobe function.

Functionally and anatomically, the prefrontal lobes can be divided into three major parallel sub-networks; the mesial frontal, the lateral frontal and the orbitofrontal systems and each of three networks appear to perform different executive functions. Goal oriented activities can be initiated by people even in the absence of any external stimuli or emotion and it is primarily the medial system, which includes the medial frontal cortex along with its connections with the basal ganglia and thalamus that is important in mediating endogenously evoked activities. Thus, patients with damage to the medial frontal cortex are impaired in the control of endogenously initiated actions, but often can initiate activities in response to external stimuli.

In contrast to the medial frontal network the lateral frontal cortex is primarily responsible for mediating activities in response to external stimuli. Deficits in this system can cause deficits where there is a failure to interact with stimuli, a failure to persist at an action directed to a stimulus as well as deficits in withholding responses, including defective response inhibition and perseveration.

The orbitofrontal cortex which has strong connections with the portions of limbic system, such as the amygdala as well as the ventral striatum play an important role in moderating actions in relation to emotional experiences as well as reward and punishment.

While many of the patients with frontal-executive deficits have bilateral hemispheric lesions, there also seems to be some left-right hemispheric asymmetries in these medial and dorsal intentional systems. Studies of patients with discrete lesions suggest that whereas the right hemisphere's frontal-subcortical networks appear to be dominant for the executive control of motor activities, the left hemisphere's frontal subcortical networks appear dominant for the executive control of cognitive activities. For example, left hemisphere frontal lesions can cause a form of speech akinesia where patients have a decrease in spontaneous speech, but can comprehend speech, name objects that are presented to these patients and when requestes repeat the words said by the examiner. This disorder is called adynamic aphasia [32].

When patients with lateral left frontal lesion are asked to produce as many different words as they can in one minute, that begin with a letter such as "F" but not to use proper names or numbers (the Controlled Oral Word Association Test) they will often start providing some words that begin with the target letter, but after they produce several words they will often stop, a form of impersistence. When given a test such as the Stroop where they are presented with words that are the names of colors that are printed in fonts that are colored, but the color of the font does not match the written word and these patient are asked to name to color of the font of each written word, but not to read the color, patients with left frontal lesions will often read the words rather than name the colors, an example of defective response inhibition. In the Wisconsin Card Sorting Task, when a patient with a left frontal lesion is presented with cards that have different shaped objects, and these objects can have one of several colors as well as a different number of objects on each card, after sorting the cards according to one of these characteristics and the examiner requests a change in sorting strategy, a patient with left frontal lesions will often continue sorting the card using the same strategy, that is a form of perseveration.

Whereas disorder of the action-intentional system are also frequently caused by bilateral hemispheric lesions, patients with right frontal and subcortical lesions may show limb akinesia or hypokinesia (slowed response times) [8, 33]. They may also show directional akinesia [14]. Kim et al. studied patients with right and left hemisphere strokes and found that the frequency of hypokinesia and impersistence was higher in the patients with right than left hemisphere strokes [34]. These investigators also found that the patients with right hemisphere strokes demonstrated left contralesional directional impersistence. Chamorro et al. found that participants with frontal or subcortical lesions were significantly more likely to demonstrate hypokinesia and impersistence than those with posterior lesions; however, limb akinesia (motor neglect) has been reported with right parietal lobe lesions [12]. Other intentional deficits associated with right frontal-subcortical disease include motor impersistence as well as perseveration [25, 27]. Studies have also shown that patients with right hemispheric lesions that involve the inferior frontal gyrus appear to impair response inhibition [35].

Functional imaging studies have provided supporting evidence for the role of right frontal lobes in mediating different elements of action-intentional activities. For example, Gusnard et al. demonstrated using functional imaging that the orbitofrontal and adjacent medial prefrontal cortex may play an important role in persistence [36]. Based on functional imaging Jung and coworkers also thought that the orbitofrontal cortex which provides top-down control over the ventral striatum was important for persistence [37]. However, Dettmers et al. using PET imaging demonstrated that during a task that a required sustained muscle activation, there was increased cerebral blood flow to the basal ganglia and right dorsolateral prefrontal cortex [38].

Other than the olfactory cortex, the prefrontal lobes do not have direct sensory input and thus information coming to the frontal lobes about the outside world comes from sensory association cortex and polymodal cortex, primarily in the parietal lobes. The parietal lobes are primarily connected with the frontal lobes by the superior longitudinal fasciculus. The anterior portion of the temporal lobes connects to the frontal lobes by means of the uncinate fasciculi and the posterior temporal lobes by means of the arcuate fasciculi. As mentioned, the frontal lobes also have critical connections with the thalamus, basal ganglia, limbic system and therefore the normal functions of the prefrontal lobes are heavily dependent on white matter connections, including the anterior limb of the internal capsule, the anterior portion of the corona radiata, the uncinate fasciculus, and the longitudinal fasciculi. These white matter pathways are important not only for connecting the frontal lobes to the sensory environment, but also for providing them with knowledge and past experience about reward and punishment. Thus, diseases that injure these pathways often lead to action intentional disorders.

Action-Intentional Disorders in Progressive Neurological Diseases

Almost any neurological disease that injures the frontal lobes, the basal ganglia, the thalamus, or the white matter pathways that connect the frontal lobes with other areas of the brain can cause action intentional disorders. Although the following is a brief discussion of some of the signs seen with progressive neurological diseases, unfortunately, most of the neuropsychological test batteries used to assess for dementia do not include tests for action intentional disorders.

Parkinson's Disease and Parkinsonian Disorders (Progressive Supranuclear Palsy, Corticobasal Degeneration, Multisystem Atrophy, Lewy Body Dementia): One of the major disorders associated with Parkinson's disease (PD) and parkinsonian disorders is akinesia. Many patients with these disorders have akinesia paradoxica where they may increase their activity with external stimuli. However, even with external stimuli patients with PD and Parkinsonian disorders are often slow to respond (hypokinesia). It has been reported that patients with Parkinsonian disorders such as corticobasal degeneration and Lewy body dementia have motor perseveration when assessed with the "applause sign" [39]. Patients with PD have also been reported to have defective response inhibition [19].

Demyelinating diseases: In regard to diseases of the white matter, one of the primary symptoms of patients with multiple sclerosis is called "fatigue" by many patients and physicians. However, many patients with white matter diseases do have trouble initiating activities, and persisting until completion as well as the signs of akinesia-hypokinesia-abulia and impersistence.

Alzheimer's disease: Mölsä et al. reported that patients with AD were often hypokinetic [40]. Pekkala et al. found that in Alzheimer's disease (AD) perseveration increases with the increasing severity of this disease and that recurrent and continuous perseverations can even appear early in AD [41]. Lopez et al. found that a small percentage of patients with AD also showed motor impersistence [42].

Vascular dementia: Cummings reported that vascular subcortical dementia was frequently associated with perseveration and impersistence [43]. In addition, Yoon et al. studied action-intentional processing (force initiation, development, maintenance, and termination) in patients with subcortical vascular mild cognitive impairment, which is a prodromal stage of subcortical vascular dementia [44]. They found that of the four motor intentional tasks, the maintenance (persistence) task proved sensitive in differentiating subcortical vascular MCI from mild cognitive from the amnestic MCI.

Frontotemporal dementia (FTD): Gustafson reported that utilization behaviors, a form of defective response inhibition is commonly associated with the FTD [45]. In addition, patients with FTD also reveal perseveration on the applause test [46].

Possible Treatments for Action Intentional Disorders

Medications

Since the classic paper by Cotzias et al. it has been noted the levodopa is able to improve the akinesia associated with Parkinson's disease and subsequently, it has been shown that other dopaminergic agonists may also be helpful [47]. In addition, levodopa treatment has also been shown to influence perseveration [48].

Whereas akinetic mutism, a severe loss of motor and speech initiation that usually results from bilateral mesial frontal lesions or medial thalamic lesions, Ross and Stewart reported a patient with a hypothalamic lesion that disrupted midbrain dopaminergic neurons as they ascended to the frontal lobes [49]. Ross and Stewart treated this akinetic and mute patient with bromocriptine, a D2 dopamine receptor agonist and found that this treatment abated the patients' akinetic mutism [49].

Similarly, Alexander treated a patient with akinetic mutism from a mesencephalic and hypothalamic infarction with levodopa and the D1/D2 receptor agonist pergolide and also found that this patient's akinetic mutism improved, but because of adverse side effects this medication is no longer available [50]. Powell et al. use bromocriptine in 8 individuals with traumatic brain injury (TBI) and found that there was a reduction of their abulia [51]. In addition, Imamura et al. found that bromocriptine reduced perseveration in patients with dementia and also reported that amantadine improved perseveration [52, 53].

Children with attentional disorders often have sign of action-intentional disorders and while medications that are norepinephrine agonists such as methylphenidate and atomoxetine (a selective norepinephrine re-uptake inhibitor) often reduce these children deficits, we could not find studies that examined these medications as treatments for the action-intentional disorders associated with degenerative or progressive neurological diseases.

Transcranial Electrical Stimulation

Transcranial direct current stimulation (tDCS): When searching Pubmed, we could find no articles that investigated the effects of transcranial direct current stimulation on akinesia, abulia, impersistence, perseveration or defective response inhibition.

Transcranial magnetic stimulation (TMS): Degardin et al. reported that TMS reduced the akinesia associated with Parkinson's disease and Pascual-Leone et al. showed that TMS improved hypokinesia (e.g., reduced reaction times) [54, 55].

Conclusion

Many of the action-intentional disorders described in this paper, have been reported for more than one half of a century; however, most of these studies have been performed in patients with strokes. Although TBI can cause damage to those same cortical and white matter pathways that have been reported to be damaged in patients with strokes who have action-intentional deficits, there has been a paucity of studies in patients with progressive neurological diseases that have investigated the signs and symptoms of motor action-intentional disorders as well as the pathophysiology of these disorders and their treatments. Since the action-intentional disorders described in this review can be a major source of disability there is a great need for further research. Hopefully, this review will help to stimulate investigators to perform research on this important topic.

REFERENCES

[1] Heilman KM, Rothi, LJG, Apraxia. In: *Clinical Neuropsychology,* 5th Edition. 2012 Eds. KM Heilman and E Valenstein, Oxford University Press, New York, pp 214-237.

[2] Heilman KM, Valenstein E, Rothi LJG, Watson RT, *Upper Limb Action-Intentional and Cognitive Apraxic Disorders.* 2008. Chapter 10, In Neurology in Clinical Practice Fifth Edition, Eds: WG Bradley, RB Daroff, GM Fenechel, J Jankovic, Phila PA Butterworth Heineman, Elsevier, Pages 121-132.

[3] Nielsen JM. The cortical components of akinetic mutism. *J Nerv Ment Dis.* 1951 Nov;114(5):459-61.

[4] Cairns H, Oldfield HC, Pennybaker JB, Whineridge D. Akinetic mutism with an epidermoid cyst of the third ventricle. *Brain,* 34 (1941), pp. 273–290.

[5] Sockeel P, Dujardin K, Devos D, Denève C, Destée A, Defebvre L. The Lille apathy rating scale (LARS), a new instrument for detecting and quantifying apathy: validation in Parkinson's disease. *J Neurol Neurosurg Psychiatry.* 2006 May;77(5):579-84.

[6] Marin RS, Biedrzycki RC, Firinciogullari S. Reliability and validity of the Apathy Evaluation Scale. *Psychiatry Res.* 1991 Aug;38(2):143-62.

[7] Heilman KM, Valenstein E. Watson RT. Neglect. In: *Clinical Neuropsychology,* 5th Edition. 2012 Eds. KM Heilman and E Valenstein, Oxford University Press, New York,

[8] Coslett HB, Bowers D, Heilman KM. Reduction in cerebral activation after right hemisphere stroke. *Neurology.* 1987 Jun;37(6):957-62.

[9] Heilman KM. Intentional neglect. Front Biosci. 2004 Jan 1;9:694-705.

[10]Watson RT, Miller BD, Heilman KM. Nonsensory neglect. *Ann Neurol.* 1978 Jun;3(6):505-8.

[11]Gold M, Adair JC, Jacobs DH, Heilman KM. Anosognosia for hemiplegia: an electrophysiologic investigation of the feed-forward hypothesis. *Neurology.* 1994 Oct;44(10):1804-8.

[12]Triggs WJ, Gold M, Gerstle G, Adair J, Heilman KM. Motor neglect associated with a discrete parietal lesion. *Neurology.* 1994 Jun;44(6):1164-6.

[13]Heilman KM, Bowers D, Watson RT. Performance on hemispatial pointing task by patients with neglect syndrome. *Neurology.* 1983 May;33(5):661-4.

[14]Heilman KM, Bowers D, Coslett HB, Whelan H, Watson RT. Directional hypokinesia: prolonged reaction times for leftward movements in patients with right hemisphere lesions and neglect. *Neurology.* 1985 Jun;35(6):855-9.

[15]De Renzi, E., Faglioni, P., and Scott, G. Hemispheric contribution to the exploration of space through the visual and tactile modality. *Cortex.* 1970 1:410- 433.

[16]Marshall CR, Maynard FM. Vestibular stimulation for supranuclear gaze palsy: case report. Arch Phys Med Rehabil. 1983 Mar;64(3):134-6.
[17]Valenstein E, Heilman KM. Unilateral hypokinesia and motor extinction. *Neurology.* 1981 Apr;31(4):445-8.
[18]Fitzgerald DB, Drago V, Jeong Y, Chang YL, White KD, Heilman KM. Asymmetrical alien hands in corticobasal degeneration. *Mov Disord.* 2007 Mar 15;22(4):581-4.
[19]Crucian GP, Heilman K, Junco E, Maraist M, Owens WE, Foote KD, Okun MS. The crossed response inhibition task in Parkinson's disease: disinhibition hyperkinesia. *Neurocase.* 2007 Jun;13(3):158-64.
[20]Denny-Brown D, Chambers RA. The parietal lobe and behavior. Res Publ Assoc Res Nerv Ment Dis. 1958;36:35-117.
[21]Riestra AR, Heilman KM. Visual facial grasp. Neurocase. 2004 Oct;10(5):363-5.
[22]Luria AR. *Higher Cortical Functions in Man.* Basic Books, 1966.
[23]Lhermitte F. 'Utilization behaviour' and its relation to lesions of the frontal lobes. *Brain.* 1983 Jun;106 (Pt 2):237-55.
[24]Fisher, CM. Left Himiplegia and motor impersistence. *The Journal of Nervous and Mental Disease.* 1956 March; Vol. 123, No. 3.
[25]Kertesz A., Nicholson I., Cancelliere A., Kassa K. and Black S. Motor impersistence: A right-hemisphere syndrome. *Neurology.* 1985 May; 35:662-666.
[26]Seo SW, Jung K, You H, Lee BH, Kim GM, Chung CS, Lee KH, Na DL. Motor-intentional disorders in right hemisphere stroke. *Cogn Behav Neurol.* 2009 Dec;22(4):242-8.
[27]Sandson J, Albert ML. Perseveration in behavioral neurology. *Neurology.* 1987 Nov;37(11):1736-41.
[28]Dubois B, Slachevsky A, Pillon B, Beato R, Villalponda JM, Litvan I. "Applause sign" helps to discriminate PSP from FTD and PD. *Neurology.* 2005 Jun 28;64(12):2132-3.
[29]Acosta LM, Goodman IJ, Heilman KM. Unilateral perseveration. *Cogn Behav Neurol.* 2013 Dec;26(4):181-8.
[30]Na DL, Adair JC, Kang Y, Chung CS, Lee KH, Heilman KM. Motor perseverative behavior on a line cancellation task. *Neurology.* 1999 May 12;52(8):1569-76.
[31]Gandola, M., Toraldo, A., Invernizzi, P., Corrado, L., Sberna, M., Santilli, I., Bottini, G., Paulesu, E. How many forms of perseveration? Evidence from cancellation tasks in right hemisphere patients. *Neuropsychologia.* 2013 Dec;51(14):2960-75.
[32]Gold M, Nadeau SE, Jacobs DH, Adair JC, Rothi LJ, Heilman KM. Adynamic aphasia: a transcortical motor aphasia with defective semantic strategy formation. *Brain Lang.* 1997 May;57(3):374-93.
[33]Howes D, Boller F. Simple reaction time: evidence for focal impairment from lesions of the right hemisphere. *Brain.* 1975 Jun;98(2):317-32.
[34]Kim EJ, Lee B, Jo MK, Jung K, You H, Lee BH, Cho HJ, Sung SM, Jung DS, Heilman KM, Na DL. Directional and spatial motor intentional disorders in patients with right versus left hemisphere strokes. *Neuropsychology.* 2013 Jul;27(4):428-37.
[35]Aron, A. R., Fletcher, P. C., Bullmore, E. T., Sahakian, B. J. and Robbins, T. W. (2003). Stop-signal inhibition disrupted by damage to right inferior frontal gyrus in humans. *Nat Neurosci,* 6, 115-116.

[36]Gusnard, D. A., Ollinger, J. M., Shulman, G. L., Cloninger, C. R., Price, J. L., Van Essen, D. C. and Raichle, M. E. (2003). Persistence and brain circuitry. *Proc Natl Acad Sci U S A,* 100, 3479-3484.

[37]Jung, Y. C., Ku, J., Namkoong, K., Lee, W., Kim, S. I. and Kim, J. J. (2010). Human orbitofrontal-striatum functional connectivity modulates behavioral persistence. *Neuroreport,* 21, 502-506.

[38]Dettmers C1, Lemon RN, Stephan KM, Fink GR, Frackowiak RS. Cerebral activation during the exertion of sustained static force in man. *Neuroreport.* 1996 Sep 2;7(13):2103-10.

[39]Isella V, Rucci F, Traficante D, Mapelli C, Ferri F, Appollonio IM The applause sign in cortical and cortical-subcortical dementia. J Neurol. 2013 Apr;260(4):1099-103.

[40]Mölsä PK, Marttila RJ, Rinne UK. Extrapyramidal signs in Alzheimer's disease. *Neurology.* 1984 Aug;34(8):1114-6.

[41]Pekkala, S., Albert, M. L., Spiro, A., 3rd, and Erkinjuntti, T. (2008). Perseveration in Alzheimer's disease. *Dement Geriatr Cogn Disord,* 25, 109-114.

[42]Lopez, O. L., Becker, J. T. and Boller, F. (1991). Motor impersistence in Alzheimer's disease. *Cortex,* 27, 93-99.

[43]Cummings JL Vascular subcortical dementias: clinical aspects. *Dementia.* 1994 May-Aug;5(3-4):177-80.

[44]Sang Yoon D, Jung K, Ha Kim G, Hui Kim S, Hwa Lee B, Won Seo S, You H, Na DL. Motor intentional disorders in vascular mild cognitive impairment and vascular dementia of subcortical type. *Neurocase.* 2014;20(1):53-60.

[45]Gustafson L. Clinical picture of frontal lobe degeneration of non-Alzheimer type. *Dementia.* 1993 May-Aug;4(3-4):143-8.

[46]Luzzi S, Fabi K, Pesallaccia M, Silvestrini M, Provinciali L. Applause sign: is it really specific for Parkinsonian disorders? Evidence from cortical dementias. *J Neurol Neurosurg Psychiatry.* 2011 Aug;82(8):830-3.

[47]Cotzias GC, Van Woert MH, Schiffer LM. Aromatic amino acids and modification of parkinsonism. *N Engl J Med* 1967;276:374-379.

[48]Hughes LE, Altena E, Barker RA, Rowe JB. Perseveration and choice in Parkinson's disease: the impact of progressive frontostriatal dysfunction on action decisions. *Cereb Cortex.* 2013 Jul;23(7):1572-81.

[49]Ross ED, Stewart RM. Akinetic mutism from hypothalamic damage: successful treatment with dopamine agonists. *Neurology.* 1981;31(11):1435-9.

[50]Alexander MP. Chronic akinetic mutism after mesencephalic-diencephalic infarction: remediated with dopaminergic medications. *Neurorehabil Neural Repair.* 2001;15(2):151-6.

[51]Powell JH, Al-adawi S, Morgan J, Greenwood RJ. Motivational deficits after brain injury: effects of bromocriptine in 11 patients. *J Neurol Neurosurg Psychiatr.* 1996;60(4):416-21.

[52]Imamura T, Takanashi M, Hattori N, Fujimori M, Yamashita H, Ishii K, Yamadori A. Bromocriptine treatment for perseveration in demented patients. *Alzheimer Dis Assoc Disord.* 1998 Jun;12(2):109-13.

[53]Imamura T1, Suzuki K, Yamadori A, Sahara M, Nagasawa H, Itoh M, Itoh H. Improved perseveration with amantadine. *No To Shinkei.* 1994 Jun;46(6):556-62.

[54]Degardin A, Devos D, Defebvre L, Destée A, Plomhause L, Derambure P, Devanne Effect of intermittent theta-burst stimulation on akinesia and sensorimotor integration in patients with Parkinson's disease. *Eur J Neurosci.* 2012 Sep;36(5):2669-78.

[55]Pascual-Leone A1, Valls-Solé J, Brasil-Neto JP, Cohen LG, Hallett M. Akinesia in Parkinson's disease. I. Shortening of simple reaction time with focal, single-pulse transcranial magnetic stimulation. *Neurology.* 1994 May;44(5):884-91.

In: Progressive Cognitive Impairment …
Editor: Gediminas Peter Gliebus
ISBN: 978-1-63485-221-0

Chapter 5

EMOTIONAL PROCESSING AND NEURODEGENERATIVE DISEASES

Peter Pressman[1,*], MD, and Elliott Ross[2], MD
[1]Department of Neurology, University of California San Francisco, San Francisco, CA, US
[2]Department of Neurology, University of Oklahoma Health Sciences Center, Oklahoma City, OK, US

1. EMOTIONAL PROCESSING OVERVIEW

As a rule, people want to be happy, and prefer to avoid sorrow, anger, or fear. Emotion is a primary motivating factor for all we do. Nevertheless, neuroscience has focused more on the investigation of motor, sensory, or cognitive systems rather than emotional processes. Neurological diseases influence several different aspects of emotional functioning, resulting in emotional deregulation, diminished empathy, depression, and anxiety, among many others. Such changes can be at least as impactful as sensory or motor lesions in regards to a patient's quality of life and ability to function in society.

Progress in emotion research has been slowed by an academic debate over a precise definition of emotion. For this chapter, we agree with Levenson's definition of emotions as "short-lived psychological-physiological phenomena that represent efficient modes of adaptation to changing environmental demands." [1] While emotional experience is ultimately a private and subjective phenomenon, one can indirectly study emotion through a variety of indicators, including neuroendocrine secretions, visceral sensations, facial and bodily reactions, language, attention and thought. Note this definition of emotion does not include long lasting (mood) states such as pervasive depression or anxiety, though these disorders may share common neuroanatomical pathways with emotions.

Neuropathology is intractably linked to neuroanatomy. This is particularly true of neurodegenerative diseases, which tend to selectively attack particular neural networks, that in some instances may be due to a prion-like mechanism of propagation [2, 3]. We cannot

* Correspondence to: Peter.Pressman@ucsf.edu.

hope to understand the effects of neurological illness on emotion without understanding the roles of different neuroanatomical structures and networks in emotional processing. Consequently, this chapter will discuss the neuroanatomy of emotion in some detail. We must also clarify what steps and functions contribute to our emotional lives. Only then can we describe how the brain's networks and structures support these emotional sub-processes and create a complete emotional experience.

There are dozens of theoretical models of emotional processing. Despite their differences, most of these models agree on some basic themes such as emotional appraisal, reactivity, recognition and regulation. Like all models, it is necessary to sacrifice some detail and accuracy in the name of conceptual clarity. In this chapter we will discuss each emotional process in turn, emphasizing key anatomical structures and respective disorders for each. While the following processes are presented separately and sequentially, it must be remembered that in actuality the brain is organized to allow parallel and dynamic interaction between systems and structures, both neuroanatomical and conceptual. Each brain region may participate in several aspects of emotional processing. While all models are ultimately wrong, we nevertheless hope the simple model presented here will be useful in emphasizing how the brain generates emotional functions, and how these functions can be disrupted by disease.

Prior to forming an emotional reaction, the brain must assign a value to the stimulus through the process of *appraisal*. Do we think this event or object is positive (e.g., candy) or negative (e.g., wasps)? What degree of arousal does the event merit? Should we be afraid, angry, joyful or embarrassed? This appraisal process may be very quick and largely subconscious, or it can incorporate higher levels of slower and more deliberate processing as we consider the context and identity of the stimulus [4-7].

After the stimulus has been appraised, a wide array of different emotional networks is called on to appropriately adjust the body's internal milieu, shift our cognitive resources towards salient stimuli, and communicate with our social peers. This process is called *emotional reactivity*. We can also become consciously aware of how we are feeling via a process sometimes called *emotion recognition* or *emotional understanding*. Our emotional understanding can extend to others through a separate act of appraisal, often involving covert simulation of the other's emotional reactivity. Finally, our immediate emotional reactions may need to be adjusted depending on the situation, which is accomplished through methods of *emotion regulation*, such as thinking about the stimulus in a more neutral or positive manner (reappraisal), for example, or by consciously suppressing emotional displays.

A) Controversy in Emotion

While a statement of ongoing controversy and need for future research is usually reserved for a chapter's end, emotion is a field where even basic neuroanatomy and terminology has major thematic debates, without understanding of which further discussion will prove difficult.

1.A.i. What Is the Extent and Role of the Limbic System in Emotional Processing?

Those who have studied emotion and the brain have likely read about the phylogenetically ancient limbic system. The limbic network has been inconsistently delineated, but is generally agreed to include allocortical and corticoid nervous tissue of the amygdala, hippocampus, and olfactory cortex. Depending on the author, the limbic system may also be said to encompass the hypothalamus, paralimbic cortical belt, limbic striatum such as the nucleus accumbens, the limbic pallidum, the ventral tegmental area, the habenula, and the limbic and paralimbic thalamic nuclei [8]. It must be emphasized, however, that the emotional components of the limbic system are also modulated by orbitofrontal, prefrontal, temporal and insular neocortices, so even an extended limbic system fails to include all structures required for healthy emotional processing. Furthermore, the limbic system also includes regions more peripherally associated with emotion, such as the hippocampus and olfactory cortex. For this reason, we will rarely discuss the limbic system as a whole in this chapter, though we will discuss many of its components, and we will extend our scope to other brain areas as well. (Figure 1)

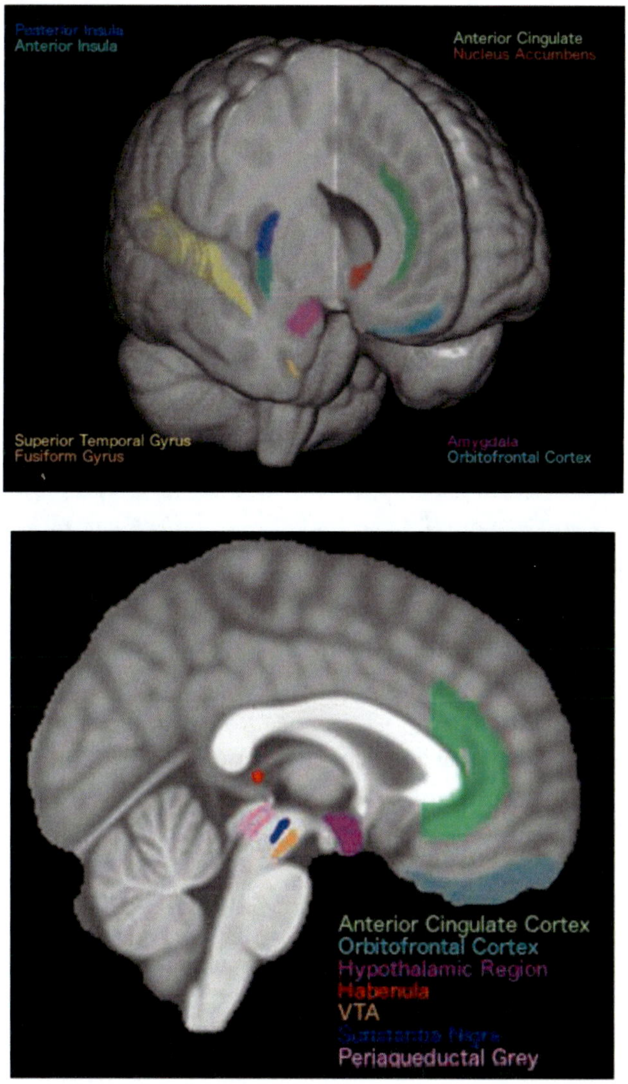

Figure 1. Cutaway and sagittal midline illustration of important neuroanatomical structures in emotion. Demonstrated on MRIcroGL. http://www.mccauslandcenter.sc.edu/mricrogl/.

1.A.ii. Is Emotional Processing Lateralized?

There are at least three models positing a relative hemispheric lateralization of emotion.

1. Right Hemisphere Hypothesis: All primary emotions (such as anger, sadness, fear, joy and disgust) are preferentially processed by the right hemisphere. Some literature extends this to more involved "secondary" emotions as well [9-14].
2. Valence Hypothesis: The right hemisphere is involved in processing "negative" emotions such as fear, sadness and disgust, and the left hemisphere mediates processes related to approach such as happiness. A variation on this hypothesis suggests the lateralization is based on approach vs. avoidance behavior, in which case anger might be left lateralized [15-21].
3. Emotion Type Hypothesis: Innate primary emotions and related displays, such as surprise, anger, fear, elation, are processed by the right hemisphere, whereas emotions that are acquired through social interactions (social emotions), such as envy, pity jealousy, admiration are processed by the left [22]. This can also be viewed as a synthesis of the previous two theories, as the right hemisphere hypothesis focuses on primary rather than social emotions and most basic emotions are negative in valence because they are related to the fight-flight response.

It is also worth mentioning that in addition to the hypotheses discussed above, many studies support a null hypothesis of no hemispheric difference. Data exist to support all of the above, and the conversation is ever evolving. Each of these hypotheses is also subject to further nuance. For example, while it has been suggested that left hemispheric damage may lead to more dysphoria due to its association with positive emotion under the valence hypothesis, damage to inhibitory circuitry in the left hemisphere may pathologically increase such positive emotion due to diminished suppression, resulting in a seemingly paradoxical euphoria [23].

1.A.iii. Are There Basic, Universal and Shared Emotions?

There are two main theories of emotion types. As is often the case with supposed antitheses, the truth is likely a synthesis between the purported opposites.

The first theory emphasizes emotional specificity, or natural forms. The theory suggests that there are core or primary emotions, which arise from evolutionarily beneficial biological systems shared across not only cultures, but often other mammalian species. This theory takes root in Darwin's "On Emotions in Man and Animals," which demonstrates several shared behaviors between man and other phylogenetically related animals [24]. Basic emotional displays and experiences have since been suggested to be shared across even geographically and culturally remote human populations [15, 25]. More nuanced emotions such as embarrassment or pride (social emotions) are then superimposed on the framework of those basic and shared emotions [26, 27].

An opposing theory is that labels such as sorrow or anger do not in fact represent fundamental and shared expressions, but are cultural constructs superimposed on much simpler physiological states. This theory suggests that all emotions can be best described dimensionally, for example falling somewhere on an axis of valence (pleasurable or aversive), arousal (high or low energy) or approach/withdrawal. Anything else is argued to the result of psychological construction. For example, anger would describe from an aversive, high arousal state, which would then be labeled "anger" only due to culturally contextualized higher-order knowledge [28-30].

One can see in these two extreme positions the perennial argument between "top-down" and "bottom-up" approaches to psychology. In actuality, of course, the brain incorporates countless neural loops permitting both paths in parallel. It is also beyond dispute that the complexity of the nervous system allows a great deal of specificity in its responses to the environment. It is heuristically simpler, however, to divide emotion and its corresponding neuroanatomy into basic functional groups or dimensions. Without swearing allegiance to any particular theory, this chapter will use these "lumping" approaches, while attempting to frequently remind the reader of the greater complexities lurking just around the corner.

For example, as the sympathetic nervous system and parasympathetic nervous system can roughly be seen as having opposing actions, so can two main neural networks that connect a stimulus with a particular emotional valence through a process of appraisal. The first, the amygdaloid limbic system, is classically associated with responses of fear and aggression. The second is the dopaminergic basal forebrain, which is historically linked to pleasure and reward. While these associations provide an aesthetically pleasing dichotomy and are supported by research, the amygdala is also involved with pleasure, and the ventral "reward" pathways have a role in aversive appraisals.

2. Appraisal

Appraisal has been summed as the comparison of an event or stimulus to an organism's goals and resources. If we are hungry, appraisal may attach a positive valence or feeling of excitement towards an apple. The valence of our appraisal quickly changes when we see a large spider crawling over the fruit. The valence may change more slowly as we eat more and more of the apple and grow tired of the taste.

Several different brain structures are likely involved with appraisal. The clearest data on emotional appraisal points to the amygdala (Figure 2) as the connection between external stimuli and alignment of internal resources towards our shifting goals. This appraisal is fast and often coursc, but ultimately coordinates an emotional reaction with great effects on both body and brain [31].

2.A. The Amygdala

The amygdala has been hailed as the epicenter of emotion. The amygdala has been most consistently associated with mediation of fear conditioning, and can underpin our tendency to develop a negative attitude towards a particular stimulus. For example, the amygdala is more activated by unpredictable sounds or potentially threatening images [32, 33]. The amygdala responds strongly to social and emotional stimuli conveyed via the face and eyes, and may alter activity when exposed to frightened faces. People whose amygdalae and surrounding structures are destroyed bilaterally may no longer be able to respond appropriately to social emotional stimuli, though these lesions were quite extensive and may not be specific to the amygdala [34, 35].

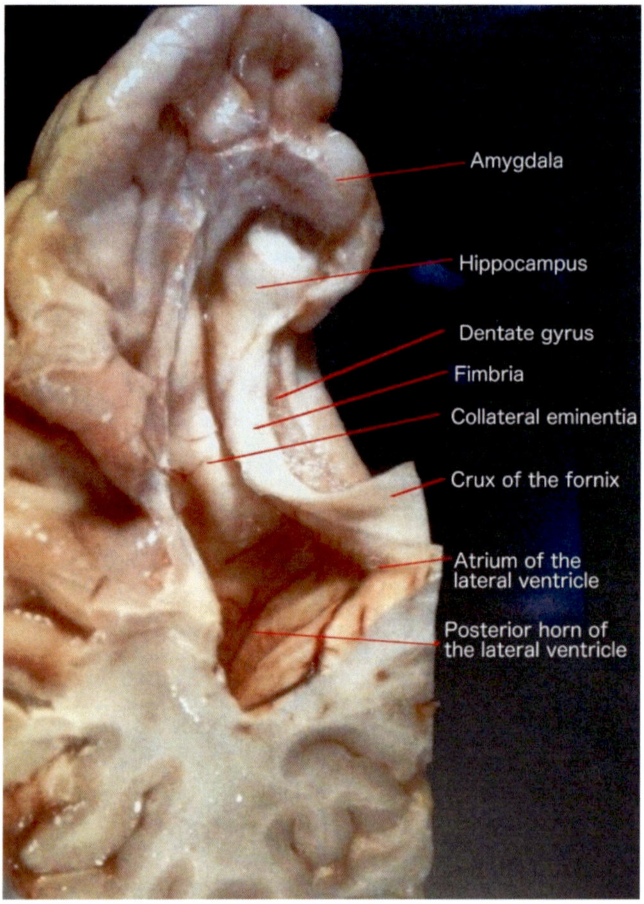

Figure 2. Anatomy of the Amygdala.
Gross anatomical axial view of the amygdala and hippocampus from the superior aspect of the temporal lobe. The amygdala closes anteriorly the inferior horn of the lateral ventricle. Posteriorly, the floor of the lateral ventricle contains 3 structures, plus the beginning fo the hippocampal fibria. The medial wall fo the inferior horn is formed only by the ependima and the pia mater. Courtesy of Juan J Cayaffa and the Northwestern Memorial Hospital Neurology Department.

Despite its strong historical association with fear and anger, the amygdala is better considered as broadly assigning an emotional and motivational valence to biological stimuli, thereby assessing the potential of a stimulus to be associated with punishment or reward [36]. It is true that lesions of the amygdala can lead to a loss of fear responses. However, people with amygdala lesions may still consciously experience "fear." The amygdala is an important part of coordinating an autonomic and behavioral response, but it is not critically necessary to consciously feel the emotion. The amygdala can coordinate an automatic and even unconscious response to a threat with or without the conscious sensation of fear. The conscious experience most likely results from a cortical integration of varying expressions of attention, memory, and interoception, resulting in a unique emotional experience, as is demonstrated by pain asymbolia as discussed later within this chapter [37].

It is also worth noting that while much has been written about the amygdala's association with negative stimuli, it has also been tied with pleasure [38]. Detoxified cocaine users respond to images of cocaine with craving as well as increased amygdala activity [39]. The amygdala also contains a high concentration of opiate receptors, suggesting a role for pleasure as well [40]. In short, while the medical lore of the amygdala and negative emotion is well-known, it may be less well-understood, and may occasionally cross the line into medical mythology. The amygdala is best understood within the context of a network dedicated to determining emotional salience.

As befits its role in emotional appraisal, the amygdala receives direct connections from sensory processing regions in the thalamus as well as cortical sensory processing regions [41]. Some have posited that crude processing of emotional stimuli can travel through a subcortical route, while cortical pathways permit more detailed assessment [42]. This rough and fast subcortical route of emotional processing is sometimes referred to as the "low road" of emotion processing, compared to the more precise, slower, cortical "high road."

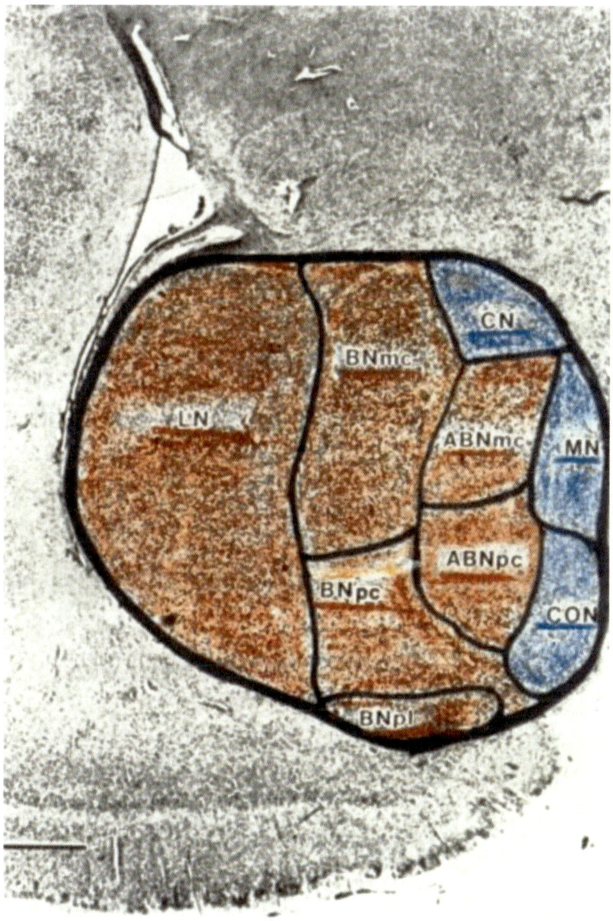

Figure 3. Subnuclei of the Amygadala.
Pathological coronal depiction of the amgydalar subnuclei. Centromedial groups is in blue, comprised of the central nucleus (CN), medial nucleus (MN), and cortical nucleus (CON). The basolateral group is in red and is comprised of – the lateral nucleus (LN), basal nucleus, which is itself subdivided into magnocellular (BNmc) and parivellular regions (BNpc), the accessory basal nucleus (subdivided into magnocellular (ABNmc) and parvocllular (ABNmp), and the basal nucleus paralaminal region (BNpl). Courtesy of Juan J Cayaffa and the Northwestern Memorial Hospital Neurology Department.

The amygdala is more accurately called the amygdaloid nuclear complex, a collection of different nuclei located in the medial portion of the temporal lobe, where it forms the anterior limit of the inferior horn of the lateral ventricle. In addition, the so-called extended amygdala includes the central amygdaloid nucleus, the bed nucleus of the striae terminalis, and part of the substantia innominata (Figure 3).

The amygdala is usually divided into the corticomedial and basolateral nuclear groups. The corticomedial group, consisting of the medial, cortical, and central nuclei, maintains prominent connections with phylogenetically older central nervous system regions such as the olfactory bulb, hypothalamus and brainstem. The central nucleus of the amygdala helps to organize behavioral reactions in the context of emotional learning. The amygdala likely does this in collaboration with the basal ganglia such as the ventral subthalamic nucleus and nucleus accumbens as part of the "low road" of emotional processing. The corticomedial group is connected with the hypothalamus via the stria terminalis, also called the dorsal amygdalofugal pathway, by which the amygdala can organize autonomic and endocrinological reactions (Figure 4).

The larger, ontogenetically and phylogenetically more recent basolateral group, consisting of the lateral, basal, and accessory basal nuclei, has extensive connections with frontal, temporal, and insular cortex, the mediodorsal nucleus of the thalamus, striatum, entorhinal cortex, subiculum, hippocampus and the cholinergic cells of the nucleus basalis of Meynert. Whereas the centromedial group can operate below the level of conscious awareness, relays from the amygdala to neocortical and mesocortical areas such as the insula likely lead to the subjective feeling of emotion. In addition to a large projection to the posterior insula, extensive amygdalo-cortical projections travel through the uncinate fasciculus to the orbitofrontal and medial aspect of the prefrontal cortex, which further help integrate sensory information prior to forming a behavioral response.

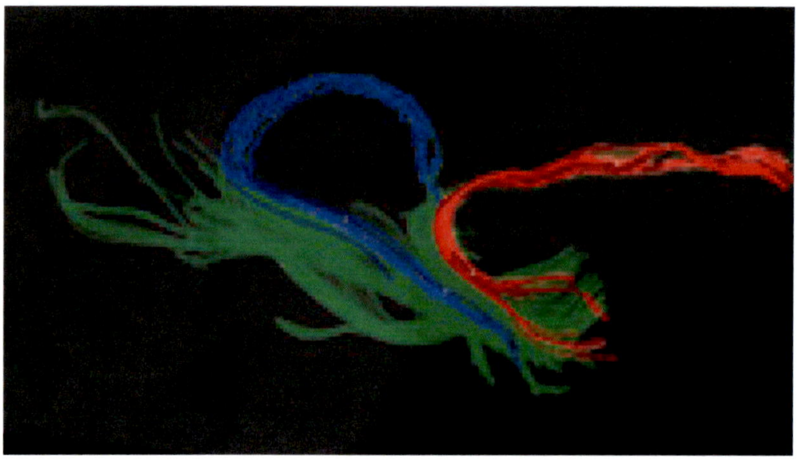

Figure 4. Major pathways to and from the amygdale.
A schematic based on diffusion tensor tractography imaging (TrackVis by Ruopeng Wang and Van WeDeen, courtesy of Dr. Patrick Simen of Princeton University) illustrating major pathways from amygdala. The stria terminalis (red) runs medial to the uncinate fasciculus (red), and the ventral amygdalofugal pathway (green). The ventral amygdalofugal pathway is actually more diffuse than depicted, the amygdala to and from the insular, frontal, temporal, and parietal cortices, as well as the basal ganglia.

2.A.i. Disorders of the Amygdala and its Connections

The best-known clinical syndrome associated with the amygdala (albeit somewhat imprecisely) is the Kluver-Bucy Syndrome. From 1937 to 1939, H. Kluver and P.J. Bucy described the results of a neurosurgical procedure in Rhesus monkeys (macacca mulata), in which the amygdala was resected along with the rest of the temporal lobe anterior to the vein of Labbe, including most of the temporal association areas, entorhinal cortex, and hippocampus. The pair described the following:

1) Visual agnosia. The monkeys handled objects in a way that suggested the simians no no longer understood the object's nature. For example, they would attempt to grasp a flame.
2) Oral tendency: The monkeys developed a strong tendency to examine objects using the mouth.
3) Hypermetamorphopsia: The animals tended to touch every object in sight.
4) Bulemia
5) Emotional placidity: The monkeys demonstrated an absence of emotional reactions, with no fear or anger. This likely resulted from the removal of the amygdala.
6) Changes in sexual behavior: The animals were markedly hypersexual.

Amygelectomized monkeys also failed to generate autonomic responses to provocative stimuli, likely because the hypothalamus and autonomic system has lost a critical source of input [43-45]. Since its first description in monkeys, Kluver-Bucy syndrome has also been described in humans. Ralph Lilly, for example, described a series of 12 patients with Kluver-Bucy in 1983, four of which had herpes encephalitis, on with posttraumatic encephalopathy, five cases of what he called Pick's disease and one with Alzheimer's disease [46]. In general, however, a complete Kluver-Bucy syndrome remains a rare diagnosis of more historical and educational than clinical interest.

The extent to which the classical symptoms of Kluver-Bucy syndrome relate to the removal of the amygdala versus the anterior temporal lobe is debated. Symptoms such as an oral tendency, hypermetamorphopsia, and visual agnosia have been associated with temporal networks. Removal of the anterior temporal lobes while leaving the amygdala or hippocampus in monkeys results in profound behavioral deficits, including hypoemotionality, leading to exclusion from their social groups [47, 48]. Furthermore, it's possible that rather than a true hypoemotionality, patients simply suffered from a visual agnosia due to disruption of the ventral visual pathways in the temporal lobes. A visual sensory-specific hypoemotionality has been demonstrated in both animals and people who have suffered damage to the temporal visual pathways, suggestive of a visuo-emotional disconnection syndrome [43, 49, 50]. That said, the amygdala may be involved with appraisal of a stimulus even before the image hits the occipital cortex and is processed along dorsal and ventral cortical pathways. Demonstrations of a subcortical pathway for comprehension of others' facial affect come from cases of "affective blindsight," in which patients suffering from cortical blindness still respond above chance to visually presented, emotional rousing stimuli. The neural substrate of affective blindsight is still being worked out, but the phenomenon is likely supported by a subcortical route from the superior collicular nucleus to the thalamic pulvinar nucleus, and then to the amygdala [51].

2.A.ii. The Dopaminergic Reward Pathway

Classically, the negative preoccupations of the amygdala are contrasted with the ventral tegmental reward and pleasure centers. In 1954, James Olds and Peter Milner from McGill University demonstrated that stimulation of the septal nuclei served as a reward in rats [52]. The rodents had electrodes implanted into the septal nuclei, which they could stimulate by pressing a lever, and would obligingly do so thousands of times an hour, ignoring trivial distractions such as food [53]. Other researchers later found similar results in monkeys [54]. This work was seminal to the delineation of a mesolimbic reward network projecting through the ventral striatum, nucleus accumbens, paralimbic areas of the prefrontal cortex (including the anterior cingulate area and the orbitofrontal cortex), the amygdala and the hippocampal formation [55]. The habenula and deep brainstem nuclei such as the parabrachial nucleus of the pons are also likely involved with reward processing [56].

As with the amygdala, these predominantly dopaminergic subcortical structures may operate on a largely unconscious level, having more to do with desire or "incentive salience" rather than liking, which may depend more on endogenous opiate receptors. The experience of enjoyment may also rely on cortical rather than subcortical structures. The medial edge of the orbitofrontal cortex (OFC) has been shown in imaging to studies to be activated in tasks related to the valence of positive events, whereas lateral portions may represent more negative and punishing events. This medial-lateral "liking" gradient coexists with an anterior-posterior abstraction gradient-- more complex reinforcers (such as monetary gain) are more anterior than less complex rewards (such as a pleasant taste) [54, 55, 57]. Debate remains, however, about the extent to which these regions represent pleasure rather than simply monitoring and predicting reward values.

Another example of the interplay between pleasure and punishment can be found in the nucleus accumbens, a structure of particular importance to reward-mediated learning. The nucleus accumbens is the ventral extension of both the caudate and putamen, sitting in the ventral aspect of the forebrain bilaterally. The nucleus accumbens receives projections from the ventral tegmental area, the paralimbic areas of the prefrontal cortex (PFC) and the amygdala. The nucleus accumbens consists of two regions, the core (NAcC) and the shell (NAcS). Lesions of the core abolish some behavioral responses to conditioned stimuli, and so appears to be related to motor activity associated with emotional significance. The core appears to amplify behavior—for example if amphetamine is infused into the NAcS, the animal is more likely to work towards a reward-conditioned stimulus. Despite its traditional association with reward-mediated learning, however, a valence of fear may be assigned to a stimulus by manipulating the circuitry of the nucleus accumbens. Recent studies have suggested that the medial shell of the nucleus is systematically arranged in terms of valence generators, so that intense dread may result depending on where the medial shell is stimulated [55].

2.A.iii. Disorders of the Reward Pathways

As has been mentioned, dopamine is a key neurotransmitter in the brain's reward pathways. Emotional processes are impaired in a number of different neurologic and psychiatric pathologies involving the dopaminergic system, including drug abuse, obsessive-compulsive disorder, attention deficit disorder, Parkinson's disease and Huntington's disease [58-61].

Of those disorders, Huntington's disease has particularly been associated with cognitive and emotional deficits. The disease is due to an autosomal-dominant cytosine-adenine-guanine trinucleotide repeat expansion on chromosome 4p16.3, within a gene encoding a protein named "huntingtin." Those with Huntington's disease have between 36 to 121 of these repeats, compared to 10 to 29 in controls. The disease causes atrophy in the basal ganglia, especially the caudate and putamen, the ventral and anterior expansion of which become the nucleus accumbens.

While Huntington's disease is best recognized as a movement disorder, predominantly involving chorea, at least 15-20% of patients may first present with psychiatric features. Those with Huntington's disease are reported to have an emotion recognition deficit, as well as difficulty controlling emotions such as anger [62, 63]. In addition, those with Huntington's can suffer from depression, executive dysfunction, and psychotic features [64-66]. As the ventral aspects of the basal ganglia are more classically associated with emotional function, the presence of early psychiatric features appeared discordant with early literature describing a dorsal to ventral wave of degeneration throughout the caudate and putamen [67]. More recent data, however, suggest that changes within the limbic system and hypothalamus can occur in early Huntington's disease [68], including early pathological and volumetric changes within the nucleus accumbens [67, 69].

Parkinson's disease is traditionally connected with dopaminergic pathways and degeneration of the substantia nigra pars compacta. While many people recognize the dopaminergic connection between the pars compacta and other basal ganglia, more than 50% of the nigral output projects to the neocortex in the rat and primates [70, 71] through the medial forebrain bundle which courses lateral to the hypothalamus and next to the nucleus accumbens to innervate the anterior cingulate and dorsomedial prefrontal cortex [72]. These dopaminergic pathways may help explain why those with Parkinson's disease sometimes experience unusual craving and addictive behavior when on dopaminergic medications, and may also explain the higher incidence of depression among people with Parkinson's [73]. Well-described loops between striatum and cortex are also likely involved [74-76].

The reward pathways incorporate neurotransmitters beyond dopamine. For example, the neurons of this reward pathway are locally inhibited by serotonergic autoreceptors. Either dopamine receptor antagonists, then, or serotonergic stimulants can inhibit this projection system, leading to reduction of drive. Strategic use of dopaminergic antagonists such as haloperidol have long been recognized as often calming agitated or violent patients (though with a significant risk of side effects). Selective serotonin reuptake inhibitors such as citalopram may be useful in reducing agitation in patients, and avoid some of the side effects of antipsychotics.

3. Emotional Reactivity

Emotional reactions provide a powerful synchronization of different biological systems towards a common goal, efficiently coordinating several aspects of physiology to respond to an environmental change. Emotion accomplishes this act of coordination on at least three levels—focusing our internal and external attention towards the emotionally provocative stimulus, adjusting our autonomic nervous system to prepare our body to better handle the change of environment, and signaling the nature of our emotion to others in our social group [1, 77].

3.A.Shifting of Attention and Cognitive Resources

Selective attention refers to our ability to focus on certain stimuli (including distinct memories or thought processes) over others, in the face of competition from a constant bombardment of both internal and external distractions. Emotion can assist in the prioritization of selective attention, as well as general alertness. For example, neuroimaging studies have demonstrated that emotionally arousing films more vigorously engage visual cortex [78]. Similar effects also exist for memory, as we recall more emotionally rousing events [79, 80].

This emotional modulation of attention is dependent on the amygdala. Lesions of the amygdala shift our perceptual bias towards the emotionally mundane [81]. When stimulated, the amygdala immediately provokes an elevated state of alertness [82, 83]. This may result from any number of amygdalar connections, including to the reticular activating system in the brainstem, from which several nuclei launch activating combinations of acetylcholine, glutamate, serotonin, dopamine and norepinephrine throughout the brain and particularly to the thalamus and hypothalamus, with which amygdala also communicates directly. While the hypothalamus primarily mediates further autonomic and endocrinological responses, the mediodorsal nucleus and anterior thalamus have been implicated in memory formation and retrieval as part of the circuit of Papez. Similarly, the lateral amygdala communicates directly with the hippocampus, facilitating both memory retrieval and consolidation [84]. Thus, the amygdala is situated both to alert the brain and play an important role in memory encoding and retrieval.

While the amygdala is able to influence cognitive resources somewhat independently, it also collaborates with other components of what has been called the salience network to identify stimuli with personal and emotional relevance. Other components of this network include the anterior cingulate cortex and anterior insula, both of which are closely integrated with autonomic and interoceptive circuitry [85]. In many ways, these paralimbic structures may represent the border between unconscious emotional processing and conscious awareness. While the bulk of the discussion in this section is reserved for anterior cingulate cortex, a brief introduction to the insula is also required. While the analogy is imperfect, the insula has been called the center of limbic sensation, as it represents a site of internal representation ultimately supportive of emotion recognition [86]. The posterior insula receives a large projection from the basolateral amygdala in primates [87], and lesions of the posterior insular have been associated with the clinical syndrome of pain asymbolia [37]. The posterior insula is also thought to have a somatopic representation of somatosensory, temperature and painful stimuli.. In addition, a large body of literature supports the functional connectivity between the anterior insula and anterior cingulate cortex (ACC). Granger causality studies suggest that the insular activity often drives the action of the ACC, reminiscent of how sensations lead to reflex action [88]. Further discussion of the insula is reserved for the section on emotion recognition.

The anterior cingulate cortex has been referred to as limbic motor cortex [88], and is especially implicated in emotional reactivity. The ACC further organizes a multitude of cognitive and autonomic responses to the changing representation of the self within an environment presented by the anterior insular cortex. While the ACC does communicate with premotor cortex, the role of the ACC is not restricted to somatic muscle movement. As befits its multifaceted roles in emotion, the ACC has many cytoarchitectonically defined sub-regions serving cognitive, autonomic and motor functions, among others. For example, different parts of the ACC influence the shifting of cognitive set, modulation of sensory processing, or control of heart rate and vasodilation [88].

The cingulate can be divided into four main regions—anterior, mid, and posterior, as well as retrosplenial. These are then further subdivided [89, 90]. Broadly speaking, the dorsal aspect of the ACC (areas 24 b-c and 32) is involved with cognitive processes such as attention modulation, error monitoring, conflict processing, and response selection. Mesulam presented the notion that the ACC was part of the cortical network directing attentional resources [91]. In particular, the ACC was thought to be concerned with assessing motivational valence, that is the potential for reward or punishment associated with different external stimuli. This region has strong interconnections with dorsolateral prefrontal cortex, well as premotor and supplementary motor areas. The rostral ventral division (24a-c and 32 and ventral 25 and 33) is more tightly connected with autonomic and emotional nuclei. There is some evidence that the two portions of the ACC may deactivate each other. For example, intense emotional states can lead to suppression of the cognitive division, and the emotional subdivision may be deactivated during divided attention, working memory, and antisaccade tasks [92].

The ACC is likely a nexus between two broader networks, dorsal and ventral, for attention in the brain. The dorsal attention network is posited to be more "top-down" in nature, allowing for a willful control of attention, whereas the ventral pathway is posited to redirect attention towards stimuli which are unexpected but behaviorally relevant. Dynamic interplay between these two systems is likely mediated by the inferior and middle frontal gyrus [93].

As the "limbic motor cortex," damage to the ACC, classically by rupture of a berry aneurysm of the anterior communicating artery, can lead to lack of motivation or abulia. In its most severe form patients can experience akinetic mutism, though this may require that other brain regions such as supplementary motor areas, basal ganglia, or the thalamus be involved [94]. These regions are also classically impacted by tauopathies such as corticobasal degeneration and progressive supranuclear palsy, which typically impact executive function and attention. Von Economo neurons in the ACC and insula are among the earliest cells to degenerate in bvFTD, helping to explain why these patients have social and emotional improprieties, as well as diminished executive function and attention [95]. Selective damage to the right ACC by behavioral variant frontotemporal dementia pathology has been particularly implicated in the loss of self-conscious emotional reactivity in this population [96]. Anterior cingulate cortical degeneration likely underlies the apathy that is one of the defining clinical characteristics of bvFTD, especially in later disease stages.

3.B. Autonomic and Endocrinologic Emotional Reactivity

The argument portraying emotional responses as simply existing on two dimensions (e.g., valence and arousal) invokes an overly simplistic view of autonomic reactivity. While it is true that, generally, the parasympathetic system allows one to "rest and digest" whereas sympathetic systems allows for "fight or flight," it is also true that each system involves several different receptor types, suggesting a systemic capacity for greater specificity in emotional reactions. For example, classically one pales with fright and reddens with anger, rather than the other way around, despite both emotions sharing a similar valence and level of arousal [97].

The expression of complex visceromotor and somatic behavior associated with emotion can be generated by subcortical regions such as the hypothalamus or amygdala with no further higher cortical input [98]. Such expressions, however, should be considered "sham" emotion, as they do not impact learning. More cortical brain regions such as the anterior cingulate cortex and insula have reciprocal connections with the autonomic nervous system, either via the hypothalamus or more directly to brainstem nuclei, and may represent a pathway to conscious emotion [86].

3.B.i. Hypothalamus

The hypothalamus is a major nexus between neural and endocrine systems. While it is important to emotional reactivity, hypothalamic functions extend beyond emotion and into more fundamental homoeostasis. A complete review of hypothalamic structure, function and connectivity is beyond the scope of this chapter. Instead, we will focus on a few points most relevant to emotional functioning.

The hypothalamus is so-named because it is located beneath the thalamus, separated from that structure by the hypothalamic sulcus. The tuber cinereum bulges from the hypothalamus between the optic chiasm and mammillary bodies. From this arises the infundibulum, which goes on to continue as the pituitary stalk. The anterior portion of this stalk is elevated and called the median eminence. The pituitary gland itself lies in the pituitary fossa, bounded by the anterior clinoid process and the posterior clinoid process, which combined form the sella turcica. Beneath this is the sphenoid sinus. Dura covering this is the diaphragma sella. The hypothalamus is bounded laterally on both sides by the cavernous sinus.

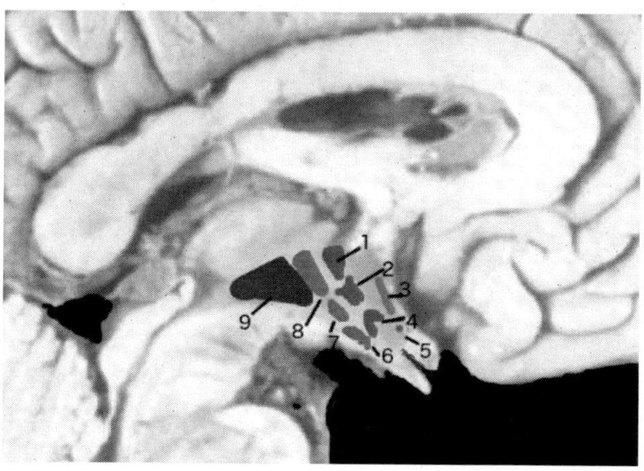

Figure 5. The hypothalamus. Schematic overlay of hypothalamic nuclei. 1. Paraventricular nucleus, 2. Anterior nucleus, 3. Medial preoptic nucleus, 4. Supraoptic nucleus, 5. Suprachiasmiatic nucleus, 6. Arcuate nucleus, 7. Ventromedial nucleus, 8. Dorsomedial nucleus, 9. The posterior hypothalamic region, including the medial mammillary nucleus, intermediate mammillary nucleus, lateral mammillary nucleus, and posterior hypothalamic nucleus. Adapted from images courtesy of Juan J Cayaffa and the Northwestern Memorial Hospital Department of Neurology.

The lateral hypothalamic nucleus is important in appetite. Lesions may lead to decreased body weight. The anterior portion may be very important to thirst. The lateral hypothalamus is permeated by the medial forebrain bundle, a tract carrying information from "reward" circuitry such as the septal nuclei, the ventral tegmental area, and the nucleus accumbens.

The medial portion of the hypothalamus contains many sub-nuclei. Most relevant to this discussion includes the paraventricular nucleus, from which descending autonomic fibers primarily originate. The paraventricular nucleus also helps create oxytocin and vasopressin for release from the posterior aspect of the pituitary gland (the neurohypophysis). Both these hormones have been implicated in social bonding. For this reason, oxytocin administration is being explored as a potential therapy in bvFTD [99].

3.B.ii. Cerebral Influence on the Autonomic Nervous System

Opportunities to influence the autonomic nervous system likely arise even in the earliest steps of appraisal. From the central nucleus of the amygdala, fibers travel to the periacqueductal grey, substantia nigra pars compacta, the parabrachial nucleus, nucleus tractus solitaries, and the dorsal motor nucleus of the vagus, among other critical brainstem nuclei. In addition, the basolateral and ventromedial amygdala communicate with the hypothalamus. Direct stimulation of the basolateral amygdala, and thereby the ventral amygdalofugal pathway, excites the medial hypothalamus. Stimulation of the ventromedial nucleus and stria terminalis inhibits these same neurons. This is likely just one of many ways that the amygdala can, via the hypothalamus, modulate the autonomic and endocrinological pathways that mediate hunger, thirst, and more [100].

The rostral ACC is heavily involved with autonomic control, being connected with autonomic nuclei in the brainstem as well as the hypothalamus [101]. The ACC communicates with the periaqueductal gray, nucleus accumbens, hippocampus and OFC, as well as anterior insula. Area 25 of the ACC, sometimes referred to as infralimbic cortex, has been associated in animal-based stimulation and lesion studies to cause changes in blood pressure and heart rate [102].

The anterior insula also mediates autonomic function [103, 104]. Insular cortex has also been implicated in heart-rate changes, for example with seizures [105]. Gustatory responses terminate in insular cortex [106]. The insula is very closely tied with emotional reactivity, particularly disgust, perhaps due to its interoceptive connections [107]. The behavioral variant of frontotemporal dementia is classically associated with loss of disgust reactions, which has been correlated with anterior insular damage [107]. Furthermore, while some of the dysautonomia classically associated with Lewy body diseases such as Parkinson's is likely peripheral in etiology, some may be centrally mediated and related to Lewy body pathology in the insula as well as early brainstem involvement [108, 109].

3.B.iii. Brainstem Structures

While it's only about as big as your thumb, the brainstem contains nuclei influencing some of the most critical functions for life, including centers for control of blood pressure, heart rate, and digestion. Autonomic pathways descend from brainstem nuclei such as the nucleus solitarius, noradrenergic nuclei, raphe nucleus, and pontomedullary reticular formation. Each of these centers receives descending fibers from the hypothalamus, particularly from the paraventricular nucleus, but also from dorsomedial, lateral and posterior hypothalamus. The fibers initially travel in the medial forebrain bundle, then in the dorsolateral brainstem and periaqueductal gray matter, where the fibers synapse on preganglionic parasympathetic nuclei in the brainstem and intermediate zone of the sacral spinal cord, as well as preganglionic sympathetics in the intermediolateral cell column of the thoracolumbar spinal cord.

The periaqueductal grey (PAG) has been particularly implicated as a rudimentary regulator of autonomic and behavioral responses to emotional events. The PAG is a tube-shaped region of the midbrain involved in survival-related responses and homeostatic regulation. The lateral/dorsolateral PAG produces active-coping responses, increasing heart rate and arterial pressure, with fast-acting nonopioid mediated analgesia. The ventrolateral portion produces passive coping, with freezing behavior, reduced heart rate, and a longer-acting opioid-mediated analgesia. MRI analysis suggests each subregion participates in distinct functional circuitry. Disorders of the PAG have been implicated in anxiety, panic, migraine and chronic pain [110, 111].

3.C. Emotional Expression

The study of emotional expression has a venerable history dating at least to Darwin's "Expression of Emotions in Man and Animals" [24]. Such emotional displays can benefit us by signaling our emotional state to peers—for example, with tears of distress. The displays likely did not evolve for this purpose originally, but were rather adopted from other organismal needs. The snarl of anger, for example, may have originally been a preparation to bite.

Studies of emotional displays have historically emphasized the face, but enormous amounts of information are available through other means as well. The voice, for example, can convey a wide range of emotions even within a single syllable. In addition, we are able to express much through our physical posture and gestures. Inability to express emotions, whether in the face, voice, or body, may have significant social and emotional consequences.

3.C.i. Face

Facial expressions depend on intact musculature and cranial nerves. Nuclei for these nerves primarily reside in the pons and midbrain. Descending fibers come from "face representation areas" in the cortex and limbic region of the brain. Traditionally, cortical control of the face is attributed to Brodmann areas 4 and 6. Lesions of this region predominantly influence lower but not upper facial control, as the pontine subnucleus for control of the upper face receives bilateral input. The locus for control for the upper half of the face has been further explored by Morecraft and colleagues in the rhesus monkey. In addition to the motor strip, premotor cortex, and supplementary motor area, Morecraft identified important regions of rostral (M3) and caudal cingulate (M4) motor cortex as well, both of which receive substantial ipsilateral amygdalar input. Primary motor and premotor cortex innervate contralateral lower face as classically described, with some slight premotor cortical innervation ipsilaterally as well. The SMA and rostral cingulate innervate the upper face somewhat symmetrically. M4 is predominantly involved with the contralateral side involved in snarling and disgust [112-115].

As is often the case in emotion, there have been ongoing debates about hemispheric dominance in facial expression. The right hemisphere has been associated with spontaneous expression of emotion using high speed videography [112], as well as lesion studies [116]. Some have posited that the left hemisphere involves more complex emotions, and the right more basic. Others have suggested that the more important facial axis of emotion may be vertical. This suggests that the upper face more commonly relay true emotional feelings, whereas the mouth can more easily "fake" emotion. The classic example is the Duchenne smile, wherein the eyes crinkle at the edges [15]. A smile without this telltale sign is more likely to be insincere.

In additional to hemispheric debates, another likely source of difference between spontaneous or calculated emotional facial production contrasts subcortical and cortical structures. For example, the basal ganglia are thought to be involved with highly routine motor patterns which occur very quickly. This "low road" of emotional expression may help explain the existence of microexpressions, flashes of emotion which can then be hidden by a more socially desirable response [117]. This may be important in diseases that predominantly impact the subcortical structures. An investigation of spontaneous versus posed facial expression in Parkinson's disease suggested that PD patients were less able to produce spontaneous emotion [118]. That said, it must also remembered that such loss of expression could relate to loss of dopaminergic innervation of cingulate and medial motor areas of the frontal lobe. Regardless of etiology, such diminished spontaneously emotional expressivity has social consequences for those with PD. Inability to convey emotion can negatively impact interpersonal relationships with both friends and caregivers [119, 120], resulting in negative first impressions of people with Parkinson's disease [121].

3.C.ii. Voice

As Charles Darwin mentioned in *Descent of Man*: "Even monkeys express strong feelings in different tones—anger and impatience by low—fear and pain by high notes."

Prosody, the melody of speech, has many different uses and components. Affective prosody includes both emotional prosody (how we feel) and attitudinal prosody (how we feel towards or about something). Sarcasm is an example of attitudinal prosody [122]. These are in contrast to linguistic prosody, which adds more grammatical and semantic meaning to literal words. Examples include the difference between a single word expressed as a statement or question, or the acoustic difference between a white house and the White House. Components of prosody include frequency measures (e.g., pitch), time measures (e.g., rhythm and tempo) and quality measures (e.g., timbre and loudness).

The same debates about primary and blended emotion in facial expression exist for prosodic expression. Debates of lateralization are likely even more heated due to the association between prosody and language, as the lexical component of language is clearly lateralized to the left hemisphere in most people. Initial studies of "dysprosody" suggested an association with the left frontal lobe, but such cases largely consisted of foreign accent syndrome due to stroke or trauma, and impacted linguistic rather than affective prosody [123].

Using examples from stroke patients, Ross and colleagues have demonstrated a relative tendency for people with the syndrome of expressive aprosodia (loss of the ability to express or repeat emotion in the voice with relatively intact comprehension of affective prosody) to have disproportionate damage to the right posterior frontal lobe [124, 125]. Since then, a strong body of literature has been published showing a relative right hemisphere lateralization for affective prosodic processing [126]. Among the neurodegenerative diseases impacting affective prosody, those considered movement disorders such as progressive supranuclear palsy and Parkinson's disease have received the most attention, with some claiming that diagnoses can be facilitated by means of prosodic analysis [127, 128]. It is doubtful, however, that such analyses are specific to affective prosody. Studies investigating expressive prosody in frontotemporal dementia are ongoing.

3.C.iii. Posture and Gesture

Posture and gesture can relay either linguistic or emotional information. Gesture particularly can have a strong linguistic component, and may be an evolutionary predecessor to verbal language. The creation of gestures relates to the study of praxis, the scope of which is beyond this chapter.

That said, most of the literature on posture, gesture and emotion must be inferred from literature on movement generally, except as it relates to emotional understanding of others. For this reason, we will discuss this further later in the chapter.

4. Emotion Recognition

4.A. Understanding Emotions in the Self

The recognition of one's own emotions allows appropriate action or regulation based on that emotion. Inability to fully appreciate one's own emotional experience has been termed alexithymia. Such a condition has been described in a wide range of neurological diseases, including frontotemporal dementia and Parkinson's disease. Both diseases involve neuropathology within several important brain regions of emotion. Alexithymia is also a symptom of certain "psychiatric" disorders such as some forms of autism.

Emotion recognition results at least in part from a process of interoception, that is the ability to recognize such internal sensations as increased heart rate and changes in the gastrointestinal tract. These physiological changes are represented in the posterior insula, relayed through the nucleus of the solitary tract an dparabrachial complex. In addition to direct communication from the amygdala, the posterior insula receives interoceptive information about the body's physiological status, thereby interpreting our own somatic reactions to stimuli [129]. According to a prominent theory of insular function, information is then moved along a gradient towards the anterior insula, where information from the frontal lobes and anterior temporal lobes interact to assigning emotional values to different stimuli [86, 130].

As has been mentioned, the insula interacts with the amygdala and ACC in a network to determine the emotional salience of a stimulus. Berthier and colleagues found the critical location of lesions causing pain asymbolia was the posterior insula, a region which receives the densest amount of amygdalar output [87]. Pain asymbolia is a lack of emotional reactivity to threatening stimuli [37, 131]. When presented with a threat, such patients fail to take defensive measures although they can describe the threat verbally in detail. As the patients still had an autonomic response to threat, it appeared the amygdala had performed an appraisal and was orchestrating an autonomic response, but that a primary output regarding conscious perception-recognition of the stimuli's emotional salience was lost.

Deterioration of the salience network may hinder patients' ability to detect relevant affective cues, monitor their own emotional behavior, respond empathically, and interact appropriately with others [132-136]. Nevertheless, neither the ACC nor insula should necessarily be considered a *sine qua non* of emotional awareness, as even those with extensive lesions in of such areas may still be able to describe emotion, perhaps by relying on alternative neural pathways [137]. Just as there are different levels of understanding, so may there be different types of emotion recognition. For example, it is one thing to know that one's heart rate has increased, another to give it the name "tachycardia, " and yet another to recognize how that increased heart rate fits into one's current social situation. To completely integrate all of these levels of recognition and understanding likely calls on significantly more cortical resources than the insula alone. For example, the left temporal lobe will be involved with the naming of the sensation, and the frontal lobes with placing it in a larger social context. Distinguishing these various degrees and sources of emotional understanding can be difficult.

4.B. Understanding Emotions in Others

If understanding emotions in oneself is so complex, how much more complicated must it be to understand others? In many ways, not much more complicated, as the pathways are often shared. When we really understand another's emotions, we reproduce them to some degree ourselves. For example, we not only blunt our ability to express emotions when we inject Botox into relevant facial muscles -- our experience of another's emotions may also be reduced, though the effect size is likely small [138, 139]. The same neuroanatomy involved with our own emotion recognition is involved with others. For example, the anterior insula, anterior cingulate cortex and amygdala are all frequently activated by emotion recognition tasks [140, 141].

To explore, then, how our ability to appreciate another's emotions may be blunted, we can follow the neural pathways from processing sensory information onward. We can do this for each of the three main ways that emotion is expressed: in the face, voice and body.

4.B.i. Comprehension of Others' Facial Affect

Recognition of facial affect necessarily begins with the visual system. In a sense, this is another form of appraisal—it's just that the stimulus is another human. As a major hub in emotional appraisal, damage to the amygdala has been associated with detecting emotion in others as well as within the self, though the extent of its involvement can be debated [142]. Affective blindsight allows better-than-chance identification of emotional faces even in those who suffer from cortical blindness, likely through an accessory visual pathway [51].

In addition to this rough and very early subcortical appraisal of another's emotions, the cortical visual association areas perform processing in the occipital, parietal and temporal lobes. A region in the fusiform gyrus, predominantly in the right hemisphere, has demonstrated enhanced activation in response to faces [143]. A lesion here will result in prosopagnosia, an inability to recognize a specific face. Some research suggests that cortical emotion recognition also begins in the fusiform gyrus, though the process likely ultimately requires a distributed network involving (not exclusively) the amygdala, medial prefrontal cortex, inferior frontal cortex, and inferior temporal cortex [144, 145]. Much of the research that established the fusiform face area made use of static images, whereas moving images have been found to activate the right superior temporal sulcus instead. The right superior temporal sulcus is involved with recognizing biological movement, such as changes in gaze [146]. There has been some debate about the degree to which this more dynamic processing is separate from the fusiform gyrus [147-149].

Regardless of the stimulus, experiments on facial emotional expression suggest a significant correlation between emotion recognition and the right temporal lobe [150]. Degenerative diseases have also demonstrated the relationship between the right temporal lobe and emotion recognition. One of the most specific examples comes from a rare disorder known as the right temporal variant of bvFTD, sometimes called the right temporal subtype of semantic variant primary progressive aphasia. While technically meeting the definition of bvFTD, this group has several distinguishing features noted by researchers across the world, including a diminished ability to recognize faces generally, as well as facial expressions of emotion [151-153]. The semantic variant is almost always related to abnormal deposits of TAR-DNA binding protein type C, and has also been associated with increased risk of autoimmune disease, making it an appealing target for clinical trials [154].

4.B.ii. Comprehension of Others' Vocal Affect

Based on the work of Ross and colleagues, the right posterior-superior temporal region appears to be the nodal point for comprehension of affective prosody [125]. Predominantly right-hemispheric regions in the auditory cortex in the superior temporal sulcus shows enhanced activity in response to human voices in contrast to other sounds [155]. This information travels to anterior temporal and medial/orbital prefrontal regions, where meaning is layered onto the social cues.

Electrophysiological literature, which is better able to track neural processing in time, supports a three phase process of emotional prosodic perception. There is no debate that sound is initially perceived bilaterally in Heschel's gyri in the superior temporal lobe. The second phase may involve more passive integration with other emotional information. There is some disagreement as to the location of this second phase. Differences in opinion stem from several causes, including imaging parameters used in each particular study [156]. One model suggests it occurs in posterior superior temporal cortex [157]. In fact, the mid-STG and its posterolateral extension have been referred to as the "emotional voice area" [158]. Another model postulates that this passive integration occurs in the anterior superior temporal sulcus [159]. The third phase involves more active and explicit evaluation of emotional processing While authors agree that this process occurs in the inferior frontal cortices, some suggest this only involves the right IFC, while others suggest the process is bilateral. In addition, the processing of emotional stimuli in the brain may follows two pathways, with relatively invariant qualia being processed more temporally, and highly variant information following a more dorsal pathway [160]. While these models also suggest that affective prosody relies on a right-hemisphere predominant processing of slower (suprasegmental) but more extreme frequency changes, most of these data were collected from non-tone languages—evidence from tone languages such as Chinese suggest that affective prosody also relies on rapid (intrasegmental) fluctuations of vocal pitch [161].

Most of the pathways described for prosodic processing thus far have been cortical in nature, but the basal ganglia likely supply a "low road" for processing vocal as well as facial signals of emotion. Some studies have implicated the globus pallidus, caudate, and claustrum.

Although models based on functional imaging have implicated the amygdala in the perception of emotional prosody [162], lesion studies have not confirmed that amygdala damage causes deficits on emotional prosodic perception tasks [163].

Atrophy of the superior temporal sulcus may be seen as part of Alzheimer's disease, and some have posited that patients with Alzheimer's disease experience a diminished ability to detect emotional prosody [164]. Such deficits may correlate with behavioral problems and dementia severity [165]. On the other hand, it is important to consider in such studies that healthy aging is also associated with a strong decline in the ability to detect emotional prosody, even after accounting for hearing loss and age-related cognitive decline [166, 167].

4.B.iii. Comprehension of Others' Postural and Gestural Affect

The whole body can convey emotional expression, with or without facial or prosodic cues [168, 169, 170]. In order to interpret this, our body may covertly simulate the observed behavior. This is also true of vocalizations and facial expressions, but has been most studied in gesture.

Again, when interpreting posture and gesture, we start with the visual system. A region in the lateral occipitotemporal cortex seems to be involved in processing visual stimuli surrounding the human body [171]. As with facial expressions, it is possible that a subcortical route processes this information even before cortex [172]. Certainly amygdala activity influences both how emotional facial and body expressions are processed [173, 174, 175].

This network was first described in macaque monkeys by a group of Italian neurophysiologists at the university of Parma. When a monkey would reach for food, a nerve cell would fire. Interestingly, the same nerve cells would fire when the monkey just watched a human pick up a piece of food. This led to experiments that found such "mirroring" in about ten percent of neurons in the inferior frontal and inferior parietal cortices of monkeys [176]. The advent of fMRI led to similar studies in humans, demonstrating regions of overlap between regions activated by watching those experiencing emotions or performing certain actions, and regions that activate when we undergo those experiences ourselves [177]. This theory was further supported by electrical measurements in humans in 2010 [178].

The significance of this network has been the subject of much speculation. Some have theorized that the network is essential in predicting others' actions or emotions. Some have speculated that disorders of the network may be involved with autism, though this is still being worked out. Others have cautioned, however, that rather than being a specific network for empathy, this neuronal activity may be an extension of more mundane neurological processes and a byproduct of everyday thought.

The inferior frontal gyrus and inferior parietal lobule are both involved in simulating other's emotional expressions as well as other motor movements. Similarly, the anterior insula is activated when seeing someone else experience disgust [141]. This overlap between regions activated by watching another's emotion or action and regions activated by direct experience of an emotion or action is sometimes referred to as shared representations [179], or a human action observation/imitation network. This influences us to automatically and somewhat covertly simulate the actions of people we observe, and may provide a basis for understanding others' intentions. It remains unclear whether these shared representations are critical for empathy or play more of a supportive role.

Recognition of postural and gestural affect has not been well explored in neurological disease. Just as the behavioral variant of FTD has been associated with declines in recognition of emotional facial expression and prosody, so it is with gesture. The comprehension deficit may relate to volume loss in the inferior frontal gyrus [180].

4.B.iv. Pathways Towards Empathy

As social animals, we need to understand and respond appropriately to the feelings of those with whom we interact. Empathy provides a bridge between focus on the self and focus on others. The ability to set aside one's own knowledge and perspective in order to better understand those of another is essential for working within a community. Not only does this allow for better empathic responses, but also it allows a perception of others objectives and to predict their future behavior.

It can be useful to distinguish between cognitive and emotional perspective taking. Cognitive perspective taking means the capacity to consider the thoughts and intentions of others. This is related to the default mode network, which has been posited to be involved with memory and internal processing, and is damaged in Alzheimer's disease [181]. Clinically, Alzheimer's disease can impair cognitive perspective taking, but patients may nevertheless remain quite empathetic with the plight of others [182].

Emotional perspective taking is the ability to empathize with others and know what they are feeling. In frontotemporal dementia, empathy may be lost even though the ability to predict another's intentions remains intact [183, 184]. The medial prefrontal cortex and adjacent paracingulate gyrus plays a role in mediating emotional perspective taking [185]. Our more instinctive and immediate emotional network can be further supplemented or regulated by other empathic abilities, such as taking the emotional perspective or another or regulating emotion to generate an appropriate response. We have attitudes, biases and stereotypes that influence our interpretation and responses to social information. Other cognitive processes facilitate empathy as well, including parietal lobes, dorsolateral prefrontal cortex, and ventrolateral prefrontal cortex [179]. Empathy may be lost in neurodegenerative diseases linked with the right temporal pole, right fusiform gyrus, right subcallosal gyrus, and right caudate, which also highlights areas involved with appraisal and regulation [186].

5. Regulation of Emotion

There are times in which emotion expressions and feelings must be regulated in order to meet social expectations, such as not laughing at a funeral, or suppressing emotional feelings to better perform a task, such as a medical student regulating feelings of disgust during their first autopsy. As regulation cannot be studied well in animals, the neuroanatomical substrate of emotion regulation has only recently been explored with the advent of neuroimaging and similar technology. That said, brain lesions have permitted some study of emotional regulation in humans since the dawn of behavioral neurology, with the misadventure of Phineas Gage and the tamping iron demonstrating the importance of the orbitofrontal cortex in these processes.

When discussing emotional regulation, we must navigate a buffet of different possible regulation strategies. Rather than attempt a comprehensive review of emotional regulation techniques, we will provide a broad overview to demonstrate some of the most important underlying neural networks. This will then allow some discussion of how such networks can be disrupted.

5.A. Emotional Reappraisal

Emotional reappraisal involves an attempt to view the original stimulus in a different manner, thereby removing some of the valence originally assigned to it. There are different methods of reappraisal. For example, in detached reappraisal, an individual focuses on non-emotional aspects of a situation to reduce an emotional response. For example, after the initial shock of seeing a dinosaur attack and try to devour someone, we may remind ourselves that dinosaurs have long been extinct and that we are in fact in a movie theater [187-189]. Or we may focus on the amazing special effects in the movie about man-eating dinosaurs, and muse about the number of artists hired by the studio for this film.

An alternative approach is positive reappraisal, wherein someone attends to positive aspects of a generally negative event. Positive reappraisal maintains focus on the emotional aspects of the situation, and is thought to demand less of executive functions normally reliant on the lateral prefrontal cortex than detached appraisal. Returning to our dinosaur movie, we could shift focus to how hungry the dinosaurs had been, and how we never liked those particular humans anyway.

Reappraisal has been tied to early responses by the dorsolateral and ventrolateral frontal cortices, with decreased subjective experience of emotional experience and decreased response by amygdala and insula, both involved with appraisal and salience. Other brain regions active during reappraisal include the subgenual anterior cingulate cortex and ventromedial prefrontal cortex. Neuroimaging literature has suggested that more active and explicit methods of reappraisal rely more on dorsolateral prefrontal cortex, whereas more implicit and automatic methods rely on structures such as the ACC and orbitofrontal cortex [190]. Within the ACC, cognitive approaches seem to activate the more rostral aspects.

The orbitofrontal cortex (OFC) and the basal ganglia also help us establish, update and reverse attitudes in response to new events. For example, the OFC is critical for the extinction phase of a learned paradigm. For example, repeated re-exposure to a condition that once provoked a fear-response (i.c., a bite from a dog) will allow us to learn that the conditioned stimulus no longer predicts an aversive outcome (we learn that not all dogs bite) [191, 192]. The OFCs role in maintaining or reducing the value of a stimulus extends to foods as well, as the pleasure response to different foods can change once we are sated [193]. Damage to the OFC can lead to fixed paradigms in which a patient cannot reappraise the value of a stimulus when conditions change. For example, in an experiment where patients must change from a type of card deck in which one results in small loss and the other a mixture of large rewards and even more catastrophic losses, these patients are unable to inhibit to drive to choose larger immediate rewards, even as they learn that this is not helpful in the long-run [194].

5.B. Selective Attention

Positive reappraisal or detached reappraisal can be viewed as a form of selective attention—we are only considering part of the stimulus presented to us. Selective attention may take even more obvious forms. For example, we might intentionally look away from the screen or plug our ears when the dinosaurs are chasing the humans. We may opt not to go to these kinds of movies in the first place. In either of these latter cases, rather than reappraising a stimulus per se, we are simply electing to restrict our exposure to the troublesome stimulus.

This shifting of attention according to emotional signals is a primary function of the anterior cingulate cortex (ACC). While we've presented a model in which the dorsal-caudal ACC is more cognitive and ventral-rostral ACC is more affective, both subdivisions do contribute to emotional processing, with dorsal caudal being involved in appraisal and expression and ventral rostral being more limbic regulatory [101]. Brassen and colleagues have correlated the anterior cingulate with such selective attention using functional connectivity [195].

In what has been called aging's "positivity effect," older adults tend to give preferential processing to positive information in memory and attention tasks [196, 197], and older adults may disengage more quickly than young adults from negative experiences [198]. For example, when shown negative or neutral stimuli, older adults tend to look away from negative images [199-201]. Elders tend to recall more positive than negative stimuli in working, short-term, and autobiographical memories [202-204]. The use of such selective attention to avoid of negative stimuli another common emotional regulatory strategy used by elderly adults, which may relate to this positivity effect [190, 195, 205, 206]. The relative preservation of the ACC has been previously connected with the emotion preservation of aging [205], and with the positivity effect in particular [195].

5.C. Emotional Suppression

Emotional suppression permits the full internal sensation of emotion, but tries to reduce the physical expression of that emotion. For example, we may simply force ourselves to sit through a movie that frightens or repulses us, and try not to reveal our discomfort in our facial expression, voice or physical movements.

Studies of emotional suppression have shown increased amygdala activation, consistent with ongoing appraisal despite masking of outward reactions [187]. Visceral reactivity is also heightened with suppression [207-209].

5.D. Disorders of Emotional Regulation

Pseudobulbar affect (PBA), sometimes referred to as involuntary emotion expression disorder, is a classical disorder of emotional regulation, associated with pseudobulbar palsy. The syndrome results in pathological laughing and crying in socially inappropriate situations. Patients with PBA may describe themselves as crying or laughing without feeling a corresponding emotion, or as responding out of proportion to the initial stimulus. The result may be socially embarrassing, e.g., laughing at a funeral.

The anatomy of PBA is thought to relate to descending white matter pathways within the pontomedullary reticular formation, an area associated with other respiratory variations such as hiccupping, coughing, sneezing and yawning. PBA may result as a consequence of several different diseases, including multiple sclerosis, infarctions, and seizure but in neurodegeneration has classically been associated with amyotrophic lateral sclerosis. Olney and colleagues showed funny and sad film clips to people with PBA due to amyotrophic lateral sclerosis, while assessing the patients' subjective emotional experience, facial behavior and autonomic responses [210]. In these subjects, pathological laughing and crying were usually associated with the appropriate subjective emotional experience. The group with PBA were less able to regulate their emotion when instructed to do so compared to controls. It should be noted, however, that previous studies have tied PBA to a wide neural network involving frontal, parietal and brainstem regions, not all of which are likely to be equally impacted by ALS [211]. It is possible that the presence or absence of corresponding subjective experience of emotion would vary depending on lesion location.

While pseudobulbar affect is often described as a disorder of pathological laughter and crying, Olney and all demonstrated that at least among those patients with amyotrophic lateral sclerosis, the subjective emotional experience was also often intact. It is uncertain if this is also true of PBA due to brainstem lesions. ALS is associated with high order cognitive dysfunction in the frontal cortex, a region at which consciousness appears. These cortical regions are also responsible for emotional regulation, which Olney et al. suggest is at the core of ALS-related PBA. On the other hand, deep brain and brainstem lesions may be able to disrupt the pathways of emotional expression without altering the subjective emotional experience of the higher cortices, as there are persistent statements of discordance between emotional experience and emotional expression by many people with PBA. PBA may respond to medical treatment, specifically a mixture of quinidine and dextromethorphan, though other medications such as tricyclic antidepressants and selective serotonin reuptake inhibitors (SSRIs) are also effective.

6. Summary: Emotion Processing, Social Function, and Frontotemporal Dementia

Although this chapter has been subdivided for conceptual clarity, we have frequently reminded the reader that in reality, regions of the brain work together, playing in parallel and in concert with each other and frequently filling similar roles. We have illustrated how neurodegenerative disease can, with some selectivity, isolate different neuronal networks in order to impact one area of emotional functioning, but the reality is not always so discrete. We have touched on bvFTD frequently throughout the chapter to illustrate separate emotional functions, but will now discuss it more in depth to illustrate how a disease specifically targeting frontal networks reduces emotional orchestration into cacophony.

Selective degeneration of the frontal lobes was first described by Czech neuropsychiatrist Arnold Pick in 1892, but remained relatively obscure through much of the 20th century [212, 213]. Within the last few decades, Pick's disease, now called frontotemporal dementia (FTD), has been recognized as the second most common neurodegenerative dementia in patients under the age of 65 [214, 215]. FTD consists of at least three separate clinical syndromes, the most common of which is the behavioral variant (bvFTD) (Figures 6 and 7). The clinical syndrome of bvFTD is associated with a number of different underlying histopathological processes including tauopathies such as Pick's disease (the term now referring to just one particular histopathological pattern) [216], progressive supranuclear palsy, or corticobasal degeneration, but can also be associated with fused in sarcoma (FUS) protein or any of four subytpes of trans-activator regulatory deoxyribonucleic acid (TAR-DNA) binding protein 43 (TDP-43) pathology (Figures 8-13) [217-219].

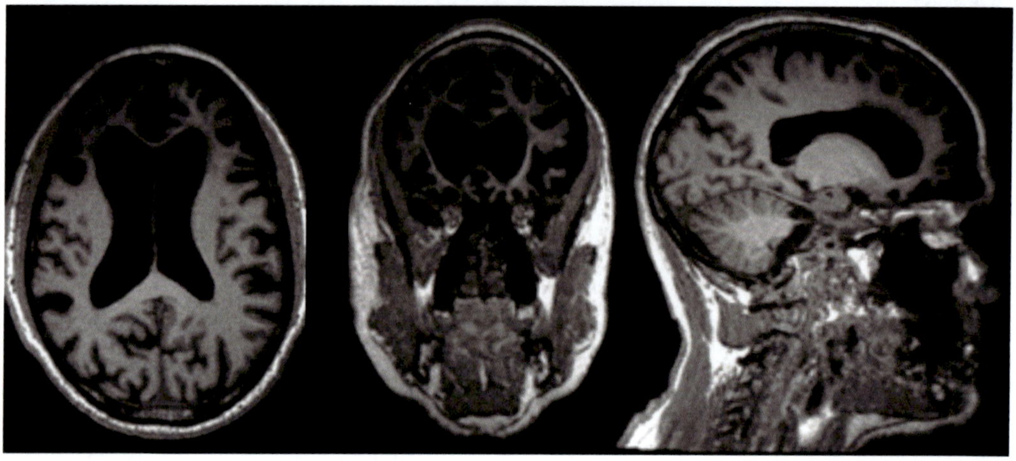

Figure 6. A T1 brain MRI in axial, corona and sagittal planes of a patient with advanced behavioral variant frontotemporal dementia (bvFTD). Shown in neurological convention. Note the severe frontal and anterior temporal atrophy. From Pressman PS, Miller BL. Diagnosis and Management of Behavioral Variant Frontotemporal Dementia. *Biological Psychiatry* 2013.

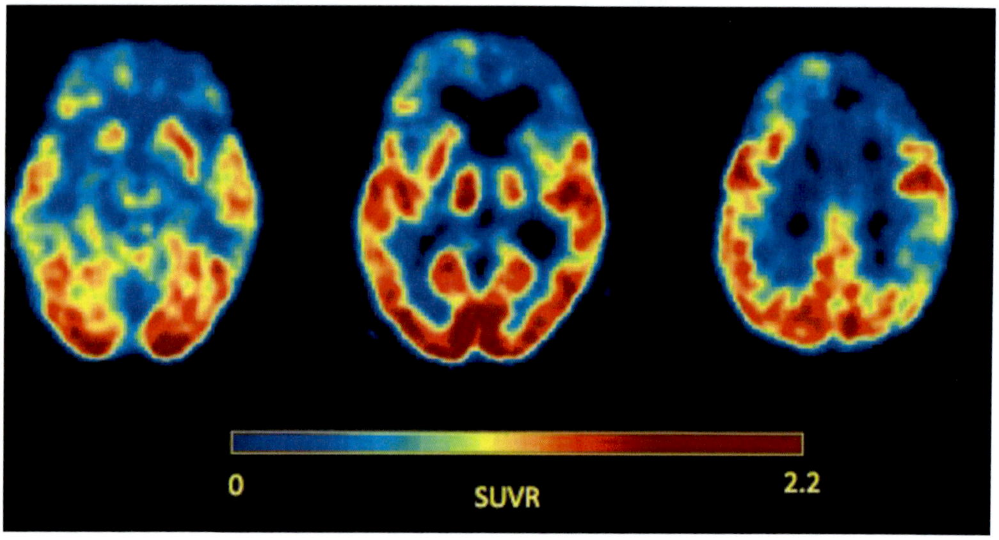

Figure 7. An axial fluorodeoxyglucose positron emission tomography (FDG-PET) of a patient with advanced bvFTD. Shown in neurological convention. Note the decreased metabolism in the bilateral anterior lobes, right more than left. Image courtesy of Pia Ghosh of the UCSF Memory and Aging Center. From Pressman PS, Miller BL. Diagnosis and Management of Behavioral Variant Frontotemporal Dementia. *Biological Psychiatry* 2013.

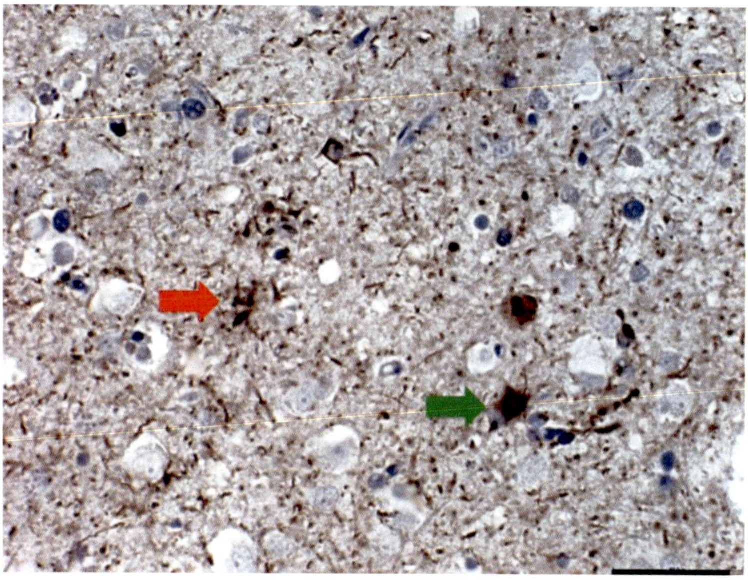

Figure 8. Pick's disease. Immunostaining of the inferior temporal cortex for phospho-tau (CP-13, courtesy of Peter Davis, NY). The red arrow indicates an astrocytic inclusion. The green arrow indicates a Pick body. Scale bar: 50 μm. Slide courtesy of Dr. Lea T. Grinberg, UCSF Memory and Aging Center. From Pressman PS, Miller BL. Diagnosis and Management of Behavioral Variant Frontotemporal Dementia. *Biological Psychiatry* 2013.

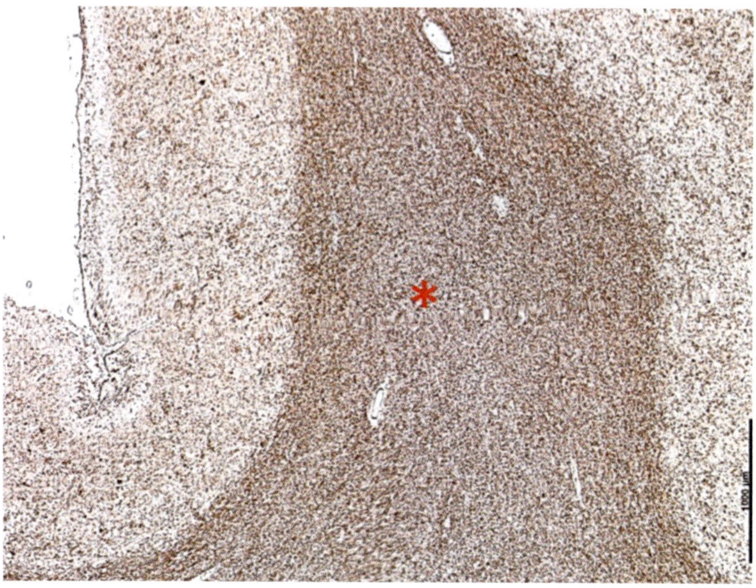

Figure 9. Corticobasal degeneration. Immunostaining of the inferior temporal cortex for phospho-tau (CP-13, courtesy of Peter Davis, NY). The asterisk indicates white matter, where tau density is higher than in gray matter. Scale bar: 1000 μm. Slides courtesy of Dr. Lea T. Grinberg, UCSF Memory and Aging Center. From Pressman PS, Miller BL. Diagnosis and Management of Behavioral Variant Frontotemporal Dementia. *Biological Psychiatry* 2013.

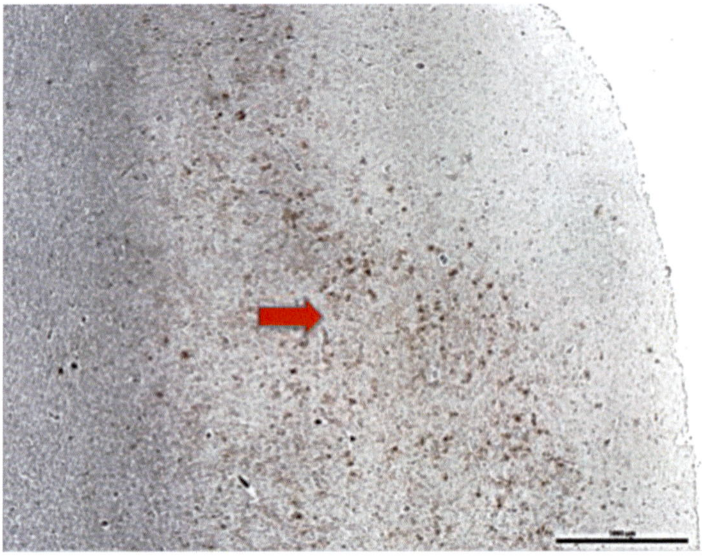

Figure 10. Progressive supranuclear palsy. Immunostaining of inferior frontal cortex for phospho-tau (CP-13, courtesy of Peter Davis, NY). The red arrow indicates a greater number of inclusion bodies (in brown) in the grey matter than white matter. Scale bar: 1000 μm. Slides courtesy of Dr. Lea T. Grinberg, UCSF Memory and Aging Center. From Pressman PS, Miller BL. Diagnosis and Management of Behavioral Variant Frontotemporal Dementia. *Biological Psychiatry* 2013.

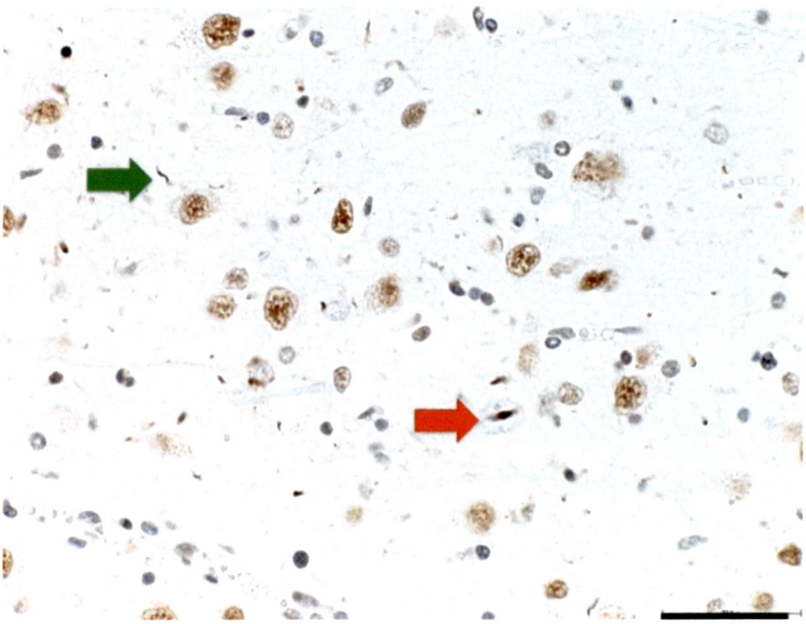

Figure 11. TDP-43 Type A. Immunostaining of inferior temporal cortex for TDP-43 (TDP-43, Proteintech). The red arrow indicates a typical "cat-eye" intranuclear inclusion. The green arrow indicates short neurites (green arrow). Scale bar: 50 μm. Slides courtesy of Dr. Lea T. Grinberg, UCSF Memory and Aging Center. From Pressman PS, Miller BL. Diagnosis and Management of Behavioral Variant Frontotemporal Dementia. *Biological Psychiatry* 2013.

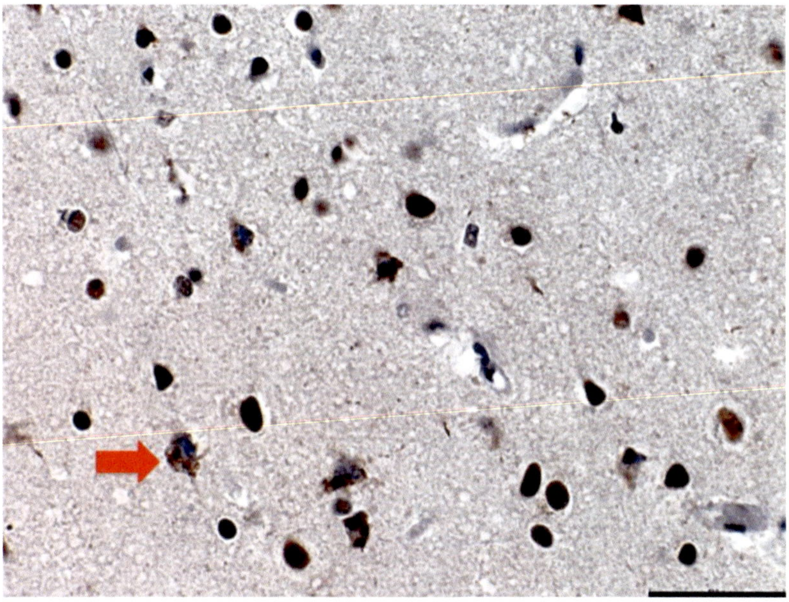

Figure 12. TDP-43 Type B. Immunostaining of inferior temporal cortex for TDP-43 (TDP-43, Proteintech). The red arrow indicates granular neuronal cytoplasmatic inclusions. Scale bar: 50 μm. Slides courtesy of Dr. Lea T. Grinberg, UCSF Memory and Aging Center. From Pressman PS, Miller BL. Diagnosis and Management of Behavioral Variant Frontotemporal Dementia. *Biological Psychiatry* 2013.

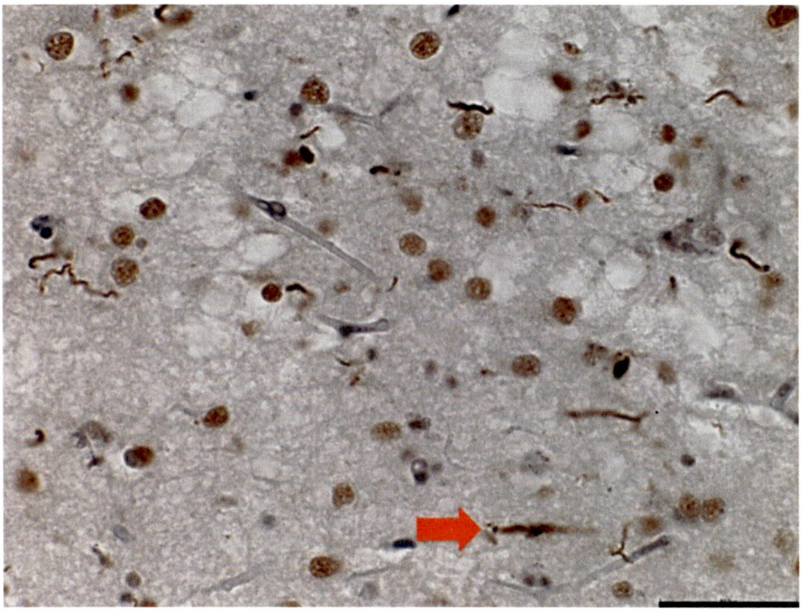

Figure 13. TDP Type C. Immunostaining of inferior temporal cortex for TDP-43 (TDP-43, Proteintech). The red arrow indicates one of many long dystrophic neurites. Scale bar: 50 μm. Slides courtesy of Dr. Lea T. Grinberg, UCSF Memory and Aging Center. From Pressman PS, Miller BL. Diagnosis and Management of Behavioral Variant Frontotemporal Dementia. *Biological Psychiatry* 2013.

Table 1. Behavioral variant frontotemporal dementia (bvFTD), 2011 criteria

Possible (3/6 of a-f)	
a.	Early disinhibition
b.	Early apathy
c.	Early loss of sympathy/empathy
d.	Early perseverative, stereotyped, or compulsive ritualistic behavior
e.	Hyperorality or dietary changes
f.	Neuropsych: Executive/generation deficits with relative sparing of memory and visuospatial
Probable	
a.	Meets criteria for possible bvFTD
b.	Exhibits significant functional decline
c.	Magnetic Resonance Imaging or Positron Emission Tomography consistent with bvFTD
Exclusion	
a.	Deficits better accounted for by other non-degenerative disorders
b.	Behavioral disturbances better accounted for by psychiatric diagnosis.
c.	Biomarkers strongly indicative of AD or other neurodegenerative process.

From Rascovsky et al., *Brain* 2011.

Each of bvFTD's underlying proteinopathies lends itself to further clinical, imaging, and genetic trends (Table 1) [220], but collectively these histopathologies can be identified with 85% sensitivity and 95% specificity using criteria devised by an international consortium in 2011 [221]. (Table 2) While some of these criteria may at first seem quite disparate, each criterion may entirely or at least in part relate to some deficit in emotional functioning described within this chapter.

As mentioned, neurodegeneration includes von Economo neurons within key regions of the salience network, particularly the insula and anterior cingulate cortex [85]. As the salience network atrophies, so to does the patient's ability to predict how their decisions will impact their social milieu. Loss of disgust, due to either insular or frontal network degeneration, can lead to poor hygiene or grooming, as well as behaviors such as flatulence, belching, spitting or more without concern for decorum [107]. In some cases, insular loss may even extend to a diminished capacity to recognize physical discomfort or pain. Degeneration of the orbitofrontal cortex and its appraisal of the potential for punishment and reward further contributes to such thoughtless behavior, as does a loss of emotional regulatory circuitry in the dorsolateral prefrontal cortex.

Both the insula and orbitofrontal cortex normally act together to change our motivation based on our internal states, essentially helping us know when enough is enough. Without such regulation, people with bvFTD can become prone to dietary changes, wherein they may eat impulsively or only eat a stereotypical object. In some cases, patients attempt to eat inedible objects, such as a banana peel in addition to a banana. In this we see further evidence of behavior harkening back to the Kluver-Bucy syndrome. Some of the perseverative and compulsive behaviors that may arise in patients with bvFTD may also result from disruption both in the orbitofrontal reward systems and in a kind of executive dysfunction (reliant on dorsolateral prefrontal cortices) that hinders the ability to "shift set."

Table 2. Clinicopathological Correlations in bvFTD

Pathological Diagnosis	Common Symptoms	Typical Neuroimaging	Common Genetics	Histopathology
Tau: Pick's	"classic" bvFTD, nfvPPA	"knife edge" bifrontal atrophy	MAPT	Pick bodies
Tau: PSP	PSP-syndrome, nfvPPA, depression	midbrain atrophy	MAPT	tufted astrocytes, globose tangles, glial threads
Tau: CBD	CBS among many others	dorsal atrophy near motor strip	MAPT	astrocytic plaques, ballooned achromatic neurons
TDP-43 A	CBS, nfvPPA	dorsal, asymmetric atrophy, frontal, inferior, parietal lobes as well as basal ganglia.	progranulin	many neurocytoplasmic inclusions and short dystrophic neurons in layer 2 of the cortex.
TDP-43 B	FTD-ALS, "psychiatric" symptoms such as delusions and hallucinations	symmetric volume loss in dorsolateral, medial, orbitofrontal, and anterior temporal cortex, cerebellum, thalamus	C9orf72	moderate numbers of neurocytoplasmic inclusions and few dystrophic neurons throughout the cortical layers
TDP-43 C	strong association with svPPA	Anterior temporal lobe atrophy	rarely genetic	few neurocytoplasmic inclusions and numerous long dystrophic neurons
TDP-43 D	strong association with inclusion body myopathy with Paget's disease of bone and FTD	Wide variety, atrophy of frontal and anterior temporal lobes, with prominent callosal and frontal white matter loss.	VCP	many lentiform intranuclear inclusions and many short dystrophic neurons throughout all of the cortical layers
FUS: aFTLD-U	younger age of onset, psychiatric symptoms	symmetric frontal lobe and caudate atrophy	FUS	fused in sarcoma protein deposits
FUS: BIBD	early-onset ALS	symmetric frontal lobe and caudate atrophy	FUS	basophilic inclusion bodies
FUS: NIFID	Parkinsonism	symmetric frontal lobe and caudate atrophy	FUS	neuronal intermediate filament inclusion
CHMP-2B	diffuse impairments in memory, calculation and praxis	Diffuse atrophy	CHMP-2B	Enlarged cortical neuronal vacuoles in the frontal, temporal, parietal and occipital cortices

Legend: An overview of clinicopathological trends in bvFTD. There is significant variation between individuals. aFTLD-U: atypical FTLD with ubiquitin, ALS: amyotrophic lateral sclerosis, BIBD: basophilic inclusion body disease, bvFTD: behavioral variant frontotemporal dementia, C9orf72: chromosome 9 open reading frame 72, CBD: corticobasal degeneration, CBS: corticobasal syndrome, CHMP-2B: chromatin modifying protein 2B, FTD: frontotemporal dementia, FUS: fused in sarcoma, MAPT: microtubule-associated protein tau, NIFID: neuronal intermediate filament inclusion disease, nfvPPA: nonfluent variant primary progressive aphasia, PSP: progressive supranuclear palsy, svPPA: semantic variant primary progressive aphasia, TDP-43: TAR-DNA binding protein 43, VCP: valosin containing protein. From Pressman PS, Miller BL. Diagnosis and Management of Behavioral Variant Frontotemporal Dementia. *Biological Psychiatry* 2013.

The insula is involved not only with recognition of the emotion within the self, but also in others, contributing to socially inappropriate and disinhibited behaviors as well as a loss of empathetic behavior. The ability to read others emotions breaks down with tissue loss in the inferior frontal cortex, and perhaps especially in the right temporal variant of frontotemporal dementia. Both complex social rules and more simple emotional expressions lose their meaning, hindering those with bvFTD from nonverbally checking their behavior against the reactions of their peers.

While at first bvFTD may spare emotional reactivity, however misdirected, ultimately this reactivity begins to fail and is replaced by apathy and inertia as the anterior cingulate cortex atrophies. Paradoxically, this sometimes leads to what appears to be a kind of clinical improvement as the disease progresses, as patients lose the desire to follow through on their poorly regulated emotions and behavior. Ultimately, though, such improvement is superficial, and those with bvFTD will be too apathetic even to leave the bed, at which point they become susceptible to diseases of inactivity such as aspiration pneumonia and pulmonary emboli.

In summary, bvFTD impacts emotion at every level of processing, including appraisal, reactivity, understanding and regulation, with profound consequences for their ability to function in society. Even so, patients with bvFTD may score highly on standardized neuropsychological screens such as the mini-mental status exam, which fail to emphasize executive functioning. Bedside tests of emotion are rarely part of the neuropsychologist's armamentarium, forcing clinicians to rely on careful extraction of clinical history from patients with limited insight, and from caregivers regarding processes that are largely unconscious.

While emotions may have been somewhat overlooked in neuroscientific research, they cannot be ignored by the many who suffer neurological diseases of emotional processing. Many important research questions remain. To what degree are emotions specific vs. coherent? How do emotions lateralize in the brain? How can we teach both patients and caregivers how to better relate in the face of emotional disorders? Recognizing the underlying neuroanatomical correlates can guide understanding not only of the location and nature of neurological disease, but of the design behind some of our most universal and unique qualities as a species.

REFERENCES

[1] Levenson, R., *Human emotion: A functional view, in The nature of emotion: Fundamental questions,* P. Ekman and R. Davidson, Editors. 1994, Oxford: New York. p. 123-126.

[2] Seeley, W.W., et al., Neurodegenerative diseases target large-scale human brain networks. *Neuron,* 2009. **62**(1): p. 42-52.

[3] Polymenidou, M. and D.W. Cleveland, Prion-like spread of protein aggregates in neurodegeneration. *J Exp Med,* 2012. **209**(5): p. 889-93.

[4] Rosen, H.J. and R.W. Levenson, The emotional brain: combining insights from patients and basic science. *Neurocase,* 2009. **15**(3): p. 173-81.

[5] Kunst-Wilson, W.R. and R.B. Zajonc, Affective discrimination of stimuli that cannot be recognized. *Science,* 1980. **207**(4430): p. 557-8.

[6] Murphy, S.T. and R.B. Zajonc, Affect, cognition, and awareness: affective priming with optimal and suboptimal stimulus exposures. *J Pers Soc Psychol,* 1993. **64**(5): p. 723-39.

[7] Ohman, A. and J.J. Soares, On the automatic nature of phobic fear: conditioned electrodermal responses to masked fear-relevant stimuli. *J Abnorm Psychol,* 1993. **102**(1): p. 121-32.

[8] Mesulam, M.-M., *Behavioral Neuroanatomy, in Principles of Behavioral and Cognitive Neurology,* M.-M. Mesulam, Editor. 2000, Oxford: New York. p. 1-120.

[9] Borod, J.C., et al., Right hemisphere specialization for the identification of emotional words and sentences: evidence from stroke patients. *Neuropsychologia,* 1992. **30**(9): p. 827-44.

[10] Borod, J.C., et al., Facial asymmetry during emotional expression: gender, valence, and measurement technique. *Neuropsychologia,* 1998. **36**(11): p. 1209-15.

[11] Gainotti, G., Emotional behavior and hemispheric side of the lesion. *Cortex,* 1972. **8**(1): p. 41-55.

[12] Ley, R.G. and M.P. Bryden, Hemispheric differences in processing emotions and faces. *Brain Lang,* 1979. **7**(1): p. 127-38.

[13] Schwartz, G.E., R.J. Davidson, and F. Maer, Right hemisphere lateralization for emotion in the human brain: interactions with cognition. *Science,* 1975. **190**(4211): p. 286-8.

[14] Suberi, M. and W.F. McKeever, Differential right hemispheric memory storage of emotional and non-emotional faces. *Neuropsychologia,* 1977. **15**(6): p. 757-68.

[15] Ekman, P., R.J. Davidson, and W.V. Friesen, The Duchenne smile: emotional expression and brain physiology. II. *J Pers Soc Psychol, 1990.* **58**(2): p. 342-53.

[16] Jones, N.A. and N.A. Fox, Electroencephalogram asymmetry during emotionally evocative films and its relation to positive and negative affectivity. *Brain Cogn,* 1992. **20**(2): p. 280-99.

[17] Ahern, G.L. and G.E. Schwartz, Differential lateralization for positive versus negative emotion. *Neuropsychologia,* 1979. **17**(6): p. 693-8.

[18] Ahern, G.L. and G.E. Schwartz, Differential lateralization for positive and negative emotion in the human brain: EEG spectral analysis. *Neuropsychologia,* 1985. **23**(6): p. 745-55.

[19] Dimond, S.J., L. Farrington, and P. Johnson, Differing emotional response from right and left hemispheres. *Nature,* 1976. **261**(5562): p. 690-2.

[20] Sackeim, H.A., et al., Hemispheric asymmetry in the expression of positive and negative emotions. Neurologic evidence. *Arch Neurol,* 1982. **39**(4): p. 210-8.

[21] Duerden, E.G., et al., Lateralization of affective processing in the insula. *Neuroimage,* 2013. **78**: p. 159-75.

[22] Ross, E.D., R.W. Homan, and R. Buck, Differential hemispheric lateralization of primary and social emotions - implications for developing a comprehensive neurology for emotions, repression, and the subconscious. *Neuropsychiatry Neuropsychology and Behavioral Neurology,* 1994. **7**(1): p. 1-19.

[23] Sturm, V.E., et al., Damage to left frontal regulatory circuits produces greater positive emotional reactivity in frontotemporal dementia. *Cortex,* 2015. **64**: p. 55-67.

[24] Darwin, C., P. Ekman, and P. Prodger, *The Expression of the Emotions in Man and Animals.* 3 ed. 1998, London: Harper Collins.

[25] Ekman, P. and D. Cordaro, What is Meant by Calling Emotions Basic. *Emotion Review,* 2011. **3**(4): p. 364-370.

[26]Levenson, R., Basic Emotion Questions. *Emotion Review,* 2011. **3**(4): p. 379-386.

[27]LeDoux, J., Rethinking the emotional brain. *Neuron,* 2012. **73**(4): p. 653-76.

[28]Barrett, L.F., et al., The experience of emotion. *Annu Rev Psychol,* 2007. **58**: p. 373-403.

[29]Lindquist, K.A. and L.F. Barrett, A functional architecture of the human brain: emerging insights from the science of emotion. *Trends Cogn Sci,* 2012. **16**(11): p. 533-40.

[30]Lindquist, K.A., et al., The brain basis of emotion: a meta-analytic review. *Behav Brain Sci,* 2012. **35**(3): p. 121-43.

[31]LeDoux, J., The emotional brain, fear, and the amygdala. *Cell Mol Neurobiol,* 2003. **23**(4-5): p. 727-38.

[32]Herry, C., et al., Processing of temporal unpredictability in human and animal amygdala. *J Neurosci,* 2007. **27**(22): p. 5958-66.

[33]Whalen, P.J., The uncertainty of it all. *Trends Cogn Sci,* 2007. **11**(12): p. 499-500.

[34]Lilly, R., et al., The human Klüver-Bucy syndrome. *Neurology,* 1983. **33**(9): p. 1141-1145.

[35]Marlowe, W., E. Mancall, and J. Thomas, Complete Klüver-Bucy syndrome in man. *Cortex,* 1975. **11**(1): p. 53-59.

[36]Johnsrude, I.S., et al., Impaired preference conditioning after anterior temporal lobe resection in humans. *J Neurosci,* 2000. **20**(7): p. 2649-56.

[37]Berthier, M., S. Starkstein, and R. Leiguarda, Asymbolia for pain: a sensory-limbic disconnection syndrome. *Ann Neurol,* 1988. **24**(1): p. 41-9.

[38]Fernando, A.B., J.E. Murray, and A.L. Milton, The amygdala: securing pleasure and avoiding pain. *Front Behav Neurosci,* 2013. **7**: p. 190.

[39]Childress, A.R., et al., Limbic activation during cue-induced cocaine craving. *Am J Psychiatry,* 1999. **156**(1): p. 11-8.

[40]Le Merrer, J., et al., Reward processing by the opioid system in the brain. *Physiol Rev,* 2009. **89**(4): p. 1379-412.

[41]Doron, N.N. and J.E. Ledoux, Organization of projections to the lateral amygdala from auditory and visual areas of the thalamus in the rat. *J Comp Neurol,* 1999. **412**(3): p. 383-409.

[42]Armony, J.L., et al., Stimulus generalization of fear responses: effects of auditory cortex lesions in a computational model and in rats. *Cereb Cortex,* 1997. **7**(2): p. 157-65.

[43]Bauer, R.M., Visual hypoemotionality as a symptom of visual-limbic disconnection in man. *Arch Neurol,* 1982. **39**(11): p. 702-8.

[44]Bagshaw, M.H. and S. Benzies, Multiple measures of the orienting reaction and their dissociation after amygdalectomy in monkeys. *Exp Neurol, 1968.* **20**(2): p. 175-87.

[45]Bagshaw, M.H. and K.H. Pribram, Effect of Amygdalectomy on Transfer of Training in Monkeys. *J Comp Physiol Psychol,* 1965. **59**: p. 118-21.

[46]Lilly, R., et al., The human Kluver-Bucy syndrome. *Neurology,* 1983. **33**(9): p. 1141-5.

[47]Franzen, E.A. and R.E. Myers, Neural control of social behavior: prefrontal and anterior temporal cortex. *Neuropsychologia*, 1973. **11**(2): p. 141-57.

[48]Akert, K., et al., Kluver-Bucy syndrome in monkeys with neocortical ablations of temporal lobe. *Brain,* 1961. **84**: p. 480-98.

[49]Horel, J., E. Keating, and L. Misantone, Partial Kluver-Bucy syndrome produced by destroying temporal neocortex or amygdala. *Brain Research, 1975.* **94**: p. 347-359.

[50]Horel, J.A. and E.G., Keating, Recovery from a partial Kluver-Bucy syndrome in the monkey produced by disconnection. *J Comp Physiol Psychol,* 1972. **79**(1): p. 105-14.

[51]Celeghin, A., B. de Gelder, and M. Tamietto, From affective blindsight to emotional consciousness. *Conscious Cogn,* 2015.

[52]Olds, J. and P. Milner, Positive reinforcement produced by electrical stimulation of septal area and other regions of rat brain. *J Comp Physiol Psychol,* 1954. **47**(6): p. 419-27.

[53]Olds, J., Pleasure centers in the brain. *Scientific American,* 1956. **195**: p. 105-116.

[54]Haber, S.N. and B. Knutson, The reward circuit: linking primate anatomy and human imaging. *Neuropsychopharmacology,* 2010. **35**(1): p. 4-26.

[55]Berridge, K.C. and M.L. Kringelbach, Neuroscience of affect: brain mechanisms of pleasure and displeasure. *Curr Opin Neurobiol,* 2013. **23**(3): p. 294-303.

[56]Scott, T.R. and D.M. Small, The role of the parabrachial nucleus in taste processing and feeding. *Ann N Y Acad Sci,* 2009. **1170**: p. 372-7.

[57]Richard, J.M. and K.C. Berridge, Prefrontal cortex modulates desire and dread generated by nucleus accumbens glutamate disruption. *Biol Psychiatry,* 2013. **73**(4): p. 360-70.

[58]Rapport, L.J., et al., Experienced emotion and affect recognition in adult attention-deficit hyperactivity disorder. *Neuropsychology,* 2002. **16**(1): p. 102-10.

[59]Figee, M., et al., Deep brain stimulation induces striatal dopamine release in obsessive-compulsive disorder. *Biol Psychiatry,* 2014. **75**(8): p. 647-52.

[60]Figee, M., et al., Neurosurgical targets for compulsivity: what can we learn from acquired brain lesions? *Neurosci Biobehav Rev,* 2013. **37**(3): p. 328-39.

[61]Pierce, R.C. and V. Kumaresan, The mesolimbic dopamine system: the final common pathway for the reinforcing effect of drugs of abuse? *Neurosci Biobehav Rev,* 2006. **30**(2): p. 215-38.

[62]Snowden, J.S., et al., Emotion recognition in Huntington's disease and frontotemporal dementia. *Neuropsychologia,* 2008. **46**(11): p. 2638-49.

[63]Henley, S.M., et al., Emotion recognition in Huntington's disease: a systematic review. *Neurosci Biobehav Rev,* 2012. **36**(1): p. 237-53.

[64]Nimmagadda, S.R., et al., Determinants of irritability in Huntington's disease. *Acta Neuropsychiatr,* 2011. **23**(6): p. 309-14.

[65]Rickards, H., et al., Discriminant analysis of Beck Depression Inventory and Hamilton Rating Scale for Depression in Huntington's disease. *J Neuropsychiatry Clin Neurosci,* 2011. **23**(4): p. 399-402.

[66]Rickards, H., et al., Factor analysis of behavioural symptoms in Huntington's disease. *J Neurol Neurosurg Psychiatry,* 2011. **82**(4): p. 411-2.

[67]Hedreen, J.C. and S.E. Folstein, Early loss of neostriatal striosome neurons in Huntington's disease. *J Neuropathol Exp Neurol,* 1995. **54**(1): p. 105-20.

[68]Petersen, A. and S. Gabery, Hypothalamic and Limbic System Changes in Huntington's Disease. *J Huntingtons Dis,* 2012. **1**(1): p. 5-16.

[69]van den Bogaard, S.J., et al., Early atrophy of pallidum and accumbens nucleus in Huntington's disease. *J Neurol,* 2011. **258**(3): p. 412-20.

[70]Lindvall, O., et al., Mesencephalic dopamine neurons projecting to neocortex. *Brain Res,* 1974. **81**(2): p. 325-31.

[71]Mishra, R.K., et al., A dopamine-sensitive adenylate cyclase in anterior limbic cortex and mesolimbic region of primate brain. *Brain Res,* 1975. **96**(2): p. 395-9.

[72]Ross, E.D. and R.M. Stewart, Akinetic mutism from hypothalamic damage: successful treatment with dopamine agonists. *Neurology,* 1981. **31**(11): p. 1435-9.

[73]Blonder, L.X. and J.T. Slevin, Emotional dysfunction in Parkinson's disease. *Behav Neurol,* 2011. **24**(3): p. 201-17.

[74]Lim, S.Y., et al., Dopamine dysregulation syndrome, impulse control disorders and punding after deep brain stimulation surgery for Parkinson's disease. *J Clin Neurosci,* 2009. **16**(9): p. 1148-52.

[75]O'Sullivan, S.S., A.H. Evans, and A.J. Lees, Dopamine dysregulation syndrome: an overview of its epidemiology, mechanisms and management. *CNS Drugs,* 2009. **23**(2): p. 157-70.

[76]Alexander, G.E., M.R. DeLong, and P.L. Strick, Parallel Organization of Functionally Segregated Circuits Linking Basal Ganglia and Cortex. *Annual Reviews in Neuroscience,* 1986. **9**: p. 357-81.

[77]Farb, N.A., H.A. Chapman, and A.K. Anderson, Emotions: form follows function. *Curr Opin Neurobiol,* 2013. **23**(3): p. 393-8.

[78]Keil, A., et al., Early modulation of visual perception by emotional arousal: evidence from steady-state visual evoked brain potentials. *Cogn Affect Behav Neurosci,* 2003. **3**(3): p. 195-206.

[79]Anderson, L. and A.P. Shimamura, Influences of emotion on context memory while viewing film clips. *Am J Psychol,* 2005. **118**(3): p. 323-37.

[80]Morris, J.S., A. Ohman, and R.J. Dolan, Conscious and unconscious emotional learning in the human amygdala. *Nature,* 1998. **393**(6684): p. 467-70.

[81]Anderson, A.K. and E.A. Phelps, Lesions of the human amygdala impair enhanced perception of emotionally salient events. *Nature,* 2001. **411**(6835): p. 305-9.

[82]Davis, M., Neurobiology of fear responses: the role of the amygdala. *J Neuropsychiatry Clin Neurosci,* 1997. **9**(3): p. 382-402.

[83]LeDoux, J., Emotional networks and motor control: a fearful view. *Prog Brain Res,* 1996. **107**: p. 437-46.

[84]McGaugh, J., *Memory and Emotion: The Making of Lasting Memories.* 2003, New York: Columbia University Press.

[85]Seeley, W.W., et al., Dissociable intrinsic connectivity networks for salience processing and executive control. *Journal of Neuroscience,* 2007. **27**(9): p. 2349-56.

[86]Craig, A.D., How do you feel — now? The anterior insula and human awareness. Nature Reviews *Neuroscience,* 2009. **10**: p. 59-70.

[87]Mufson, E.J., M.M. Mesulam, and D.N. Pandya, Insular interconnections with the amygdala in the rhesus monkey. *Neuroscience,* 1981. **6**(7): p. 1231-48.

[88]Medford, N. and H.D. Critchley, Conjoint activity of anterior insular and anterior cingulate cortex: awareness and response. *Brain Struct Funct,* 2010. **214**(5-6): p. 535-49.

[89]Vogt, B.A., Regions and subregions of the cingulate cortex, in Cingulate neurobiology and disease, B.A. Vogt, Editor. 2009, Oxford University Press: UK. p. 3-30.

[90]Vogt, B.A., Pain and emotion interactions in subregions of the cingulate gyrus. *Nat Rev Neurosci,* 2005. **6**(7): p. 533-44.

[91]Mesulam, M.M., A cortical network for directed attention and unilateral neglect. *Ann Neurol,* 1981. **10**(4): p. 309-25.

[92]Bush, G., P. Luu, and M.I. Posner, Cognitive and emotional influences in anterior cingulate cortex. *Trends Cogn Sci, 2000.* **4**(6): p. 215-222.

[93]Vossel, S., J.J. Geng, and G.R. Fink, Dorsal and ventral attention systems: distinct neural circuits but collaborative roles. *Neuroscientist,* 2014. **20**(2): p. 150-9.

[94]Nagaratnam, N., et al., Akinetic mutism following stroke. *J Clin Neurosci,* 2004. **11**(1): p. 25-30.

[95]Seeley, W., et al., Frontal paralimbic network atrophy in very mild behavioral variant frontotemporal dementia *Archives of Neurology,* 2008. **65**(2): p. 249-255.

[96]Sturm, V.E., et al., Role of right pregenual anterior cingulate cortex in self-conscious emotional reactivity. *Soc Cogn Affect Neurosci,* 2013. **8**(4): p. 468-74.

[97]Levenson, R.W., The Autonomic Nervous System and Emotion. *Emotion Review,* 2014. **6**(2): p. 100-112.

[98]Bard, P., A diencephalic mechanism for the expression of rage wtih special reference ot the sympathetic nervous system. *American Journal of Physiology* 1928. **84**: p. 490-515.

[99]Jesso, S., et al., The effects of oxytocin on social cognition and behaviour in frontotemporal dementia. *Brain,* 2011. **134**(Pt 9): p. 2493-501.

[100] Dreifuss, J.J., J.T. Murphy, and P. Gloor, Contrasting effects of two identified amygdaloid efferent pathways on single hypothalamic neurons. *J Neurophysiol,* 1968. **31**(2): p. 237-48.

[101] Etkin, A., T. Egner, and R. Kalisch, Emotional processing in anterior cingulate and medial prefrontal cortex. *Trends Cogn Sci,* 2011. **15**(2): p. 85-93.

[102] Cechetto, D.F., Cortical control of the autonomic nervous system. *Exp Physiol,* 2014. **99**(2): p. 326-31.

[103] Augustine, J.R., Circuitry and functional aspects of the insular lobe in primates including humans. *Brain Res Brain Res Rev,* 1996. **22**(3): p. 229-44.

[104] Cheung, R.T. and V. Hachinski, The insula and cerebrogenic sudden death. *Arch Neurol,* 2000. **57**(12): p. 1685-8.

[105] Tayah, T., et al., Ictal bradycardia and asystole in an adult with a focal left insular lesion. *Clin Neurol Neurosurg,* 2013.

[106] Yamamoto, T., et al., Gustatory responses of cortical neurons in rats. I. Response characteristics. *J Neurophysiol,* 1984. **51**(4): p. 616-35.

[107] Eckart, J.A., et al., Diminished disgust reactivity in behavioral variant frontotemporal dementia. *Neuropsychologia,* 2012. **50**(5): p. 786-90.

[108] Kim, J.B., et al., Autonomic dysfunction according to disease progression in Parkinson's disease. *Parkinsonism Relat Disord,* 2014. **20**(3): p. 303-7.

[109] Braak, H., et al., Staging of brain pathology related to sporadic Parkinson's disease. *Neurobiol Aging,* 2003. **24**(2): p. 197-211.

[110] Amorapanth, P., K. Nader, and J.E. LeDoux, Lesions of periaqueductal gray dissociate-conditioned freezing from conditioned suppression behavior in rats. *Learn Mem,* 1999. **6**(5): p. 491-9.

[111] Satpute, A.B., et al., Identification of discrete functional subregions of the human periaqueductal gray. *Proc Natl Acad Sci U S A,* 2013. **110**(42): p. 17101-6.

[112] Ross, E.D. and V.K. Pulusu, Posed versus spontaneous facial expressions are modulated by opposite cerebral hemispheres. *Cortex,* 2013. **49**(5): p. 1280-91.

[113] Morecraft, R.J., et al., Cortical innervation of the facial nucleus in the non-human primate: a new interpretation of the effects of stroke and related subtotal brain trauma on the muscles of facial expression. *Brain,* 2001. **124**(Pt 1): p. 176-208.

[114] Morecraft, R.J., et al., Amygdala interconnections with the cingulate motor cortex in the rhesus monkey. *J Comp Neurol,* 2007. **500**(1): p. 134-65.

[115] Morecraft, R.J., K.S. Stilwell-Morecraft, and W.R. Rossing, The motor cortex and facial expression: new insights from neuroscience. *Neurologist,* 2004. **10**(5): p. 235-49.

[116] Buck, R. and R.J. Duffy, Nonverbal communication of affect in brain-damaged patients. *Cortex,* 1980. **16**(3): p. 351-62.

[117] Porter, S. and L. ten Brinke, Reading between the lies: Identifying concealed and falsified emotions in universal facial expressions. *Psychological Science,* 2008. **19**(5): p. 508-514.

[118] Smith, M.C., M.K. Smith, and H. Ellgring, Spontaneous and posed facial expression in Parkinson's disease. *J Int Neuropsychol Soc,* 1996. **2**(5): p. 383-91.

[119] Pentland, B., et al., The effects of reduced expression in Parkinson's disease on impression formation by health professionals. *Clinical Rehabilitation,* 1987. **1**(4): p. 307-312.

[120] Pitcairn, T.K., et al., Non-verbal cues in the self-presentation of parkinsonian patients. *Br J Clin Psychol*, 1990. **29 (Pt 2)**: p. 177-84.

[121] Hemmesch, A.R., The detrimental effects of atypical nonverbal behavior on older adults' first impressions of individuals with Parkinson's disease. *Psychol Aging,* 2014. **29**(3): p. 521-7.

[122] Ross, E.D. and M. Monnot, Neurology of affective prosody and its functional-anatomic organization in right hemisphere. *Brain Lang,* 2008. **104**(1): p. 51-74.

[123] Monrad-Krohn, G., 1947. **70**(4): p. 405-415.

[124] Ross, E.D. and M.M. Mesulam, Dominant language functions of the right hemisphere? Prosody and emotional gesturing. *Arch Neurol,* 1979. **36**(3): p. 144-8.

[125] Ross, E.D., *Affective Prosody and the Aprosodias, in Principles of Behavioral and Cognitive Neurology,* M.-M. Mesulam, Editor. 2000, Oxford University Press: New York, New York. p. 316-331.

[126] Witteman, J., V.J. Van Heuven, and N.O. Schiller, Hearing feelings: a quantitative meta-analysis on the neuroimaging literature of emotional prosody perception. *Neuropsychologia*, 2012. **50**(12): p. 2752-63.

[127] Saxena, M., et al., Assessing speech dysfunction using BOLD and acoustic analysis in parkinsonism. Parkinsonism Relat Disord, 2014.

[128] Rusz, J., et al., Quantitative acoustic measurements for characterization of speech and voice disorders in early untreated Parkinson's disease. *J Acoust Soc Am,* 2011. **129**(1): p. 350-67.

[129] Nieuwenhuys, R., The insular cortex: a review. *Prog Brain Res,* 2012. **195**: p. 123-63.

[130] Critchley, H.D., et al., Neural systems supporting interoceptive awareness. *Nat Neurosci*, 2004. **7**(2): p. 189-95.

[131] Ross, E.D., Sensory-specific amnesia and hypoemotionality in humans and monkeys: gateway for developing a hodology of memory. *Cortex,* 2008. **44**(8): p. 1010-22.

[132] Banks, S.J. and S. Weintraub, Neuropsychiatric symptoms in behavioral variant frontotemporal dementia and primary progressive aphasia. *J Geriatr Psychiatry Neurol,* 2008. **21**(2): p. 133-41.

[133] Eslinger, P.J., et al., Metacognitive deficits in frontotemporal dementia. *J Neurol Neurosurg Psychiatry,* 2005. **76**(12): p. 1630-5.

[134] Sorg, C., J. Schlegel, and H. Forstl, [Von Economo neurons and insular cortex - the bridge between soma and psyche]. *Neuropsychiatrie*, 2010. **24**(1): p. 64-6.

[135] Santillo, A.F., C. Nilsson, and E. Englund, Von Economo neurons are selectively targeted in frontotemporal dementia. *Neuropathol Appl Neurobiol,* 2013.

[136] Allman, J.M., et al., The von Economo neurons in the frontoinsular and anterior cingulate cortex. *Ann N Y Acad Sci,* 2011. **1225**: p. 59-71.

[137] Damasio, A., H. Damasio, and D. Tranel, Persistence of feelings and sentience after bilateral damage of the insula. *Cereb Cortex,* 2013. **23**(4): p. 833-46.

[138] Davis, J.I., et al., The Effects of BOTOX Injections on Emotional Experience. *Emotion,* 2010. **10**(3): p. 433-440.

[139] Neal, D.T. and T.L. Chartrand, Embodied Emotion Perception: Amplifying and Dampening Facial Feedback Modulates Emotion Perception Accuracy. *Social Psychological and Personality Science,* 2011. **2**(6): p. 673-678.

[140] Hein, G. and T. Singer, I feel how you feel but not always: the empathic brain and its modulation. *Curr Opin Neurobiol,* 2008. **18**(2): p. 153-8.

[141] Jabbi, M., M. Swart, and C. Keysers, Empathy for positive and negative emotions in the gustatory cortex. *Neuroimage,* 2007. **34**(4): p. 1744-53.

[142] Adolphs, R., et al., Impaired recognition of emotion in facial expressions following bilateral damage to the human amygdala. *Nature,* 1994. **372**(6507): p. 669-72.

[143] Kanwisher, N. and G. Yovel, The fusiform face area: a cortical region specialized for the perception of faces. *Philos Trans R Soc Lond B Biol Sci*, 2006. **361**(1476): p. 2109-28.

[144] Sabatinelli, D., et al., Emotional perception: meta-analyses of face and natural scene processing. *Neuroimage,* 2011. **54**(3): p. 2524-33.

[145] Adolphs, R., Neural systems for recognizing emotion. *Curr Opin Neurobiol,* 2002. **12**(2): p. 169-77.

[146] Puce, A., A. Smith, and T. Allison, Erps evoked by viewing facial movements. *Cogn Neuropsychol,* 2000. **17**(1): p. 221-39.

[147] Richoz, A.R., et al., Reconstructing dynamic mental models of facial expressions in prosopagnosia reveals distinct representations for identity and expression. *Cortex,* 2015. **65**: p. 50-64.

[148] Kawasaki, H., et al., Processing of facial emotion in the human fusiform gyrus. *J Cogn Neurosci,* 2012. **24**(6): p. 1358-70.

[149] Calder, A.J. and A.W. Young, Understanding the recognition of facial identity and facial expression. *Nat Rev Neurosci,* 2005. **6**(8): p. 641-51.

[150] Campanella, F., et al., Impact of brain tumour location on emotion and personality: a voxel-based lesion-symptom mapping study on mentalization processes. *Brain*, 2014. **137**(Pt 9): p. 2532-45.

[151] Ranasinghe, K.G., et al., Clinical characteristics of behavioral-variant frontotemporal dementia across stages of disease severity. in process.

[152] Thompson, S.A., K. Patterson, and J.R. Hodges, Left/right asymmetry of atrophy in semantic dementia: behavioral-cognitive implications. *Neurology,* 2003. **61**(9): p. 1196-203.

[153] Irish, M., J.R. Hodges, and O. Piguet, Right anterior temporal lobe dysfunction underlies theory of mind impairments in semantic dementia. *Brain,* 2014. **137**(Pt 4): p. 1241-53.

[154] Miller, Z., et al., TDP-43 frontotemporal lobar degeneration and autoimmune disease. *Journal of Neurology, Neurosurgery and Psychiatry,* 2013.

[155] Belin, P., Voice processing in human and non-human primates. *Philos Trans R Soc Lond B Biol Sci,* 2006. **361**(1476): p. 2091-107.

[156] Bennett, C.M. and M.B. Miller, How reliable are the results from functional magnetic resonance imaging? *Ann N Y Acad Sci,* 2010. **1191**: p. 133-55.

[157] Bruck, C., B. Kreifelts, and D. Wildgruber, Emotional voices in context: a neurobiological model of multimodal affective information processing. *Phys Life Rev,* 2011. **8**(4): p. 383-403.

[158] Ethofer, T., et al., Emotional voice areas: anatomic location, functional properties, and structural connections revealed by combined fMRI/DTI. *Cereb Cortex,* 2012. **22**(1): p. 191-200.

[159] Kotz, S.A. and S. Paulmann, Emotion, Language, and the Brain. *Language and Linguistics Compass,* 2011. **5**(3): p. 108-125.

[160] Fruhholz, S. and D. Grandjean, Processing of emotional vocalizations in bilateral inferior frontal cortex. *Neurosci Biobehav Rev,* 2013. **37**(10 Pt 2): p. 2847-55.

[161] Edmondson, J.A., et al., The effect of right-brain damage on acoustical measures of affective prosody in taiwanese patients. *Journal of Phonetics,* 1987. **15**(3): p. 219-233.

[162] Paulmann, S., D.V. Ott, and S.A. Kotz, Emotional speech perception unfolding in time: the role of the basal ganglia. *PLoS One,* 2011. **6**(3): p. e17694.

[163] Adolphs, R., D. Tranel, and H. Damasio, Emotion recognition from faces and prosody following temporal lobectomy. *Neuropsychology,* 2001. **15**(3): p. 396-404.

[164] Horley, K., A. Reid, and D. Burnham, Emotional prosody perception and production in dementia of the Alzheimer's type. *J Speech Lang Hear Res,* 2010. **53**(5): p. 1132-46.

[165] J.A. Testa, P.W.W.B., PhD; A.C. Gleason, BA; D.M. Orbelo, BA; E.D. Ross, MD, Impaired affective prosody in AD Relationship to aphasic deficits and emotional behaviors. *Neurology,* 2001. **57**: p. 1474-1481.

[166] Diana M. Orbelo, P., P. Julie A. Testa, and M. Elliott D. Ross, Age-Related Impairments in Comprehending Affective Prosody With Comparison to Brain-Damaged Subjects. *Journal of Geriatric Psychiatry and Neurology,* 2003. **16**(1): p. 44-52.

[167] Diana M. Orbelo, P., et al., Impaired Comprehension of Affective Prosody in Elderly Subjects Is Not Predicted by Age-Related Hearing Loss or Age-Related Cognitive Decline. *Journal of Geriatric Psychiatry and Neurology, 2005.* **18**(1): p. 26-32.

[168] Aviezer, H., Y. Trope, and A. Todorov, Body cues, not facial expressions, discriminate between intense positive and negative emotions. *Science,* 2012. **338**(6111): p. 1225-9.

[169] Aviezer, H., Y. Trope, and A. Todorov, Holistic person processing: faces with bodies tell the whole story. *J Pers Soc Psychol,* 2012. **103**(1): p. 20-37.

[170] Kret, M.E., et al., Perception of face and body expressions using electromyography, pupillometry and gaze measures. *Front Psychol,* 2013. **4**: p. 28.

[171] Downing, P.E., et al., A cortical area selective for visual processing of the human body. *Science,* 2001. **293**(5539): p. 2470-3.

[172] Van den Stock, J., et al., Cortico-subcortical visual, somatosensory, and motor activations for perceiving dynamic whole-body emotional expressions with and without striate cortex (V1). *Proceedings of the National Academy of Sciences of the United States of America,* 2011. **108**(39): p. 16188-16193.

[173] Vuilleumier, P. and S. Schwartz, Emotional facial expressions capture attention. *Neurology,* 2001. **56**(2): p. 153-8.

[174] Zald, D.H., The human amygdala and the emotional evaluation of sensory stimuli. *Brain Res Brain Res Rev,* 2003. **41**(1): p. 88-123.
[175] Peelen, M.V., et al., Emotional modulation of body-selective visual areas. *Soc Cogn Affect Neurosci,* 2007. **2**(4): p. 274-83.
[176] Rizzolatti, G. and L. Craighero, The mirror-neuron system. *Annu Rev Neurosci,* 2004. **27**: p. 169-92.
[177] Iacoboni, M., et al., Cortical mechanisms of human imitation. *Science,* 1999. **286**(5449): p. 2526-8.
[178] Mukamel, R., et al., Single-neuron responses in humans during execution and observation of actions. Curr Biol, 2010. **20**(8): p. 750-6.
[179] Decety, J. and P.L. Jackson, The functional architecture of human empathy. *Behav Cogn Neurosci Rev,* 2004. **3**(2): p. 71-100.
[180] Van den Stock, J., et al., Impaired recognition of body expressions in the behavioral variant of frontotemporal dementia. *Neuropsychologia,* 2015. **75**: p. 496-504.
[181] Greicius, M.D., et al., Default-mode network activity distinguishes Alzheimer's disease from healthy aging: evidence from functional MRI. *Procedures of the National Academy of Science U S A,* 2004. **101**(13): p. 4637-42.
[182] Sturm, V.E., et al., Heightened emotional contagion in mild cognitive impairment and Alzheimer's disease is associated with temporal lobe degeneration. *Proc Natl Acad Sci U S A,* 2013. **110**(24): p. 9944-9.
[183] Fernandez-Duque, D., J.A. Baird, and S.E. Black, False-belief understanding in frontotemporal dementia and Alzheimer's disease. *J Clin Exp Neuropsychol,* 2009. **31**(4): p. 489-97.
[184] Gregory, C., et al., Theory of mind in patients with frontal variant frontotemporal dementia and Alzheimer's disease: theoretical and practical implications. *Brain,* 2002. **125**(Pt 4): p. 752-64.
[185] Hynes, C.A., A.A. Baird, and S.T. Grafton, Differential role of the orbital frontal lobe in emotional versus cognitive perspective-taking. *Neuropsychologia,* 2006. **44**(3): p. 374-83.
[186] Rankin, K.P., et al., Structural anatomy of empathy in neurodegenerative disease. *Brain,* 2006. **129**(Pt 11): p. 2945-56.
[187] Goldin, P.R., et al., The neural bases of emotion regulation: reappraisal and suppression of negative emotion. *Biol Psychiatry,* 2008. **63**(6): p. 577-86.
[188] Gross, J.J. and O.P. John, Individual differences in two emotion regulation processes: implications for affect, relationships, and well-being. *J Pers Soc Psychol,* 2003. **85**(2): p. 348-62.
[189] Ochsner, K.N., et al., For better or for worse: neural systems supporting the cognitive down- and up-regulation of negative emotion. *Neuroimage,* 2004. **23**(2): p. 483-99.
[190] Gyurak, A., J.J. Gross, and A. Etkin, Explicit and implicit emotion regulation: a dual-process framework. *Cogn Emot,* 2011. **25**(3): p. 400-12.
[191] Morgan, M.A., L.M. Romanski, and J.E. LeDoux, Extinction of emotional learning: contribution of medial prefrontal cortex. *Neurosci Lett,* 1993. **163**(1): p. 109-13.
[192] Cardinal, R.N., et al., Emotion and motivation: the role of the amygdala, ventral striatum, and prefrontal cortex. *Neurosci Biobehav Rev,* 2002. **26**(3): p. 321-52.
[193] Ward, J., J. Simner, and V. Auyeung, A comparison of lexical-gustatory and grapheme-colour synaesthesia. *Cogn Neuropsychol,* 2005. **22**(1): p. 28-41.

[194] Bechara, A., et al., Failure to respond autonomically to anticipated future outcomes following damage to prefrontal cortex. *Cereb Cortex,* 1996. **6**(2): p. 215-25.

In: Progressive Cognitive Impairment …
Editor: Gediminas Peter Gliebus
ISBN: 978-1-63485-221-0

Chapter 6

MEMORY DISORDERS IN NEURODEGENERATIVE DISEASES

Gediminas Peter Gliebus*, MD
Drexel Neurosciences Institute
Drexel University College of Medicine, Philadelphia, PA, US

ABSTRACT

The ability to form memories is a process in the brain that is vital for the functioning of humans and other species. Memory enables information and experiences to be registered and later retrieved. This ability relies on many anatomically interconnected brain structures. Genetically programmed but activity-dependent interactions between nerve cells at the molecular level support lasting connectivity at the brain network level. Some brain structures are more involved in the memory registration stage, whereas others are more active during the storage and retrieval stages. Distinctive neurodegenerative conditions have a predilection for specific brain networks; identifying the cognitive impairment pattern thus helps determine the underlying process causing it. Non-degenerative conditions can also affect the same brain networks and should be considered when formulating a differential diagnosis.

CLASSIFICATION

There are several memory classifications. The most widely used classification divides memory into declarative or explicit memory and nondeclarative or implicit memory as demonstrated in Figure 1 [1]. The difference between these two memory types lies in whether consciousness is involved in the learning and retrieval of information. Conscious learning is involved in declarative memory formation but is not involved in nondeclarative memory formation.

* Correspondence to: GGliebus@DrexelMed.edu.

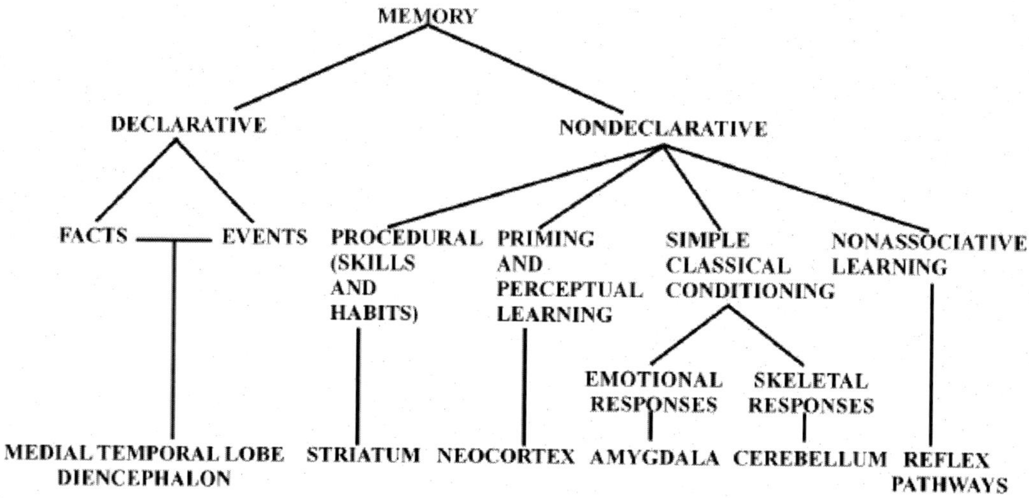

Figure 1. Long-term memory classification. The classification lists brain regions thought to be important in each memory subtype formation. (With permission from Gazzaniga MS, The cognitive Neurosciences III. 2004).

Declarative memory is further classified into episodic and semantic memories, the functions of which rely on the medial temporal lobe structures. Episodic memory is composed of experiences and events that were acquired through multiple sensory modalities. The semantic memory system retains facts.

Nondeclarative memories are more diverse and include a memory system for motor performance (procedural memory), priming, conditioning and non-associative memories. Procedural memory encompasses memories associated with skills and habits. Priming refers to an implicit mental process when exposure to prior stimulus affects the characteristics of perception during subsequent exposures to similar or related stimuli. Conditioning is a learning process during which initially a previously neutral stimulus is paired with a specific reaction-inducing stimulus. Later, the original neutral stimulus upon recurrent presentation can induces the same specific reaction in the absence of secondary stimulus.

A different memory classification takes into account time-dependent factors and broadly divides memory into short- and long-term memories. Sensory memory, such as “iconic” for visual stimuli, “echoic” for auditory stimuli or “haptic” memory for touch, is included in this group. This memory usually lasts only milliseconds after stimulus presentation and is either passed to the short-term memory system or is ignored.

Working memory refers to the system that enables information to be held and manipulated at a conscious level [2]. The term working memory is sometimes used interchangeably with short-term memory. The memories that are registered and recalled after a delay of minutes to hours are called long-term memories. The long-term memories that have been consolidated and stored for months and years become remote memories.

Memory can also be classified according to the events or facts that have been tested in relation to a chosen moment of reference. Retrograde memory is referred to as a memory that was formed prior to the time point of reference (for example, brain injury). Anterograde memory includes memories formed after the chosen time point of reference.

Due to the complexity of memory formation, it is not surprising that multiple brain regions are involved in this process.

Declarative memory function and dysfunction will be the primary focus of this chapter.

Molecular Mechanism

The mechanisms of declarative memory formation have been widely studied. These memories are formed when the connections between the neurons in a given network become stronger. The underlying biochemical mechanism for neuronal connectivity is believed to rely on synaptic plasticity that is based on the long-term potentiation (LTP) process.

Synaptic plasticity refers to both the modification of connection strength between the neurons and synaptic remodeling, what forms the basis of learning. N-methyl-D-aspartate (NMDA) receptors play an important role in LTP. Multiple studies (with some exceptions) demonstrated that blocking NMDA receptors impairs new learning. LTP was initially demonstrated in medial temporal lobe structure neurons [3]. Hippocampal neurons are highly plastic and play a crucial role in learning. The same processes were also demonstrated in cortical neurons.

The changes in gene expression enable synaptic plasticity and reorganization, which facilitate learning [4].

Plasticity enables the connection of multiple senses streaming through different channels from the surrounding environment to form one cohesive experience.

Neuroanatomy and Functional Connectivity of Declarative Memory Formation

Memory is a complex process that involves multiple brain regions and occurs in several steps. The memory formation steps include the acquisition or encoding of new information, retention and consolidation, as well as the subsequent retrieval of information. Different brain regions and neural networks are involved in the various steps, and the limbic system represents the nexus of this process. Limbic system refers to closely interconnected cortical and subcortical structures located in telencephalon and diencephalon. The name originates from Latin word *limbus*, which roughly means "border," referring to inner border of the cortex. The different regions involved in memory function are summarized in Figure 2.

Limbic structures are at the core of the process of transitioning memory from short- to long-term storage. The information processed from the external world (via the heteromodal cortical areas) accesses the limbic structures through the entorhinal cortex, which is located in the parahippocampal gyrus. The entorhinal cortex also receives inputs from the cingulate gyrus via the cingulate bundle. The entorhinal cortex projects to the dentate gyrus via the perforant pathway, which in turn projects to CA3 pyramidal hippocampal cells and further to CA1 pyramidal hippocampal cells. The hippocampus is considered the central structure in the transition of short-term memories to long-term memories. The hippocampal cells have connections with cells in the mamillary nuclei, which project to the anterior thalamic nuclei and back to the hippocampus through cingulate cortical connections. This circuit (hippocampus - mamillary bodies - thalamus - cingulated gyrus - entorhinal cortex - hippocampus) is called the Papez circuit and is important in long-term memory formation

[5, 6]. Limbic structures located in the left hemisphere are more involved in verbally-based memory formation, whereas the structures on the right are more involved in visually-based memory formation [7].

The emotional enhancement of memories depends on a network consisting of amygdaloid nuclear complex (ANC), orbitofrontal cortex and insula [8], with the ANC playing a central role in this process. ANC consists of more than 10 structurally distinguishable nuclei which are located in the anterior medial temporal lobe regions, next to the hippocampal complex. ANC has extensive afferent and efferent connections with multiple brain regions. It receives inputs from all external and internal sensory systems. It primarily (with minor exceptions) connects to cortical regions via ventral amygdalofugal pathway (VAP), and to subcortical regions – via stria terminalis. The VAP connects amygdala to orbitofrontal cortex, prefrontal cortex, anterior cingulate gyrus, olfactory cortex, insula, nucleus accumbens, ventral striatum, hypothalamus and septal regions. The stria terminalis connects the ANC with hypothalamus, thalamus, septal region and contralateral amygdala structures. Amygdala also has direct connections with entorhinal cortex – hippocampus complex. These connections allow amygdala to be involved in combining the factual memory with emotions. In other words, it participates in supplying the color to the picture.

The functioning of the limbic system is crucial not only in the memory storage process but also in information encoding and retrieval, though the latter two processes also involve other brain regions.

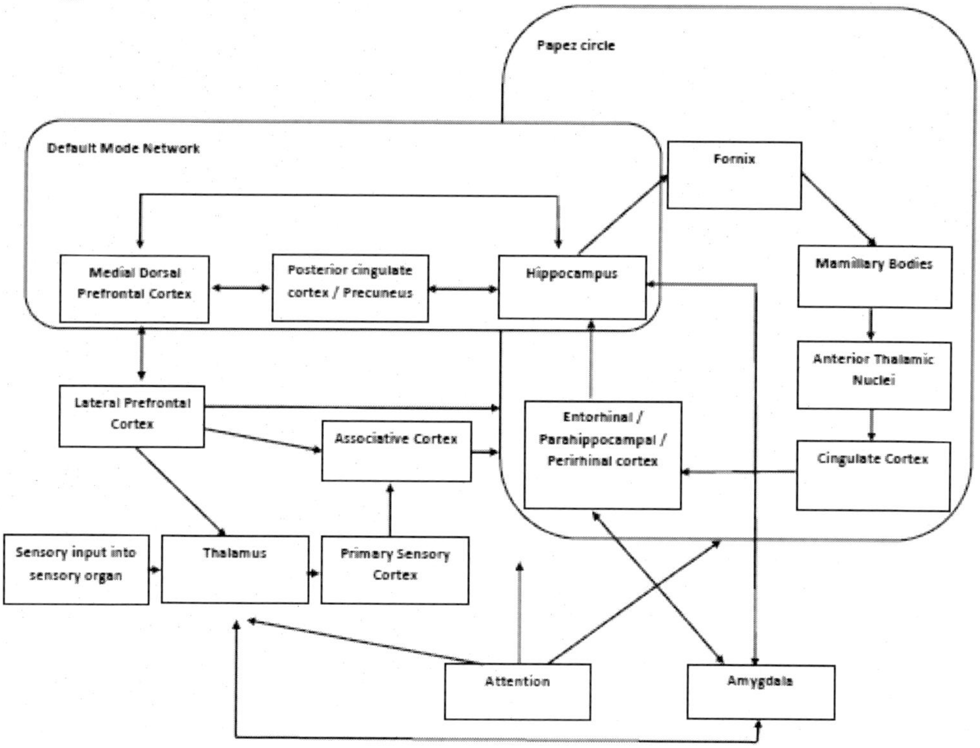

Figure 2. Schematic presentation of brain regions involved in memory function.

The successful encoding (acquisition) process is dependent on the interactions between prefrontal cortex (PFC) and medial temporal lobe structures (MTL) [9, 10]. PFC is involved in working memory and executive control functions. These two functions are important during memory encoding by allowing the target information to stay "active" in consciousness. Studies indicate that left PFC becomes preferentially activated during word encoding, while right PFC - during nonverbal item encoding. The PFC activity increases with increased effort to register information, though its sole activity does not guarantee successful information encoding. The different sub-regions of PFC possibly play a different role during encoding process: ventrolateral PFC is important in directing attention to relevant information and inhibiting irrelevant information (information "selection") [11], while dorsolateral PFC is thought to be involved in information organization [12]. PFC connections with MTL and heteromodal cortical regions allow simultaneous influence on multiple brain regions.

Multiple cortical regions are activated during stimulus processing, for example, object visual features are processed in primary and higher order visual regions, while auditory information – in auditory regions, which later converge in heteromodal cortical areas. These separate brain regions are linked during encoding process by MTL structures. The PFC may modulate MTL activity, which is crucial in the information storage process.

Successful memory retrieval can be viewed as information allocation and reconstruction. The central coordination of conscious retrieval depends on PFC. Lateral PFC demonstrates posterior to anterior gradient with anterior regions participating in higher-level control processes [13]. Successful autobiographical memory retrieval depends on simultaneous activation of brain areas overlapping with the posterior regions of default mode network (DMN) and MTL structures. The DMN is active during autobiographical memory retrieval and internal mental processing, which takes place during restful thinking without external stimulation. The DMN consists of the medial prefrontal cortex, retrosplenial cortex, ventral posterior parietal cortex and medial temporal lobe structures, temporal lobe cortex and certain regions of the lateral parietal cortex. The right anterior prefrontal cortex is activated more than the left during retrieval [14-16]. Successful DMN deactivation was demonstrated to guarantee successful encoding [17]. While central control of retrieval relies on PFC, MTL structures play a crucial role in reconstructing the episode. This is achieved through several back-projection steps activating specific cortical regions believed to store target information [18, 19]. These are the same cortical regions that take part in processing separate features during encoding process. The hippocampus has regional specialization in allocating certain information, for example left anterior hippocampus becomes active during retrieval of verbal information, while right posterior hippocampus – pictorial information [20].

The memory consolidation process guarantees the stabilization of a memory trace. Neurobiologists distinguish between consolidation occurring at the synaptic level and consolidation occurring at the system level. Synaptic consolidation occurs over a few hours and includes structural changes in synapses to establish memory traces, whereas system-level consolidation is slower and changes the overall connection in neuronal networks [21]. Though the timeline and mechanism are not completely clear, many scientists agree that memories become less dependent on the hippocampus during the long-term consolidation process likely due to strengthened cortico-cortical connections, which could take months to years to occur [22]. Memory consolidation is dependent on memory reactivations that occur during active (conscious) or passive (e.g., during sleep) retrieval [23].

An integral part of long-term memory function is adequate short-term (working) memory function, which is the ability to hold information active "on line." Working memory is a part of the central executive control system. The networks involving the frontal, parietal and temporal lobes play a crucial role in working memory. Verbally-based working memory function relies on the left dorsolateral prefrontal cortex connections with the left parietal (supramarginal) regions. Similar connections on the right primarily act as a basis network for visual-spatial working memory, and frontal-temporal connections - for object features such as shape [24, 25]. On the contrary, patients with abnormal limbic system function can have an adequately functioning working memory system [26].

The semantic memory system, a form of declarative memory, supports factual knowledge of the world. The semantic memory system is less anatomically defined than episodic memory. The knowledge of facts is allocated through several regions of the brain. The epicenter of the semantic system is thought to be in the anterior temporal cortex [27].

Certain other brain regions also play an important role in memory function. These include the basal forebrain with its cholinergic projections, such as nucleus basalis of Meynert, substantia innominata, the septal area, and diagonal band of Broca. The cholinergic pathways project to all regions of cerebral cortex and amygdala through discreet white matter tracts [28]. The cholinergic system is involved in enhancing information registration, especially for novel stimuli.

In summary, functionally and anatomically memory system is well connected to both, stimulus-driven (executive, fronto-parietal) and self-referential (default mode network based) systems. This allows both of these main state-dependent systems access past experiences and knowledge.

Memory Evaluation

Many tests are used to evaluate memory function. Memory evaluation can be organized by (1) evaluations for the steps used in declarative memory formation, (2) evaluations of semantic knowledge and (3) tests that are used to evaluate other types of memory.

Memory system functioning is dependent on the more general functions of the brain, such as arousal and attention, and on language and higher visually-based functions. The impairment of any of these functions could adversely affect memory formation and its evaluation.

The memory domain can be tested according to its classification, for example, short-term, long-term and remote memories. More tailored testing can be used to evaluate the retrograde and anterograde components of memories. More detailed testing is required to evaluate verbally- and visually-based memories.

Retrograde memory can be evaluated by asking the person about recent events, current knowledge, autobiographical facts, and knowledge of famous personalities. The examiner has to ensure that the person being tested was at some point aware of the event or subject in question.

Anterograde memory evaluation could be surveyed by asking about the events that took place after the time reference point (for example brain injury). Anterograde memory could also be evaluated when asking a subject to remember a story, words or figures. This testing helps evaluate the ability to encode, store and retrieve new information.

The memory evaluation can be as simple as asking the subject to remember three unrelated words, shapes or object locations and after some period of time asking the subject to recall them. When evaluating long-term memory, it is important to allow sufficient time to pass (usually at least 10 minutes) before inquiring.

The Three Words Three Shapes test is another versatile and easy test that can be used to assess verbal and non-verbal memory [29]. During this test, the subject is provided with three words and three shapes and is asked to copy them on a sheet of paper without any further instructions. Figure 3 demonstrates an example of three words and three shapes taken from original test. The six items are then removed, and the subject is asked to write those 3 words and draw those 3 shapes from memory (incidental recall). If the subject is not able to recall at least 5 items correctly, then the same items are presented again and the subject is asked to memorize them without further copying (effortful encoding). The stimuli are then removed, and the subject is asked to write and draw all of the items that he or she is able to remember. This step could be repeated up to 3 times. A delay of 10 - 15 minutes is allowed, and the subject is asked to write and draw the words and shapes from memory (delayed recall). If some of the items are missing or are incorrect, then the subject is presented with multiple choices of words and shapes (which include the correct words/shapes). The subject is then asked to identify the 3 words and 3 shapes that they were originally asked to remember (recognition).

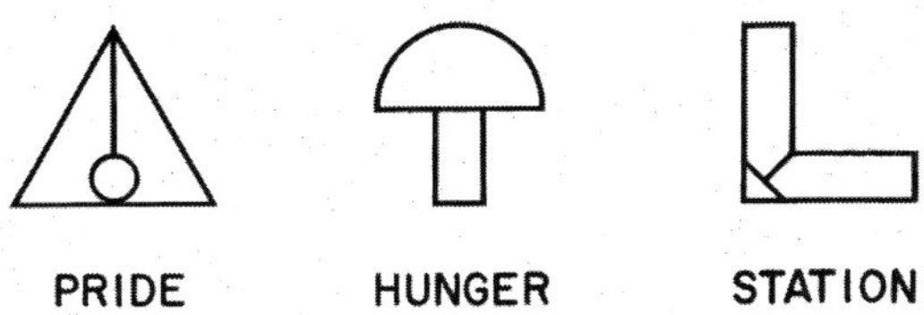

Figure 3.

This test, though seemingly simple, can be used to evaluate several aspects of memory. The inclusion of verbal and nonverbal items enables the evaluation of verbal and nonverbal memory. Immediate (working memory) recall is tested when the subject is asked to present the items immediately after being exposed to them. The ability to register (encode) information is evaluated according to the number of times that the subject must be exposed to the items to register them. The ability to store and retrieve the information is tested when the subject is asked to actively recall the items that the subject was given, and storage is being tested by evaluating recognition ability. One should remember that this test does not replace standardized memory tests used by neuropsychologists.

Neuropsychological tests are designed to assess the integrity of neuroanatomical systems by evaluating the specific steps of the memory process. A detailed overview of these tests is beyond the scope of this chapter. These tests are complex and the following highlights the principles. Working memory can be evaluated using digit span or visual span tests of the Wechsler Intelligence and Memory Scales [30]. A digit span test is generally comprised of forwards, backwards, and sometimes sequential sequencing. For the forward task, a string of numbers of increasing length is read aloud to the subject. The subject is then immediately asked to repeat the numbers back in the same order. Backward and sequential span tasks are similar in that the subject is also provided with strings of numbers of increasing length; however, the subject is directed to repeat the same numbers in reverse sequence or in order from smallest to largest, respectively. The former task requires more passive attention, whereas the latter two involve complex mental tracking and control. Younger individuals will recall approximately seven numbers forwards and six backwards. Expectations differ with age. The average range after 70 years of age is 6 forward and 5 backward. There are also visual span tasks that measure passive attention and active concentration for visually mediated stimuli.

The neuropsychological memory evaluation addresses several aspects of memory, including verbal and nonverbal memory, immediate and delayed recall and recognition. While many different formats capture verbal memory, the tests most commonly used in the context of a neuropsychological assessment typically include both word list learning tasks (California Verbal Learning Test - Second Edition [31], Rey Auditory Verbal Learning Test [32]) and narrative/story memory tasks (WMS-IV logical memory test [30]).

Several memory tests have been created to evaluate nonverbal memory. Some examples include the Rey-Osterrieth Complex Figure Test [33] and the visual reproduction test from the Wechsler Memory Scale [30]. This test indicates memory impairment only if visually-based functions (construction, spatial functions) are preserved. Most frequently used neuropsychological tests for memory evaluation are summarized in Table 1.

As noted, the acquisition of new information is also dependent on several non-memory brain functions, including arousal, alertness, language ability (for verbal information), and visuospatial skills (for nonverbal information). Frontal-executive functions are also essential in encoding and retrieving new memories, both for maintaining focus, as well as organizing the information in a manner that is meaningful and facilitates learning. Cuing and recognition formats are included in several memory tests to help distinguish between storage/retention deficits, which often reflect medial temporal lobe impairment, and retrieval deficits, which may be more related to frontal-subcortical dysfunction.

Table 1. Frequently used neuropsychological tests to assess memory function

Neuropsychological test	Area of evaluation
Wechsler Digit Span and Spatial Span Tasks	Auditory and visual working memory
Wechsler Memory Test – Fourth edition	Verbal and visual working and long term memory
Wide Range Assessment of Memory and Learning – Second edition	Verbal and visual working and long term memory
California Verbal Learning Test – Second edition	Verbal learning and long term memory
Hopkins Verbal Learning Test - Revised	Verbal learning and long term memory
Rey Auditory Verbal Learning Test	Verbal learning and long term memory
Benton Visual Retention Test	Visual long term memory
Rey – Osterrieth Complex FigureTest	Visual long term memory
Brief Visuospatial Memory Test - Revised	Visual learning and long term memory
Recognition Memory Test	Verbal and visual delayed recognition/long term memory

Memory Impairment

In general terms, memory impairment is called amnesia (from the Greek word *αμνησία* meaning "without memory").

Forgetfulness is likely the most frequent complaint encountered in cognitive neurology clinics. When referring to forgetfulness, patients most frequently refer to episodic memory impairment.

When evaluating a patient with forgetfulness, it is important to determine which processing stage(s) are involved in causing clinically palpable memory impairment. The simplified approach for this involves dividing the process into memory formation stages. Forgetfulness could be due to working memory (short-term memory), encoding, retention or retrieval deficits. It is important to understand that this separation is not absolute in the majority of cases, and patients frequently have impairment in several or all of these steps. This is explained by the understanding of memory formation process and the structures that are involved. While the declarative memory epicenter consists of limbic system structures, intact interactions between the limbic system, prefrontal and parietal cortices guarantee adequate memory functionality.

Amnesia can also be classified as anterograde or retrograde. Anterograde amnesia refers to memory impairment, which presents with difficulty forming new memories. Anterograde amnesia could present with impaired encoding, retention and retrieval. Retrograde amnesia refers to the deficient recall of past events that occurred prior to the event of reference (head injury, the beginning of the disease, etc.). Retrograde amnesia refers to faulty retrieval either due to the damaged retention of previously acquired memories or faulty retrieval mechanism. Retrograde amnesia is not uniform for all past events and frequently has a temporal gradient. A temporal gradient refers to a time span at which the events are defectively recalled and is a reflection of the consolidation process. More recent memories are more easily forgotten than memories formed earlier.

The sub-classification of amnesia into anterograde and retrograde forms is based on the point of reference (event) and not on the underlying biological systems damaged; thus, both types could be present in the same patient. For example, patients with limbic system damage demonstrate deficiencies in new memory formation (anterograde amnesia) and deficiencies in recalling episodic events prior to the event of reference (retrograde amnesia). Anterograde amnesia can occur without retrograde amnesia in some patients (for example a patient who presents with transient global amnesia).

One should remember that in a very simplified way, memory encoding and retrieval depend on optimal functioning of the limbic system, prefrontal and parietal cortices, and the interactions between these structures. Certain regions of these structures are active during encoding, deactivated during retrieval, and vise versa. The retention stage is primarily dependent on the optimal functioning of limbic system structures.

To simplify the practical approach to declarative amnesia, we will classify it into two groups: amnesia that primarily presents with faulty retention and amnesia that results from inadequate memory encoding or retrieval. This is an artificial classification; it is rarely absolute and in clinical contexts should be used only as a guideline.

IMPAIRED MEMORY RETENTION

The effective retention of information is primarily dependent on intact limbic system structures and the interactions between them. The structures, which are important in declarative information retention, include the hippocampi with surrounding parahippocampal cortical regions, fornix, mamillary bodies, anterior and mediodorsal thalamic nuclei and cingulate cortex.

Impaired retention can be recognized during testing by the rapid decay of new information after ensuring that the information was (at least partially) encoded.

There are multiple etiologies for retention deficits. These etiologies vary from focal lesions in the above specific areas to progressive pathologies that tend to develop in these areas.

The causes of this syndrome include:

1. *Alzheimer's disease.* Alzheimer's disease (AD) is the most prevalent age-related neurodegenerative condition. The majority of cases occur after age 65.

   Typical AD presents with progressive amnestic syndrome. Histopathologically, AD is characterized by extracellular fibrillary amyloid deposition and intraneuronal neurofibrillary tangle (NFT) aggregation. NFTs are formed from abnormally hyperphosphorylated microtubule-associated tau protein. The abnormally hyperphosphorylated tau causes microtubule aggregation into neurofibrillary tangles, which inhibits intracellular microtubule function and thus cell functioning in general, thereby resulting in degeneration [34].

   These two histological disease markers initially occur in different brain regions. Fibrillary amyloid initially deposits in the posterior cingulate cortex and precuneus, which are areas that overlap with the posterior regions of the human DMN [35]. Neuropathological studies demonstrated that NFTs are found in subcortical nuclei before its cortical appearance, including basal nucleus of Meynart and other cholinergic nuclei responsible for cholinergic deficiency [36]. The cortical NFTs initially aggregate in the neurons of medial temporal lobe structures, specifically in entorhinal cortex and hippocampal neurons [37].

   There are several methods to clinically evaluate fibrillary amyloid deposition. A direct evaluation can be performed using amyloid positron emission tomography (PET) imaging. The specificity of this study decreases with age due to the fact that some older asymptomatic individuals can harbor amyloid plaques [38]. Studies have also determined that when fibrillary amyloid deposition occurs, the soluble amyloid (amyloid β 42) concentration in the cerebrospinal fluid (CSF) diminishes [39]. The decrease in the CSF concentration of amyloid β 42 is thought to occur due to its diminished clearance from the brain into the CSF. The concentration of amyloid β 42 in CSF cannot be solely used for diagnosis and is used in combination with other biomarkers. The existing amyloid burden does not correlate with cognitive impairment level, although it is a predictor of future cognitive decline [40].

   There is currently no clinically validated method to demonstrate *in vivo* NFT accumulation. Intracellular NFT aggregation causes cell death, which could be indirectly evaluated using structural and functional imaging studies. The usual atrophy pattern observed via structural imaging (such as magnetic resonance imaging (MRI) or computed tomography) in AD demonstrates generalized brain atrophy including MTL structures (see Figure 4), and can be evaluated with volumetric analysis. The neurodegeneration level correlates with memory dysfunction in AD [40]. Volumetric analysis can be semi-quantitative (visual rating), or quantitative (automated). The MTL subcomponent analysis demonstrated that volumes of entorhinal cortex were better predictors of future cognitive decline than hippocampal volumes, though hippocampus and amygdale were affected as disease progressed [41, 42]. The studies also demonstrated that patients with AD have thinner cortex in the bilateral frontal, parietal, temporal and occipital lobes; cognitive performance negatively correlates with cortical thickness of the frontal, temporal and parietal lobes [43]. Measurements of cortical thickness require further validation and cannot yet be used in clinical practice.

The total and phosphorylated tau (at 181 phosphorylation site) levels in the CSF are elevated in patients with AD and can be measured for disease confirmation [44]. The total tau level is believed to be a marker of nerve cell death. It is highly sensitive but not very specific marker for AD. The levels of phosphorylated tau reflect NFTs, and is a more specific marker of an underlying Alzheimer-type pathology.

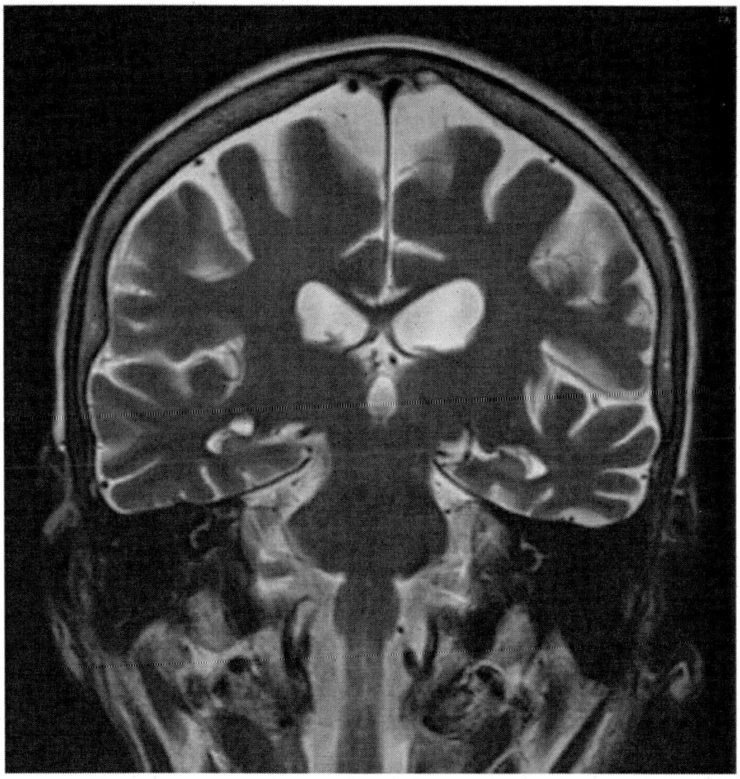

Figure 4. MRI T2 Coronal section of 68 year old female with progressive amnestic+ cognitive impairment demonstrating CSF biomarker profile compatible with AD: ATI of 0.32, Ab 42 397.4 pg/ml, P-tau 102.8 pg/ml.

Synaptic dysfunction and loss are associated with cognitive impairment in AD [45]. This change can be detected in a clinical setting using fludeoxyglucose positron emission tomography (FDG-PET) imaging to evaluate glucose metabolism as a proxy of neuronal and synaptic function. Diminished glucose metabolism in the medial parietal and lateral parietal-temporal regions is initially observed in patients with AD. FDG-PET scan carries sensitivity of over 90% and specificity of over 70% in diagnosing AD [46]. Similar findings were discovered using single-photon emission computed tomography (SPECT), which assesses changes in regional blood flow reflecting diminished metabolic demands in those regions [47]. Initial functional changes (changes in blood flow) can also be detected in the posterior regions of the DMN using arterial spin labeling imaging [48]. This functional change is due to the loss of connections (deafferentation) between the limbic structures, DMN and temporal-parietal associative cortices. The hypometabolism of the regions increases as the disease progresses. Tests evaluating direct connectivity (diffusion tensor imaging and functional magnetic resonance imaging) have not been validated for use in clinical practice; notably, data from studies on these methods increasingly demonstrate a similar deafferentation pattern.

There are also genetic AD markers. Autosomal dominant AD constitutes less than 1% of all the cases. There are 3 genes implicated in developing disease: Presenilin 1 (located on chromosome 14), Presenilin 2 (located on chromosome 1) and amyloid precursor protein (located on chromosome 21). Random search for these mutations is discouraged in clinical practice, and should be reserved for the patients with strong family history of younger onset progressive cognitive disorder.

2. *Suspected non-Alzheimer's pathophysiology* involves patients whose clinical presentation is similar to those of AD (progressive amnestic cognitive decline, similar neurodegeneration patterns on structural imaging involving medial temporal lobe structures or on functional (FDG-PET) imaging) but do not demonstrate amyloid deposition via *in-vivo* amyloid imaging [49]. This group of diseases includes pathological entities such as medial temporal tauopathy without amyloidosis, late-onset hippocampal sclerosis, argyrophilic grain disease, or other conditions that could affect these regions (vascular disease, Lewy body pathology). All of these conditions have distinct pathological abnormalities; however, it is not yet possible to clinically distinguish these pathologies using currently approved imaging techniques or biochemical analyses.
    - Medial temporal tauopathy without amyloidosis (sometimes also referred to as primary age related tauopathy). This condition is histopathologically characterized by the presence of neurofibrillary tangles in the medial temporal lobe structures, basal forebrain, brainstem and olfactory areas and the absence of fibrillary amyloid plaques. Clinical presentations in post-mortem confirmed cases varied from having no symptoms to having profound amnestic syndrome [50].
    - Late-onset hippocampal sclerosis. This condition should not be confused with hippocampal sclerosis, which typically presents with partial seizures in younger patients and demonstrates FLAIR/T2 signal abnormalities in hippocampal regions on brain MRI imaging. Late-onset hippocampal sclerosis usually presents as a progressive amnestic disorder without seizures. Late-onset

hippocampal sclerosis can be definitively diagnosed during autopsy (or biopsy, if performed) upon finding neuronal loss and gliosis in the CA1 and subiculum sections of the hippocampus, and in 85% of cases there is associated medial temporal TDP-43 deposition [51, 52]. Clinically, this condition usually cannot be distinguished from typical AD.

- Argyrophilic grain disease. This condition is frequently found in association with other neurodegenerative conditions (such as the 4-repeat tauopathies FTLD-tau (CBD) and FTLD-tau (PSP), AD, dementia with Lewy bodies and others); this raises the question of it being a truly separate disease entity. Some autopsy results have reported a predominance of this pathology. Clinically, this condition presents with a progressive amnestic disorder that is frequently associated with behavioral and neuropsychiatric symptoms but it occurs with similar frequency in elderly individuals with and without dementia [53]. Histopathologically, this condition is characterized by argyrophilic grains in the transentorhinal and entorhinal cortex, CA1 area of the hippocampus, amygdala, temporal lobe cortex and other regions of the brain, cytoplasmic tau in hippocampal dentate gyrus granular neurons, and coiled bodies are frequently found in oligodendrocytes [54].

3. *Vascular cognitive impairment.* Amnestic syndrome due to acute vascular impairment, such as ischemic stroke or hemorrhage, usually has an abrupt onset, which differentiates it from progressive conditions. Vascular cognitive impairment could present with amnestic syndrome with pronounced retention deficit if there is a vascular lesion in the limbic structures. There have been few reports of significant amnestic syndromes occurring after ischemic strokes in the regions supplied by the paramedian or polar thalamic arteries [55]. The polar thalamic artery also produces symptoms of dysphagia, hemineglect and visuospatial disturbance. Various diencephalic infarcts could cause amnestic syndrome. More pronounced deficits are observed in bilateral lesions. Verbal memory could be affected if the lesion is on the left, whereas the lesions on the right could affect more visually-based functions [56]. The sudden disruption of blood supply to the hippocampi due to the occlusion of posterior cerebral artery can produce a similar amnestic syndrome [57, 58]. This type of infarction also usually presents with visual field deficits. Vascular cognitive impairment, which is referred to as microvascular ischemic brain disease, will be discussed in more detail in later sections of this chapter.
4. *Other neurodegenerative disorders.* Many other neurodegenerative disorders can present with amnestic syndromes; however, amnesia is often not the most salient feature of the syndrome. Any progressive neurodegenerative disease involves multiple cognitive domains including memory. These diseases include but are not limited to frontotemporal dementia, Lewy body disease, corticobasal syndrome and others.
5. *Thiamine deficiency.* Thiamine deficiency has been long known to cause amnestic syndrome. Typical amnestic syndrome due to thiamine deficiency is called Korsakoff syndrome. Classic symptoms of Korsakoff syndrome consist of anterograde and retrograde amnesia, disorientation and confabulations. These patients display difficulties with declarative memory and event temporal order. The regions implicated in Korsakoff syndrome include anterior (and mediodorsal) thalamic nuclei

and mamillary bodies, which affect the diencephalic - hippocampal circuits [59]. Frontal lobe damage also contributes to the cognitive impairment associated with this syndrome [60]. Usually, Korsakoff amnestic syndrome is preceded by Wernicke's encephalopathy, which presents with abrupt-onset confusion associated with occulomotor impairment and cerebellar dysfunction. If this condition is not promptly treated with thiamine supplementation, when the acute stage passes, patients are usually left with structural brain damage in previously mentioned brain regions that results in significant amnestic disorder. This syndrome was initially described in chronically malnourished alcoholics, though any patient population with malnutrition could develop it, including patients with advanced cancer, gastrointestinal diseases affecting absorption, anorexia nervosa and others.

6. *Traumatic brain injury.* Traumatic brain injury can cause disconnection within and between brain networks secondary to diffuse axonal injury or focal injuries, both of which may affect memory. The focal lesions occurring in the limbic system may cause retention deficits, as was previously demonstrated after traumatic fornix damage or injury/hemorrhage in other associated regions such as the mediodorsal thalamus [61, 62]. Diffuse axonal injuries are discussed in more detail in the paragraphs on memory encoding and retrieval deficits.
7. *Hypoxic brain injury.* Generalized hypoxic brain injury occurs when blood flow or the oxygen supply falls below the threshold required to support neuronal metabolism. All nerve cells are affected by a lack of oxygen. Hippocampal pyramidal CA1 cells are among the most sensitive to a lack of oxygen and could be irreversibly damaged after 3 to 5 minutes of ischemia [63]. This circumscribed injury can cause significant amnestic syndrome.
8. *Inflammatory or infectious limbic encephalitis.* Several infectious and inflammatory conditions cause prominent amnestic syndrome. These include encephalitidis with a predilection for limbic structures. The most widely known and encountered limbic encephalitis is caused by Herpes simplex - 1 virus (HSV-1), which has an affinity for limbic system structures and causes pronounced amnesia and global cognitive impairment.

   Limbic encephalitis due to immune-mediated mechanisms could be paraneoplastic or idiopathic autoimmune. Both types are immune-mediated; however, the underlying pathogenetic mechanism differs. Autoimmune idiopathic encephalitis more frequently develops as an immune reaction to cell surface antigens. This type has a more favorable prognosis and is more responsive to immunosuppressive treatment [64]. Paraneoplastic encephalitis usually develops against intracellular antigens, inducing brain cell and tissue destruction with a poorer outcome and poorer response to treatment. Paraneoplastic encephalitis can be observed in cases of small cell lung, testicular and breast cancers, ovarian teratoma and thymoma. Certain specific antibodies are found in the serum and CSF of these patients and are directed against different cellular targets. These antibodies include anti-Hu, anti-CV2, PCA-2, ANNA-3, anti-amphiphysin, anti-VGKC, anti-VGCC, anti-Zic4, anti-GluR, anti-GABAR, anti-AMPAR, anti-GAD, anti-Ri, anti-Ma2, anti-GluR1/2 and anti-NMDAR [65]. Patients can be diagnosed with limbic encephalitis upon finding elevated inflammatory markers in the blood or elevated CSF white cell counts and protein levels. It can be difficult to distinguish between infectious and inflammatory encephalitis; however, specific infectious and immunological assessments can be used to distinguish between them, for example detecting HSV-1 genetic material in the CSF in cases involving herpes encephalitis, as well as specific autoimmune antibodies in cases involving autoimmune encephalitidis. In general, limbic encephalitis does not present with an isolated amnestic syndrome; it is usually accompanied by general cognitive decline, personality changes, psychiatric symptoms and seizures. The symptoms in these conditions usually develop fairly abruptly, which is a feature that distinguishes limbic encephalitis from slowly progressing neurodegenerative conditions.

9. *Space-occupying lesions*, including tumors, inflammatory or infectious lesions, cause amnestic syndrome with impaired retention if located in any of the limbic structures or associated regions.
10. *Transient global amnesia*. Transient global amnesia (TGA) is a pathological condition during which the patient is unable to form new declarative memories. TGA usually resolves in 24 hours. This condition usually develops in the elderly and can be recurrent [66]. The syndrome should not have any other accompanying neurological symptoms. The etiology of this syndrome is still not completely known. Several theories have been put forth to explain this syndrome. The theories range from focal transient hippocampal hypoperfusion to functional dysregulation in memory areas. Functional imaging, including positron emission tomography and single-photon emission tomography, scan demonstrated diminished metabolism and perfusion in the temporal lobe, diencephalic structures and cortex [67-69]. No specific intervention is necessary during the episode of TGA.

IMPAIRED MEMORY ENCODING AND RETRIEVAL

Memory encoding refers to the brain's ability to incorporate an information trace in neuronal networks, whereas retrieval refers to the ability to allocate correct information after it was successfully stored.

Encoding comprises the initial steps of the memory formation process, and intact encoding is crucial in determining whether the episode will be registered. As discussed earlier in this chapter, the activation of the prefrontal cortex and limbic system structures is necessary for successful encoding. The malfunction of either of these structures affects this memory formation step. Data from functional imaging studies demonstrate that executive control of episode encoding process is more lateralized to left prefrontal cortex [70].

The episode retrieval process involves the recall (reconstruction) of past experiences. Data demonstrates that the lateral prefrontal cortex and regions coinciding with DMN are activated during the retrieval process. On a functional level, it remains unclear if and how the lateral and medial prefrontal cortices play different roles in the retrieval process.

Any pathology affecting the limbic system and its associated structures could affect encoding, retrieval and retention.

The pathological processes that could affect successful encoding and retrieval include the following:

1. *Alzheimer's disease.* AD is characterized by the deficient retention and encoding/retrieval of information.
2. *Lewy Body spectrum disorders.* Lewy body spectrum disorders include Parkinson's disease with or without dementia, as well as dementia with Lewy bodies (DLB). Following AD, these disorders constitute the second most common cause of neurodegenerative cognitive diseases. There is an overlap in the underlying histopathology and clinical presentation of both of these diseases, and the clinical distinction is frequently based solely on the timing of occurrence of motor and cognitive symptoms. DLB is diagnosed when cognitive symptoms occur in conjunction with or prior to motor symptoms. Parkinson's disease dementia begins with motor symptoms occurring at least one year prior to cognitive impairment. In cases when the distinction is not clear, a diagnosis of Lewy Body spectrum disorder could be made.

   Histopathologically, Lewy Body disorders are characterized by the presence of intraneuronal Lewy bodies and Lewy neurites. Biochemically, Lewy bodies and neurites consist of pathologically misfolded α-synuclein toxic aggregates. There are two types of Lewy bodies: brainstem (found in the substantia nigra and locus ceruleum) and cortical. The brainstem-associated Lewy body pathology predominantly presents with motor involvement, as in classical Parkinson's disease. If Lewy bodies are primarily affecting cortical neurons, patients present with a distinct cognitive DLB profile. The same pathology frequently affects autonomic functions regulating centers. Fibrillary amyloid and hyperphosphorylated tau are also frequently observed in these patients as a secondary pathology. Biochemically, Lewy body disorders are characterized by dopaminergic and cholinergic deficiencies.

   Clinically, DLB is characterized by 1) fluctuating cognition, 2) cognitive impairment, 3) psychotic symptoms (most frequently visual hallucinations), and 4) Parkinsonism. These patients also frequently have rapid eye movement sleep behavior disorder and are highly sensitive to neuroleptics.

   The cognitive profile in DLB demonstrates impairment in multiple cognitive domains, though the most striking deficits are frequently in higher visually-based functions [71]. Memory is also frequently affected in DLB, and studies have demonstrated that amnestic syndrome in DLB is primarily due to inefficient retrieval [72].

   DLB diagnosis is made when patients have a cluster of specific clinical symptoms. There are no specific clinical tests available to directly identify Lewy bodies or Lewy neurites.

   Structural brain imaging (using MRI or CT imaging modalities) in patients with DLB demonstrates generalized brain atrophy. Relative preservation of MTL structures could serve as a suggestive marker for DLB when differentiating from AD [73]. Brain SPECT and PET imaging modalities demonstrate occipital lobe hypoperfusion and hypometabolism respectively, which are the distinct findings if compared to patients with AD [74, 75]. The SPECT imaging (using ligand (123)I-2beta-carbometoxy-3beta-(4-iodophenyl)-N-(3-fluoropropyl) nortropane ((123)I-FP-CIT) or PET imaging (using ligand (18F)Fluorodopa) for dopamine uptake is used to identify deficient dopamine re-uptake in the basal ganglia as an indirect and supplemental marker to aid the diagnosis [76, 77].

Peripheral autonomic involvement can be assessed by evaluating cardiac sympathetic denervation by using 123I-Metaiodo-benzylguanidine (MIBG) myocardial scintigraphy [78].

3. *Vascular pathology.* Vascular insults to the brain occur due to ischemic or hemorrhagic mechanisms. Specifically located vascular lesions in the limbic system that result in retention deficits were previously discussed. Specifically located injuries in the brain can also result in deficient memory encoding and retrieval mechanisms. In clinical practice, one frequently encounters subcortical ischemic changes that are located in a more diffuse distribution periventricularly and subcortically (see Figure 5). A portion of these patients present with step-wise deterioration, usually signifying more distinct ischemic events; however, some patients present with slow clinical worsening, which likely signifies a growing burden of brain white matter lesions. These ischemic changes are responsible for the more generalized disruption of cortical-subcortical circuits involved in cognitive functioning. Multiple studies demonstrated that subcortical white matter lesions correlate with a more widespread diminished cortical metabolism that signifies diminished synaptic connectivity [79]. Subcortical white matter changes affect executive functioning, as well as the encoding and retrieval processes, and the increasing burden of white matter signal changes correlates with worse performance on executive and visual construction tasks. Studies have determined that a neuropsychological profile of equal impairment on tests of executive control and memory function and radiological evidence involving approximately one-fourth of the cerebral white matter are sufficient for a diagnosis of subcortical vascular neurocognitive disorder [80]. Multiple studies also demonstrated that while memory is affected in subcortical ischemic white matter disease, these patients usually do better on memory tasks compared with patients with AD [81].
4. *Traumatic brain injury.* Patients with prefrontal cortex damage have the most difficulty with the free recall of information, whereas cued recall and recognition are less impaired or function fairly well [82, 83]. Patients with prefrontal region damage could also display difficulties with temporal sequences of the events or in identifying the correct memory source [84, 85]; these patients can present with confabulations, distortions and false memories.

Mild traumatic brain injury (mTBI) is indicated when transient alterations in the sensorium (loss of consciousness or confusion) is present. Structural brain imaging frequently does not demonstrate any changes; however, accumulating data indicate that changes could be demonstrated using functional and connectivity brain imaging modalities. The basis for cognitive impairment after mTBI could be rooted in abnormal functional and structural connectivity and the interactions between the default mode and task-related (frontal-parietal) networks [16]. Changes in task-related cortical activation were also demonstrated in certain patients with persistent post-concussive cognitive symptoms. In these cases, an increase in activation was demonstrated in areas associated with attention; decreases in activation were noted in the areas that are important in declarative memory [86].

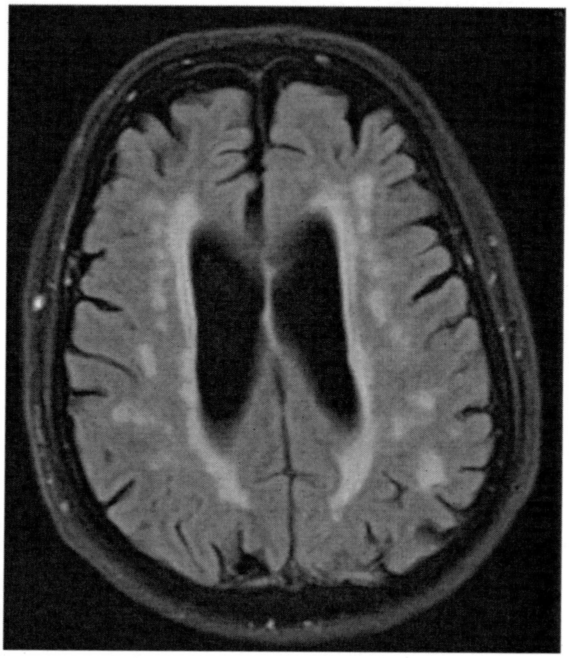

Figure 5. MRI axial FLAIR image of 75 year old male presenting with cognitive impairment. Neuropsychological testing demonstrated dysexecutive = amnestic impairment profile.

5. *Space-occupying lesions* can affect memory encoding and retrieval if located in relevant brain regions.
6. *Hydrocephalus*. Hydrocephalus is a condition that presents with an increased ventricle size due to intraventricular CSF accumulation either due to outflow obstruction or overproduction.

   Obstructive hydrocephalus is usually a medical emergency and is outside the scope of this chapter.

   Normal pressure hydrocephalus (NPH) is an idiopathic condition that is characterized by communicating hydrocephalus associated with a normal intracranial pressure. The etiological mechanism of this condition is not entirely clear. The classical triad of symptoms (cognitive impairment, ataxia and urinary incontinence) is not always present in its entirety. Neuropsychological testing demonstrates impairment across multiple cognitive domains, including memory, which is never in isolation and could be involved to a lesser degree than other cognitive domains [87]. Working memory is also frequently affected [88]. There is no single test to confirm the diagnosis of NPH. Structural imaging usually demonstrates a symmetrical widening of the lateral and third ventricles. Focal sulcal atrophy and the widening of Sylvian fissures may indicate external hydrocephalus [89]. CSF dynamics monitoring have thus far not significantly contributed to diagnosing this condition. Clinically, the response to CSF removal (via a single lumbar puncture, lumbar drainage or intraventricular drainage) is measured to predict whether a permanent intracranial CSF shunt would be effective. Gait impairment is usually the most likely to improve with CSF drainage; however, only a proportion of patients with cognitive impairment improve after treatment.

7. *Demyelinating disorders*. Multiple sclerosis (MS) is one of the most prevalent demyelinating disorders. Approximately half of the patients with multiple sclerosis demonstrate cognitive impairment. Memory is among the cognitive domains most frequently affected in patients with multiple sclerosis. Encoding and recall are frequently affected [90, 91].

Other conditions have been also demonstrated to induce memory impairment, for example human immunodeficiency virus-associated neurocognitive disorder among others [92].

SEMANTIC MEMORY DISORDERS

Semantic memory is a form of memory that involves the meaning of objects. Semantic memory is heavily interconnected with language function and is discussed in the chapter on language.

MEMORY ENHANCEMENT BY EMOTIONAL STIMULI AND ITS IMPAIRMENT

The registration and survival of memories are enhanced by emotions. This ability plays significant function through the evolutionary adaptation of any species. Emotional memories refers to a subgroup of memories which arouse specific emotions when recalled. The capacity of the emotional enhancement of memory (EEM) system is frequently overlooked when gathering a history from the patient, and there are no clinically validated methods for this enhancement mechanism to be evaluated in the office. Although the census in the field is that EEM plays a significant role in overall memory formation and function, only limited research was performed in order to clarify the mechanism of this phenomenon.

It is known that memories which have attached emotions (either positive or negative) are more likely to be incorporated into the long term memory storage system compared to memories without attached emotions [93]. This influence increases the focus and registration of the gist and details associated with the emotion arousing event or object, at the same time diminishing memories for details not associated with the main event [93, 94]. It is not completely clear whether this influence is exerted mainly by amygdala direct influence on entorhinal cortex – hippocampus complex, or is due to involvement of additional mechanisms, such as redistribution of attention, amygdalocentric system influences on vast cortical regions and effect of increased levels of stress hormones.

This section will be reviewing emotional enhancement of memories rather than investigating the biology of emotions and emotion processing. These topics are covered in the separate chapter of the book.

Studies support the idea that amygdaloid complex plays a role in enhancing memories for positive and negative emotional stimuli, which increases the chance for the memory to "survive" when compared to neutral memories. Amygdala was demonstrated to enhance memory encoding and consolidation, and is also activated during the retrieval of these memories [95, 96, 97]. Functional imaging studies also demonstrated that the orbitofrontal cortex may play a significant role in EEM [98].

It is rare to encounter patients who have isolated impairment of enhancement of declarative and non-declarative memories by emotional stimuli because even isolated amygdala lesions manifest with the whole gamma of emotional disorders. Patients with a rare Urbach-Wiethe disease who among other findings have calcified lesions in bilateral amygdala do not demonstrate expected enhancement of declarative memories by emotions [99].

The growing evidence suggests that certain neurodegenerative conditions can also demonstrate impairment in EEM. This mechanism was demonstrated to be impaired in patients with AD despite preserved emotional reactions, and this effect was more pronounced for unpleasant stimuli [100]. Further studies demonstrated possible dissociation between the ability to register emotionally enhanced verbal vs. non-verbal memories in patients with AD. In this case, the EEM mechanism was less effective for verbally based information [101]. Mori et al. demonstrated that a chance recall of emotional memories best correlated with amygdala volumes rather than hippocampal volumes or the degree of generalized brain atrophy in patients with Alzheimer's disease [102].

Behavioral variant Frontotemporal dementia (bvFTD) is in many ways different from AD. One of the differences include early impairment in recognition and processing of emotions. This also affects the ability of these patients to enhance their memory performance by emotions. It was demonstrated that the impairment of emotional enhancement was not simply due to impaired emotional processing in these patients but also due to impaired enhancement mechanism *per se* [8]. EEM mechanism was demonstrated to be impaired to a greater degree in patients with bvFTD when compared to AD [98, 8].

TREATMENT

Treatment modalities of memory disorders can be classified into the following categories:

4. *Disease-specific treatment.* This treatment includes any modality that affects the pathogenetic mechanisms of the disease by curing it, stopping or slowing its progression, or changing the disease pathogenesis in any other way. Examples of disease-specific treatments include ventriculo-peritoneal shunt placement for NPH, disease-modifying treatment for MS, and immunosuppressive therapy for autoimmune cognitive disorders.
5. *Symptomatic treatment of cognitive deficits.* This treatment group includes pharmacologic agents that improve memory and cognition and/or reduce functional decline via mechanisms other than directly affecting the disease pathogenesis. This group includes pharmacological therapies used for neurocognitive syndrome that are not specific to disease processes. The associated medication groups include centrally acting acetylcholine esterase inhibitors, which could be prescribed in conditions of cholinergic deficiency (AD, DLB/Parkinson disease dementia and vascular cognitive impairment). This medication group includes donepezil, rivastigmine and galantamine. The other group of medications blocks NMDA receptors and includes the single agent memantine, which has an approval for the treatment of AD only.

Medications that enhance or modulate attention could also be assigned to this group. This includes stimulants (e.g., amphetamine and derivates) and non-stimulants (e.g., adrenergic drugs and antidepressants, especially those associated with higher dopaminergic stimulation) medications. These medications are frequently used to treat attention deficit disorder but have also been used off-label for other cognitive disorders.

6. *Memory-specific cognitive rehabilitation.* Memory-specific cognitive rehabilitation attempts to restore lost memory capacity by facilitating acquisition. This technique capitalizes on the subject's retained strengths and teaches compensatory techniques and the use of external aids. This rehabilitation should not be confused with cognitive behavior therapy, a form of psychotherapy.

Several experimental modalities are used to study and treat memory impairment. Repetitive transcranial magnetic stimulation (rTMS) is one of them. During TMS transitory magnetic fields are generated over the scalp that in turn generate electric currents in cortical surface either inhibiting or stimulating selected cortical region. Initially rTMS effect is short lived, but with repeat exposure the effect can last from weeks to months. This is thought to be due to LTP or long term depression processes. The studies indicate that stimulation of dorsolateral PFC can enhance memory function. Drumond Marra et al. reported that high frequency rTMS delivered over 10 sessions on the left dorsolateral PFC enhanced memory in elderly patients with mild cognitive impairment (MCI) [103]. An improvement in amnestic MCI was also demonstrated after repeat high frequency rTMS was applied to the left parietal cortex supporting the findings from other studies that parietal regions are also involved in certain aspects of memory function [104].

CONCLUSION

Evolutionary processes have shaped the human brain to develop an intricate mechanism of storing experiences and information. Different types of memory have distinct processes that guarantee optimal functioning. Declarative memory impairment is one of the most common complaints in cognitive neurology clinics, and understanding the functional anatomy, testing and possible underlying pathology enables the examiner to formulate an approach for selecting targeted diagnostic procedures and treatments.

ACKNOWLEDGMENTS

Prof. Janice Jurkus, Dr. Kathryn Lester, Dr. Esther Nemchinsky, Daniel Eichorn, Alexandra Potts, Christina Maxwell.

REFERENCES

[1] Squire LR, Zola SM. Structure and function of declarative and nondeclarative memory systems. *Proc Natl Acad Sci USA.* 1996 Nov;93:13515-13522.

[2] Baddeley A. Working memory. *Science.* 1992 Jan 31;255(5044):556-559.

[3] Bliss TV, Gardner-Medwin AR. Long-lasting potentiation of synaptic transmission in the dentate area of the unanaestetized rabbit following stimulation of the perforant path. *J Physiol.* 1973 Jul;232(2):357-374.

[4] Kandel ER, Bartsch D, Bailey CH. Toward a molecular definition of long-term memory storage. *Proc Natl Acad Sci USA.* 1996 Nov;93:13445-13452.

[5] Papez J. A proposed mechanism of emotion. *Arch NeurPsych.* 1937;38(4):725-743.

[6] Hebb DO. *The organization of behavior.* Wiley, New York, 1949.

[7] Bohbot VD, Kalina M, Stepankova K, Spackova N, Petrides M, Nadel L. Spatial memory deficits in patients with lesions to the right hippocampus and to the right parahippocampal cortex. *Neuropsychologia.* 1998 Nov;36(11):1217-1238.

[8] Kumfor F, Irish M, Hodges JR, Piguet O. Frontal and temporal lobe contributions to emotional enhancement of memory in behavioral-variant frontotemporal dementia and Alzheimer's disease. *Front Behav Neurosci.* 2014 Jun 24;8:225.

[9] Floel A, Poeppel D, Buffalo EA, Braun A, Wu CWH, Seo1 HJ, et al. Prefrontal Cortex Asymmetry for Memory Encoding of Words and Abstract Shapes. *Cereb. Cortex* (2004) 14 (4): 404-409.

[10]Reber PJ, Siwiec RM, Gitelman DR, Parrish TB, Mesulam MM, Paller KA. Neural correlates of successful encoding identified using functional magnetic resonance imaging. *J Neurosci.* 2002 Nov 1;22(21):9541-8. Erratum in: J Neurosci. 2003 Jan 1;23(1):1a.

[11]Jonides J, Nee DE. Brain mechanisms of proactive interference in working memory. *Neuroscience.* 2006 Apr 28;139(1):181-93.

[12]Postle BR, Berger JS, D'Esposito M. Functional neuroanatomical double dissociation of mnemonic and executive control processes contributing to working memory performance. *Proc Natl Acad Sci USA.* 1999 Oct 26; 96(22): 12959–12964.

[13]Buckner, RL. Functional-anatomic correlates of control processes in memory. J Neurosci. 2003 May;23(10):3999-4004.

[14]Vincent JL, Snyder AZ, Fox MD, Shannon BJ, Andrews JR, Raichle ME, Buckner RL. Coherent spontaneous activity identifies a hippocampal-parietal memory network. *J Neurophysiol.* 2006 Dec;96(6):3517-3531.

[15]Nyberg L, Persson J, Habib R, Tulving E, McIntosh AR, Cabeza R, et al. Large scale neurocognitive networks underlying episodic memory. *J Cogn Neurosci.* 2000 Jan;12(1):163-173.

[16]Mayer AR, Mannell MV, Ling J, Gasparovic C, Yeo RA. Functional connectivity in mild traumatic brain injury. *Hum Brain Mapp.* 2011 Nov;32(11):1825-1835.

[17]Huijbers W, Pennartz CM, Cabeza R, Daselaar SM. The hippocampus is coupled with the default network during memory retrieval but not during memory encoding. *PLoS One.* 2011 Apr 11;6(4):e17463.

[18]Shapiro ML, Eichenbaum H. Hippocampus as a memory map: synaptic plasticity and memory encoding by hippocampal neurons. *Hippocampus.* 1999;9(4):365-384.

[19]Rolls ET. Diluted connectivity in pattern association networks facilitates the recall of information from the hippocampus to the neocortex. *Prog Brain Res.* 2015;219:21-43.

[20]Persson J, Soderlund H. Hippocampal hemispheric and long-axis differentiation of stimulus content during episodic memory encoding and retrieval: An activation likelihood estimation meta-analysis. *Hippocampus.* 2015 Jun 25.

[21]Frankland PW, Bontempi B. The organization of recent and remote memories. *Nat Rev Neurosci.* 2005 Feb;6(2):119-130. Review.

[22]Squire LR, Alvarez P. Retrograde amnesia and memory consolidation: a neurobiological perspective. *Curr Opin Neurobiol.* 1995 Apr;5(2):169-177. Review.

[23]Gais S, Born J. Low acetylcholine during slow-wave sleep is critical for declarative memory consolidation. *Proc Natl Acad Sci U S A.* 2004 Feb 17;101(7):2140-2144.

[24]Smith EE, Jonides J, Koeppe RA. Dissociating verbal and spatial working memory using PET. *Cereb Cortex.* 1996 Jan-Feb;6(1):11-20.

[25]Pessoa L, Gutierrez E, Bandettini PA, Ungerleider LG. Neural correlates of visual working memory: fMRI amplitude predicts task performance. *Neuron.* 2002 Aug 29;35:975-987.

[26]Feinstein JS, Rudrauf D, Khalsa SS, Cassell MD, Bruss J, Grabowski TJ, et al. Bilateral limbic system destruction in man. *J Clin Exp Neuropsychol.* 2010 Jan;32(1):88-106.

[27]Rogers TT, Hocking J, Noppeney U, Mechelli A, Gorno-Tempini ML, Patterson K, et al. Anterior temporal cortex and semantic memory: reconciling findings from neuropsychology and functional imaging. *Cogn Affect Behav Neurosci.* 2006 Sep;6(3):201-213.

[28]Selden NR, Gitelman DR, Salamon-Murayama N, Parrish TB, Mesulam MM. Trajectories of cholinergic pathways within the cerebral hemispheres of the human brain. *Brain.* 1998 Dec;121 (Pt 12):2249-2257.

[29]Weintraub S, Mesulam MM. Mental state assessment of young and elderly adults in behavioral neurology. *Principles of behavioral neurology.* FA Davis, Philadelphia, 1985.

[30]Wechsler D (2009). *Wechsler memory scale: forth edition.* Pearson. San Antonio, TX

[31]CVLT-2: Delis DC, Kramer JH, Kaplan E, Ober BA. (2000). California verbal learning test: second edition. *Psychological corporation.* San Antonio, TX.

[32]Schmidt M (1996). Rey auditory and verbal learning test. *A handbook. Western psychological services.* Los Angeles.

[33]Osterrieth PA (1944). Le test de copie d'une figure complex: contribution a l'etude de la perception et de la memoire. *Archives de psychologie,* 30, 286-356.

[34]Iqbal K, Alonso AC, Chen S, Chohan MO, El-Akkad E, Gong CX, et al. Tau pathology in Alzheimer disease and other tauopathies. *Biochim Biophys Acta.* 2005 Jan 3;1739(2-3):198-210.

[35]Sperling RA, Laviolette PS, O'Keefe K, O'Brien J, Rentz DM, Pihlajamaki M, et al. Amyloid deposition is associated with impaired default network function in older persons without dementia. *Neuron.* 2009 Jul 30;63(2):178-188.

[36]Stratmann K, Heinsen H, Korf HW, Del Turco D, Ghebremedhin E, Seidel K, et al. Precortical phase of Alzheimer's disease (AD)-related tau cytoskeletal pathology. *Brain Pathol.* 2015 Jul 20.

[37]Braak H, Braak E. Staging of Alzheimer's disease-related neurofibrillary changes. *Neurobiol Aging.* 1995 May-Jun;16(3):271-278.

[38]Johnson KA, Minoshima S, Bohnen NI, Donohoe KJ, Foster NL, Herscovitch P, et al. Update on appropriate use criteria for amyloid PET imaging: dementia experts, mild cognitive impairment, and education. *J Nucl Med.* 2013 Jul;54(7):1011-3.

[39]Motter R, Vigo-Pelfrey C, Kholodenko D, Barbour R, Johnson-Wood K, Galasko D, et al. Reduction of beta-amyloid peptide42 in the cerebrospinal fluid of patients with Alzheimer's disease. *Ann Neurol.* 1995 Oct;38(4):643-648.

[40]Ossenkoppele R, van der Flier WM, Verfaillie SC, Vrenken H, Versteeg A, van Schijndel RA, et al. Long-term effects of amyloid, hypometabolism, and atrophy on neuropsychological functions. *Neurology.* 2014 May 20;82(20):1768-1775.

[41]Killiany RJ, Hyman BT, Gomez-Isla T, Moss MB, Kikinis R, Jolesz F, et al. MRI measures of entorhinal cortex vs hippocampus in preclinical AD. *Neurology.* 2002 Apr 23;58(8):1188-96.

[42]Basso M, Yang J, Warren L, MacAvoy MG, Varma P, Bronen RA, et al. Volumetry of amygdala and hippocampus and memory performance in Alzheimer's disease. *Psychiatry Res.* 2006 Apr 30;146(3):251-61.

[43]Du AT, Schuff N, Kramer JH, Rosen HJ, Gorno-Tempini ML, Rankin K, et al. Different regional patterns of cortical thinning in Alzheimer's disease and frontotemporal dementia. *Brain.* 2007 Apr;130(4):1159-1166.

[44]Blennow K, Hampel H. CSF markers for incipient Alzheimer's disease. *Lancet Neurol.* 2003;2(10):605-13.

[45]Terry RD, Masliah E, Salmon DP, Butters N, DeTeresa R, Hill R, et al. Physical basis of cognitive alterations in Alzheimer's disease: synapse loss is the major correlate of cognitive impairment. *Ann Neurol.* 1991 Oct;30(4):572-580.

[46]Silverman DH, Small GW, Chang CY, Lu CS, Kung De Aburto MA, Chen W, Czernin J, et al. Positron emission tomography in evaluation of dementia: Regional brain metabolism and long-term outcome. *JAMA.* 2001 Nov 7;286(17):2120-7.

[47]Jagust WJ, Budinger TF, Reed BR. The diagnosis of dementia with single photon emission computed tomography. *Arch Neurol.* 1987 Mar;44(3):258-262.

[48]Xekardaki A, Rodriguez C, Montandon ML, Toma S, Tombeur E, Herrmann FR, et al. Arterial spin labeling may contribute to the prediction of cognitive deterioration in healthy elderly individuals. *Radiology.* 2015 Feb;274(2):490-499.

[49]Jack CR Jr, Wiste HJ, Knopman DS, Vemuri P, Mielke MM, Weigand SD, et al. Rates of β-amyloid accumulation are independent of hippocampal neurodegeneration. *Neurology.* 2014 May 6;82(18):1605-1612.

[50]Crary JF, Trojanowski JQ, Schneider JA, Abisambra JF, Abner EL, Alafuzoff I, et al. Primary age-related tauopathy (PART): a common pathology associated with human aging. *Acta Neuropathol.* 2014 Dec;128(6):755-766.

[51]Leverenz JB, Agustin CM, Tsuang D, Peskind ER, Edland SD, Nochlin D, et al. Clinical and neuropathological characteristics of hippocampal sclerosis: a community-based study. *Arch Neurol.* 2002 Jul;59(7):1099-1106.

[52]Amador-Ortiz C, Lin W-L, Ahmed Z, Personett D, Davies P, Duara R, et al. TDP-43 immunoreactivity in hippocampal sclerosis and Alzheimer's disease. *Ann Neurol* 62:435-445;2007.

[53]Togo T, Cookson N, Dickson DW. Argyrophilic grain disease: Neuropathology, frequency in a dementia brain bank and lack of relationship with apolipoprotein E. *Brain Pathol* 12:45-52;2002.
[54]Ferrer I, Santpere G, van Leeuwen FW. Argyrophilic grain disease. *Brain.* 2008 Jun;131(6):1416-1432.
[55]Graff-Radford NR, Damasio H, Yamada T, Eslinger PJ, Damasio AR. Nonhaemorrhagic thalamic infarction. Clinical, neuropsychological and electrophysiological findings in four anatomical groups defined by computerized tomography. *Brain.* 1985 Jun;108(2):485-516.
[56]Clarke S, Assal G, Bogousslavsky J, Regli F, Townsend DW, Leenders KL, Blecic S. Pure amnesia after unilateral left polar thalamic infarct: topographic and sequential neuropsychological and metabolic (PET) correlations. *J Neurol Neurosurg Psychiatry.* 1994 Jan;57(1):27-34.
[57]Benson DF, Marsden CD, Meadows JC. The amnesic syndrome of posterior cerebral artery occlusion. *Acta Neurol Scand.* 1974;50(2):133-145.
[58]Maeshima S, Osawa A, Yamane F, Shimaguchi H, Ochiai I, Yoshihara T. Memory impairment caused by cerebral hematoma in the left medial temporal lobe due to ruptured posterior cerebral artery aneurysm. *BMC Neurol.* 2014 Mar 7;14:44.
[59]Nardone R, Höller Y, Storti M, Christova M, Tezzon F, Golaszewski S, et al. Thiamine deficiency induced neurochemical, neuroanatomical, and neuropsychological alterations: a reappraisal. *Scientific World Journal.* 2013 Oct 21;2013:309143.
[60]Shimamura AP, Jernigan TL, Squire LR. Korsakoff's syndrome: radiological (CT) findings and neuropsychological correlates. *J Neurosci.* 1988 Nov;8(11):4400-4410.
[61]D'Esposito M, Verfaellie M, Alexander MP, Katz DI. Amnesia following traumatic bilateral fornix transection. *Neurology.* 1995 Aug;45(8):1546-1550.
[62]Teuber HL, Milner B, Vaughan HG. Persistent anterograde amnesia after stab wound of the basal forebrain. *Neuropsychologia.* 1968 Sept;6(3):267-282.
[63]Gee CE, Benquet P, Raineteau O, Rietschin L, Kirbach SW, Gerber U. NMDA receptors and the differential ischemic vulnerability of hippocampal neurons. *Eur J Neurosci.* 2006 May;23(10):2595-2603.
[64]Rosenfeld MR, Dalmau JO. Paraneoplastic disorders of the CNS and autoimmune synaptic encephalitis. *Continuum.* 2012 Apr;18(2):366-383.
[65]Dalmau J, Rosenfeld MR. Paraneoplastic syndromes of the CNS. *Lancet Neurol.* 2008 Apr;7(4):327-340.
[66]Markowitsch HJ. Transient global amnesia. *Neurosci Biobehav Rev.* 1983 Spring;7(1):35-43.
[67]Gonzalez-Martinez V, Comte F, de Verbizier D, Carlander B. Transient global amnesia: concordant hippocampal abnormalities on positron emission tomography and magnetic resonance imaging. *Arch Neurol.* 2010 Apr;67(4):510-511.
[68]Evans J, Wilson B, Wraight EP, Hodges JR. Neuropsychological and SPECT scan findings during and after transient global amnesia: evidence for the differential impairment of remote episodic memory. *J Neurol Neurosurg Psychiatry.* 1993 Nov;56(11):1227-1230.

[69]Yamane Y, Ishii K, Shimizu K, Sofue K, Yoshikawa T, Miyamoto N, et al. Global cerebral hypoperfusion in a patient with transient global amnesia. *J Comput Assist Tomogr.* 2008 May-Jun;32(3):415-417.

[70]Nyberg L, Cabeza R, Tulving E. PET studies of encoding and retrieval: The HERA model. *Psychon Bull Rev.* 1996 Jun;3(2):135-148.

[71]Salmon DP, Galasko D, Hansen LA, Masliah E, Butters N, Thal LJ, et al. Neuropsychological deficits associated with diffuse Lewy body disease. *Brain Cogn.* 1996 Jul;31(2):148-165.

[72]Hamilton JM, Salmon DP, Galasko D, Delis DC, Hansen LA, Masliah E, et al. A comparison of episodic memory deficits in neuropathologically-confirmed Dementia with Lewy bodies and Alzheimer's disease. *J Int Neuropsychol Soc.* 2004 Sep;10(5):689-697.

[73]Barber R, Ballard C, McKeith IG, Gholkar A, O'Brien JT. MRI volumetric study of dementia with Lewy bodies: a comparison with AD and vascular dementia. *Neurology.* 2000 Mar 28;54(6):1304-9.

[74]Ishii K, Yamaji S, Kitagaki H, Imamura T, Hirono N, Mori E. Regional cerebral blood flow difference between dementia with Lewy bodies and AD. *Neurology.* 1999 Jul 22;53(2):413-416.

[75]Tateno M, Kobayashi S, Saito T. Imaging improves diagnosis of dementia with lewy bodies. *Psychiatry Investig.* 2009 Dec;6(4):233-240.

[76]Ransmayr G, Seppi K, Donnemiller E, Luginger E, Marksteiner J, Riccabona G, et al. Striatal dopamine transporter function in dementia with Lewy bodies and Parkinson's disease. *Eur J Nucl Med.* 2001 Oct;28(10):1523-1528.

[77]Hu XS, Okamura N, Arai H, Higuchi M, Matsui T, Tashiro M, et al. 18F-fluorodopa PET study of striatal dopamine uptake in the diagnosis of dementia with Lewy bodies. *Neurology.* 2000 Nov 28;55(10):1575-7.

[78]Yoshita M, Taki J, Yamada M. A clinical role for [(123)I]MIBG myocardial scintigraphy in the distinction between dementia of the Alzheimer's-type and dementia with Lewy bodies. *J Neurol Neurosurg Psychiatry.* 2001 Nov;71(5):583-8.

[79]Tullberg M, Fletcher E, DeCarli C, Mungas D, Reed BR, Harvey DJ, et al. White matter lesions impair frontal lobe function regardless of their location. *Neurology.* 2004 Jul 27;63(2):246-253.

[80]Price CC, Jefferson AL, Merino JG, Heilman KM, Libon DJ. Subcortical vascular dementia: integrating neuropsychological and neuroradiologic data. *Neurology.* 2005 Aug 9;65(3):376-382.

[81]Hassing L, Bäckman L. Episodic memory functioning in population-based samples of very old adults with Alzheimer's disease and vascular dementia. *Dement Geriatr Cogn Disord.* 1997 Nov-Dec;8(6):376-383.

[82]Gershberg FB, Shimamura AP. Impaired use of organizational strategies in free recall following frontal lobe damage. *Neuropsychologia.* 1995 Oct;33(10):1305-1333.

[83]Wheeler MA, Stuss DT, Tulving E. Frontal lobe damage produces episodic memory impairment. *J Int Neuropsychol Soc.* 1995 Nov;1(6):525-536.

[84]Kopelman MD, Stanhope N, Kingsley D. Temporal and spatial context memory in patients with focal frontal, temporal lobe, and diencephalic lesions. *Neuropsychologia.* 1997 Dec;35(12):1533-1545.

[85]Janowsky JS, Shimamura AP, Squire LR. Source memory impairment in patients with frontal lobe lesions. *Neuropsychologia.* 1989;27(8):1043-1056.

[86]Dean PJ, Sato JR, Vieira G, McNamara A, Sterr A. Multimodal imaging of mild traumatic brain injury and persistent postconcussion syndrome. *Brain Behav.* 2015 Jan;5(1):45-61.

[87]Saito M, Nishio Y, Kanno S, Uchiyama M, Hayashi A, Takagi M, et al. Cognitive profile of idiopathic normal pressure hydrocephalus. *Dement Geriatr Cogn Dis Extra.* 2011 Jan;1(1):202-211.

[88]Kazui H. Cognitive impairment in patients with idiopathic normal pressure hydrocephalus. *Brain Nerve.* 2008 Mar;60(3):225-231.

[89]Holodny AI, George AE, de Leon MJ, Golomb J, Kalnin AJ, Cooper PR. Focal dilation and paradoxical collapse of cortical fissures and sulci in patients with normal-pressure hydrocephalus. *J Neurosurg.* 1998 Nov;89(5):742-747.

[90]Rao SM, Leo GJ, Bernardin L, Unverzagt F. Cognitive dysfunction in multiple sclerosis. I. Frequency, patterns, and prediction. *Neurology.* 1991 May;41(5):685-691.

[91]DeLuca J, Barbieri-Berger S, Johnson SK. The nature of memory impairments in multiple sclerosis: acquisition versus retrieval. *J Clin Exp Neuropsychol.* 1994 Apr;16(2):183-189.

[92]Robertson K, Liner J, Heaton R. Neuropsychological assessment of HIV-infected populations in international settings. *Neuropsychol Rev.* 2009 Jun;19(2):232-249.

[93]Burke A, Heuer F, Reisberg D. Remembering emotional events. *Mem Cognit. 1992* May;20(3):277-290.

[94]Adolphs R, Tranel D, Buchanan TW. Amygdala damage impairs emotional memory for gist but not details of complex stimuli. *Nat Neurosci.* 2005 Apr;8(4):512-518.

[95]Hamann SB, Ely TD, Grafton ST, Kilts CD. Amygdala activity related to enhanced memory for pleasant and aversive stimuli. *Nat Neurosci.* 1999 Mar;2(3):289-293.

[96]Hamann SB, Mao H. Neural correlates of emotional memory and reactions to verbal and nonverbal emotional stimuli: an fMRI study. *J Cogn Neurosci.* 2001; 30.

[97]Dolan RJ, Lane R, Chua P, Fletcher P. Dissociable temporal lobe activations during emotional episodic memory retrieval. *Neuroimage.* 2000 Mar;11(3):203-209.

[98]Kumfor F, Irish M, Hodges JR, Piguet O. The orbitofrontal cortex is involved in emotional enhancement of memory: evidence from the dementias. *Brain.* 2013 Oct;136(Pt 10):2992-3003.

[99]Cahill L, Babinsky R, Markowitsch HJ, McGaugh JL. The amygdala and emotional memory. *Nature.* 1995 Sep 28;377(6547):295-296.

[100] Hamann SB, Monarch ES, Goldstein FC. Memory enhancement for emotional stimuli is impaired in early Alzheimer's disease. *Neuropsychology.* 2000 Jan;14(1):82-92.

[101] Baran Z, Cangöz B, Ozel-Kizil ET. The impact of aging and Alzheimer's disease on emotional enhancement of memory. *Eur Neurol.* 2014;72(1-2):30-37.

[102] Mori E, Ikeda M, Hirono N, Kitagaki H, Imamura T, Shimomura T. Amygdalar volume and emotional memory in Alzheimer's disease. *Am J Psychiatry.* 1999 Feb;156(2):216-222.

[103] Drumond Marra HL, Myczkowski ML, Maia Memória C, Arnaut D, Leite Ribeiro P, Sardinha Mansur CG, et al. Transcranial Magnetic Stimulation to Address Mild

Cognitive Impairment in the Elderly: A Randomized Controlled Study. *Behav Neurol.* 2015;2015:287843.

[104] Cotelli M, Calabria M, Manenti R, Rosini S, Maioli C, Zanetti O, et al. Brain stimulation improves associative memory in an individual with amnestic mild cognitive impairment. *Neurocase.* 2012 Jun;18(3):217-23.

In: Progressive Cognitive Impairment …
Editor: Gediminas Peter Gliebus

ISBN: 978-1-63485-221-0

Chapter 7

LANGUAGE DISORDERS IN NEURODEGENERATIVE DISEASES

Borna Bonakdarpour*, MD
Cognitive Neurology and Alzheimer Disease Center
Davee Department of Neurology
Northwestern University Feinberg School of Medicine, Chicago, IL, US

ABSTRACT

The goal of this chapter is to discuss neuroanatomy of normal language function, and review clinical evaluation and management of progressive aphasias. Systematic use of neuroimaging, laboratory work up, and pharmacological, neuromodulatory, and non-pharmacological interventions including speech-language therapy, and psychosocial remediation will be reviewed. Based on recent neuroimaging studies, language network is studied based on neuroanatomically distinct *ventral* and *dorsal* pathways. These pathways contribute to lexical and phonological/syntactic processing respectively. Gradual impairment in these pathways, in the absence of significant decline in other cognitive networks will result in syndromes of primary progressive aphasia (PPA). Meticulous evaluation of word comprehension, fluency and grammaticality, repetition, naming, reading and writing, helps with further subtyping PPA. Following formulation of the clinical syndrome, structural and functional neuroimaging (topographical or progression biomarkers) are helpful tools to further specify the clinical phenotype as a guide to determine the underlying neuropathological process. Currently analysis of the cerebrospinal fluid and amyloid positron emission tomography (PET) can help with diagnosis of the neuropathological process (etiologic or state biomarkers). Based on diagnosis of the underlying neuropathology decision regarding appropriate pharmacological intervention will be possible. Comprehensive management of PPA involves utilization of both pharmacological and non-pharmacological intervention which include speech-language therapy, and psychosocial remediations.

* Correspondence to: bbk@northwestern.edu.

Introduction

The earliest archeological evidence of a written language traces back to the Cuneiform Sumerian language 3000 year before present time (BP) [1]. However, origin of spoken language stems from much earlier time. There is no direct evidence to relate us to the speech of our ancestors. Human's first attempt to represent information visually as cave drawings came about around 35,000 BP [2]. Traces of modern human life dates back to about 200,000 BP [3]. Anthropologic evidence to suggest origins of spoken language focuses on some of the physical aspect of humans that are not shared with any other creatures, such as upright posture, bipedal locomotion, and revised role for the front limbs and development of dominance in using limbs as evidenced by asymmetry in hypertrophic bones seen in remains of modern humans. The form of Neanderthal man from around 300,000 BP suggests that some consonant-like sound distinctions would have been possible [4]. Therefore it has taken few hundred thousands of years for our head and neck and brain anatomy to acquire linguistic capabilities.

First systematic approach to study of language was performed by Panini in India the 5th century BC, and Plato in Greece around the same time. Modern linguistics has shaped up thanks to works of Saussure, Boas, and Sapir, and later with outstanding works of Naom Chomsky [5]. Our understanding of language, however, is not limited to linguists, and has become a multidisciplinary field with contributions from archeologists, anthropologists, psychologists, cognitive neuroscientists, neuropsychologists, and investigators in the fields of speech-language pathology and neurology.

Linguistics has sub-fields that focus on different aspects of language structure. Cognitive neuroscientists and neurolinguists have attempted to determine the underlying neural mechanisms of these sub-fields and speech-language pathologists and neurologists study mechanisms of their disintegration and rehabilitation. Linguistic sub-fields for our purposes include the following structures:

- *Phonemes:* the smallest units of sound recognizable as spoken language (/g/, /m/)
- *Morphemes:* the smallest meaningful units of a word (/dys-/, /-ing/)
- *Graphemes:* the smallest unit of written language (pre-, -ing)
- *Lexical/semantics:* words and their meanings
- *Syntax:* sentence structure = grammar

Language, Speech, and Other Brain Cognitive Domains

In neurology language and speech have different meanings. Language is a systematic means of communication by the use of sounds or conventional symbols. Speech is the vocalized form of human communication and involves all steps from programming to final production of language units, or words.

It is also important to know that the neural network underlying language is not independent of other cognitive brain network. Therefore disruption other networks can secondarily affect the language and vice versa. For example, impairment in visual processing, known as agnosias, can affect picture naming and reading, or difficulty with word retrieval, or anomia can affect evaluation of verbal memory.

FUNCTIONAL NEUROANATOMY OF LANGUAGE

Language network is the most asymmetric network in the brain. Marc Dax was first to describe left hemisphere dominance for language (1836) [6], however his report remained unknown until after Paul Broca reported his cases of patients with aphasia and lesion in the *left posterior inferior frontal gyrus (IFG)* in 1865 report [6]. Following Broca's report, Karl Wernicke described a patient with fluent aphasia and impairment in language comprehension in 1874. Wernicke's patient had a lesion in the *posterior aspect of the superior temporal gyrus* [7]. In 1908 Lichtheim introduced the *arcuate fasciculus* as the connection bundle between the above two areas now known as *Broca's* and *Wernicke's areas* (Wernicke-Lichtheim model). It was not until 1965, when Norman Geschwind presented his model of language network that encompassed seven components [8]. Based his model, now known as *Wernicke-Geschwind* model in addition to the three above components, angular gyrus, motor cortex, and visual cortex, contribute to language processing. Language, similar to other cognitive domains, is an input-output system, and in this manner the Wernicke-Geschwind model takes the sensory-motor interface into consideration.

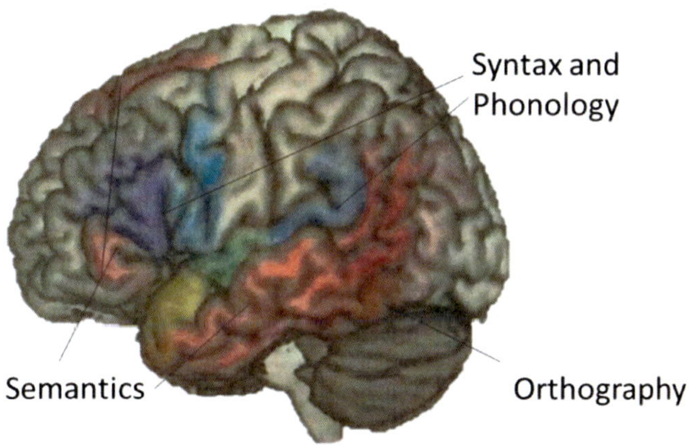

Figure 1. Key left hemisphere areas involved in language processing based on a broad survey of PET, fMRI, and lesion-deficit correlation studies. Adapted from Binder (2008) and Rapcsak and Beeson (2011) [11].

Until late 1980s most of our understanding of the language network relied on lesion-deficit correlations, and heavily reliant on stroke-induced aphasias. Introduction of Positron Emission Tomography (PET), functional Magnetic Resonance Imaging (fMRI), and Diffusion Tensor Imaging (DTI) to language network research of both normal and aphasic individuals have revolutionized our understanding of language neuroanatomy and physiology. In addition, progress in investigation of pathophysiology of progressive aphasias has contributed significantly to our knowledge of the language network. Based on the above mentioned structural, functional and diffusion weighted imaging techniques we now know that the language network consists of a core perisylvian component which has interface with extrasylvian (contributory) areas (Figure 1) [9]. The core perisylvian components of the language network are divided into two pathways: dorsal, and ventral, which are discussed below [10]. The ventral pathway is mostly dedicated to processing language at lexical level and the dorsal pathway is mostly involved in sentence level processing.

Dorsal Language Pathway

This pathway consists of two major fiber bundles: Arcuate fasciculus (AF) which was mentioned above, and parts of the superior longitudinal fascicle (SLF). AF connects posterior aspect of Broca's area (BA 44, pars opercularis) and Wernicke's area. SLF connects middle temporal gyrus (MTG) and superior temporal gyrus (STG) with the dorsal premotor cortex (PMC), via parietal cortex (PC) [12]. Figure 2 depicts the two language pathways.

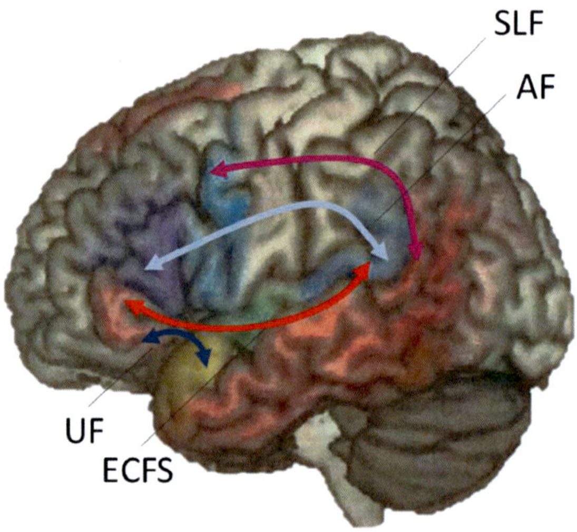

Figure 2. Dorsal and ventral language pathways. Superior longitudinal fasciculus (SLF) and arcuate fasciculus (AF) are the fiber tracts of the dorsal pathway, and extreme capsule fiber system (ECFS) and uncinated fasciculus (UF) form the ventral pathway.

Syntactic and phonological processing: The AF pathway supports complex syntactic and phonological processes. Processing of complex syntactic structures involve posterior Broca's area (BA 44) and posterior STG [13]. Verb and sentence production relies on both Broca's area and STG [14], with processing of arguments assigned to a verb (e.g., object and subject) supported by supramarginal gyrus (SMG) and angular gyrus (AG) [15, 16].

It is important to note that additional syntactic processes may require involvement of extrasylvian areas. For example addition of reflexives, which needs the BIND operation (Nick looked at *himself*) requires recruitment of SFG, or addition of past tense –ed, or –s plural/third person (agreement), recruit premotor and association parietal cortices [17]. Movement of sentence components such as verbs (MOVE $_{V}$) requires SFG and MFG recruitment, while movement of nouns (MOVE $_{XP}$) would rely on Broca's area [18]. A limited part of syntactic processing also relies on the ventral pathway which will be covered below. Figure 3 demonstrates the relationship between major nodes involved in processing of syntax.

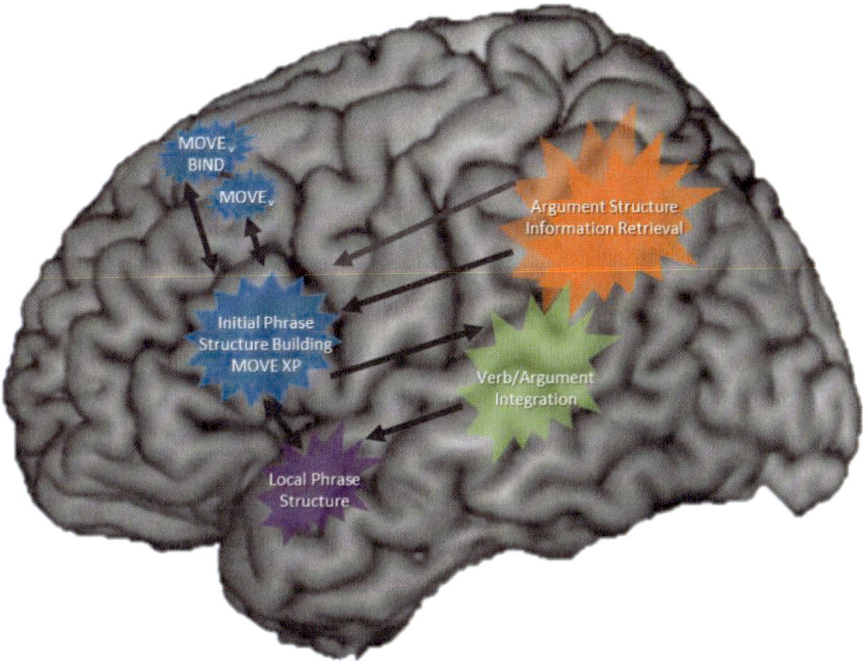

Figure 3. Major cortical areas supporting syntactic processing. Adapted from Grozinsky and Friederici (2006) [18], and Metzler and Thompson [131].

Speech repetition: SLF pathway supports speech repetition. The underlying cognitive components of speech repetition include perception of spoken language (Heschl's gyrus, and planum temporale), phonological working memory (ventral PC), and articulatory planning and execution (PMC). This extensive input-output (auditory-to-motor mapping) is supported by the SLF [19].

Ventral Language Pathway

The ventral pathway is built upon two major tracts: the uncinate fascicle (UF) and the extreme capsule fiber system (ECFS), or the inferior-fronto-occipital fascicle (ECFS) which runs through the ECFS. The major function of the ventral pathway is its role in semantic processing which is accomplished through the ECFS. UF supports basic syntactic processes.

Semantic processing: The ECFS connects the MTG with anterior aspect of Broca's area (BA 45/47) through anterior temporal lobe (ATL). This stream of the ventral pathway supports comprehension, lexical retrieval, and naming [10]. Although Wernicke's area historically was localized to posterior aspect of STG, lesion-deficit and functional imaging studies have shown that a wide area of posterior temporal cortex (posterior STG, posterior MTG and posterior ITG) and inferior parietal lobule (IPL, including AG and SMG) are involved in its main function, sentence comprehension [20]. In Figure 4 these posterior temporal areas (IPL, and posterior aspects of STG, MTG and ITG) have been demonstrated separately. Anterior aspect of Broca's area (BA 45/47) in particular, has a role in semantic judgment and categorization, lexical semantic access, and sentence level semantic plausibility [12].

Investigations of semantic dementia and PPA have revealed the major role of the left ATL in labeling of unique and specific entities in all modalities, including auditory (musical passages and famous voices), visual (objects, faces and landmarks), and odors [21]. Both resting state functional MRI (rs-fMRI) and lesion-symptom mapping point to a stronger connectivity of the left ATL with the language network, suggesting inclusion of this area in the language network [22].

Based on current evidence, it seems that comprehension of sentences and words, contrary to old beliefs, are not both processed in the Wernicke's area. Rather, ATL supports comprehension of words, and the extended Wernicke's are seems to support sentence comprehension in conjunction with anterior aspect of Broca's area (Mesulam et al., 2015). As in dorsal pathway, extrasylvian supportive areas interact with the perisylvian semantic system. For example SFG, also plays a role in semantic retrieval [23].

Syntactic processing: As mentioned above, the anterior STG through the UF connects with the posterior Broca's area. This pathway seems to be involved in local phrase structure building. For example construction of a propositional, noun, or verb phrase (PP, NP, and VP). In the sentence: "the boy kicked the ball at the park," "the boy" in an NP, "kicked the ball" is a VP, and "near the tree" is considered a PP. The operation of combining words to make phrases is called *BIND*. Phrases are then combined to form more complex sentences using *MERGE* [18].

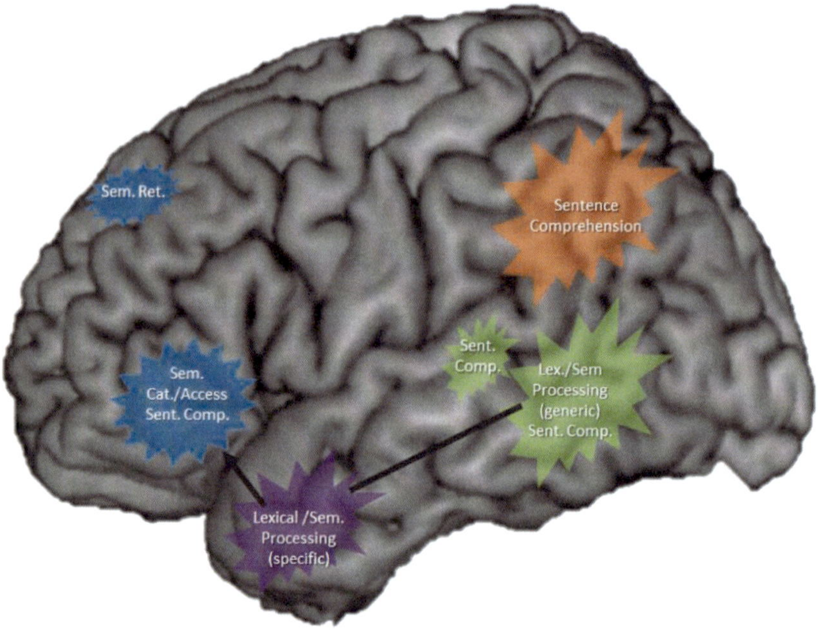

Figure 4. Major cortical areas supporting semantic processing. Sem. Ret. = Semantic retrieval, Setm. Cat. = Semantic category, Sent. Comp. = Sentence comprehension, Lex./Sem. Processing = Lexical/semantic processin.

Functional Neuroanatomy of Reading and Writing

Writing: In general there is a significant overlap between the neural circuitry involved in oral and written production of words and sentences. Based on the dual-route model of written word production, there are two pathways that contribute to writing of words. Motivation to write can originate via activation of a concept in the semantic system or through auditory pathway (writing to dictation). Both the semantic system and the phonological system can provide access to the written form of a word. Semantic system (the ventral pathway) provides the written representation of the "whole word" (lexical approach) based on formed semantic knowledge (orthographic lexicon). The phonological (sublexical) system, however, relies knowledge of sound-to-letter correspondences.

The semantic or lexical route, relies on the left extrasylvian areas such as occipito-temporal cortex, including a portion of the fusiform gyrus known as the visual word form area (VWFA). VWFA may be the neural substrate of orthographic lexicon. Posterior left MTG/ITG, angular gyrus, and anterior temporal lobe, all components of the ventral semantic system, also contribute to the process of lexical pathway of writing.

The phonological or sublexical route, relies on the perisylvian areas such as Broca's area, precentral gyrus, insula, and Wernicke's area and left SMG.

Reading: reading and writing share the same cognitive representations and neural substrates. Therefore aside from motoric processing involved in writing, phonological and semantic pathways recruited for reading involves the same areas mentioned above for writing.

CLINICAL SYNDROMES

Stroke-induced aphasias, the most common form of aphasias, usually present with an acute onset of impairment in production or comprehension of words and sentences. Progressive aphasias, however, have an insidious onset over months or years. The main focus in this chapter is aphasias caused by neurodegenerative diseases, and are therefore progressive. When aphasia is the major clinical presentation and is associated with less prominent impairment in other cognitive domains the aphasia is usually referred to as primary progressive aphasia (PPA). However, when language impairment is less prominent that other cognitive functions the aphasia is referred to as non-primary progressive aphasia (nPPA), and is usually mentioned in conjunction with the primary cognitive syndrome (e.g., behavioral variant frontotemporal dementia syndrome *with* progressive aphasia).

Primary Progressive Aphasia (PPA)

Aphasia secondary to neurodegenerative disease was first described in the 19th century by Pick, Serieux, Franceschi, and Rosenfeld [24]. However, it was not until 1982 when Mesulam characterized the syndrome as an isolated language impairment [25]. PPA usually presents before 65 year of age. Its prevalence is approximately the same across men and women. Aside from some genetic risk factors (see below), it has been seen in men with history of vasectomy, suggesting an autoimmune component [26]. Some individuals with PPA have a family history of learning disability or dyslexia suggesting of cognitive/language vulnerability. This susceptibility seems to be mostly associated with logopenic variant of PPA [27, 28]. It has also been shown that non-right handedness has been associated with semantic variant of PPA [28]. The criteria for the diagnosis of PPA and its variants are discussed below:

Core Criteria

The three core criteria for the diagnosis of PPA include [24, 29]:

7. *Gradual impairment of language*: at lexical level this usually involves difficulty with word finding or word comprehension. Inability to retrieve words can make spontaneous speech "dysfluent" due to word finding pauses. At sentence level, patients may have difficulty with producing sentences with more complex structure, making the utterances short with simplified structure. Language in these patients becomes effortful and non-fluent. As mentioned above, aphasia is a disorder of language, therefore motor speech disorders, such as dysarthria and apraxia do not fulfill this criterion.
8. *Confirmed neurodegenerative etiology*: to fulfill this criterion other causes of aphasia (e.g., neoplasm and stroke) need be ruled out using structural and/or functional neuroimaging.
9. *Prominence of aphasic symptoms*: aphasia should be the prominent part of patient's presentation, and major factor affecting activities of daily living. This can be established through interview with the patient, through peripheral information, and with formal cognitive testing. Recent diagnostic criteria does not specify the duration of isolated language impairment, which used to b 1-2 years [30].

Primary Progressive Aphasia Subtypes

Nonfluent/Agrammatic PPA (PPA-G)

Individuals with PPA-G usually present with an insidious onset of difficulty in words or sentence production with minimal or absent impairment in other areas of cognition. Similar to classic stroke induced Broca's aphasia, they may present as part of a spectrum with a pure impairment in phonological planning, also called primary progressive apraxia of speech (PPAOS), being on one end, and pure agrammatic language output being on the other, with many cases demonstrating both features with different degrees of impairment [29]. The first time PPA-G was classified as a separate entity in the literature was in 1998, where it was called Progressive Non-fluent Aphasia (PNFA), one of three phenotypes of frontotemporal lobar degenerations (FTLDs) [31]. In 2011 consensus paper it was referred to as nonfluent/agrammatic PPA to represent both motor and language impairment. Here our focus is only on language impairment and therefore PPA-G acronym will be used.

At the agrammatic end, similar to stroke-induced Broca's aphasia, PPA-G can be a non-fluent aphasia, which is characterized by decreased production of words per minute (due to prolonged word retrieval) and reduction in mean length of phrases. However, in contrast to stroke-induced Broca's aphasia agrammatism can exist in the absence of non-fluency [32].

This difference between stroke-induced aphasia and PPA is due to differences in variability of cortical atrophy in PPA patients. In stroke-induced aphasic patients the lesion always follows the vascular territory (inferior branch of middle cerebral artery stroke in case of Broca's aphasia), however, in PPA widespread non-overlapping regions have been shown to be involved in impairment of grammatical processing [33]. Many, but not all of these affected regions are in fact the same as ones demonstrated in Figure 3. Therefore an individual with early stage PPA-G may have a fluent language in the presence of agrammatic output and incorrect word order or use of grammatical morphemes.

In PPA-G naming is usually impaired, however, in the mild stages anomia may be very mild or non-existent. Impaired naming is usually due to post-semantic retrieval of names and associated with phonemic paraphasias. Naming of verbs tends to be more impaired that naming of nouns/objects [34]. However, word recognition is usually intact. Repetition is usually abnormal, for more complex sentences first (e.g.: Nick was the boy who carried the box.) and then later for less complex sentences and words. As in Broca's aphasia, comprehension is only impaired for more syntactically complex sentences.

Patients with PPA-G, usually have errors in their written language, which may even precede oral language. Friends or family members may report errors in emails. The clinical picture is that of deep dysgraphia/dyslexia type (e.g., "stool fall," instead of "the stool is falling" on Cookie Theft picture description). As in oral language, agraphia and alexia is usually worse for grammatical morphemes ("-s" plural/third person, or past tense "–ed"), less worse for verbs and least worse for nouns [35]. Impairment in reading/writing is due to disruption of the dorsal language pathway which was described above [36].

Semantic PPA (PPA-S)

Individuals with PPA-S usually present with insidious onset of difficulty with object naming. During the prodromal phase, aside from mild difficulty with object naming there is no other language impairment. Hence, word and sentence comprehension are intact. Language output is fluent and grammatical. During this period since word recognition is not impaired the term anomic PPA may fit the clinical picture better (PPA-A) [37]. Over time anomia becomes progressively worse causing profound impairment in object naming and impairment in word recognition start to emerge. This picture is referred to as the PPA-S syndrome. Other areas of language processing remain intact. In contrast to PPA-G, in this group of patients, anomia is mostly due to difficulty with naming concrete nouns, such as names of animals, fruits, and vegetables. Interestingly ability to comprehend sentences remains intact until very late stages of the disease. This is due to involvement of ATL earlier in the disease and that of extended Wernicke's area and frontal semantic regions, later in the course. The patient may be able to answer to a sentence "Why should virtuous people be rewarded?", but has tremendous difficulty understanding what "lion" is [38]. This seems to be due to "taxonomic interference," where words are recognized and objects are named at a generic, but not specific level. Communication usually consists of semantic paraphasias (versus phonemic paraphasias in PPA-G) and circumlocutions, which make the speech content impoverished. It is important to note that individuals with PPA-S, in contrast to individuals with semantic dementia, do not have difficulty with object or face recognition. A PPA-S patient with severe naming and word recognition difficulty may still be able to use tools in a workshop with no problem.

Patients with PPA-S may have degrees of surface dyslexia/dysgraphia due to disruption in the ventral language pathway involved in reading and writing of irregular words as mentioned above [36].

Logopenic PPA (PPA-L)

Individuals with PPA-L usually experience an insidious onset of difficulty with word finding which makes their language output dysfluent. This happens in the absence of overt impairment in grammar and comprehension. Impaired fluency becomes evident especially if the patient tries to access a less familiar, or less frequent word. Speech output consists of many circumlocutions as the patient tries to "talk around" the word. Object naming is usually abnormal, however, compared to PPA-S it is milder. Attempts to name an object may elicit phonemic paraphasias. During the early, prodromal stage object naming may be absent, while number of words per minute and mean length of utterance, and semantic fluency is diminished. This points to the notion that "internal naming" may have a different mechanism than "sensory-based" naming. During the initial stages of PPA-L patients have difficulty with "internal" word generation.

Abnormal repetition has been included as a major criterion for the clinical diagnosis of PPA-L. However, based on localization of atrophy repetition may not be present in some patients [39, 40]. Comprehension syntax can be impaired in patients with PPA-L and the degree of impairment may be more severe than patients with PPA-G as the atrophy affects the posterior aspect of the syntax network [41].

Patients with PPA-L may have associated cognitive findings. Cortical atrophy within the left temporoparietal regions may cause impairment in calculation, working memory, writing, finger gnosis and left-right orientation. Therefore association with a full or partial Gerstmann syndrome is possible [36]. Higher incidence of impairment in memory tasks and limb praxis has also been reported [42].

Non-Primary Progressive Aphasia (nPPA)

In neurodegenerative diseases the disease usually starts from one network and damages that network. With progression, the disease progresses to involve other networks in parallel to the primary one. For example, Alzheimer disease typically starts in hippocampus and entorhinal cortex and presents with a primary amnestic syndrome. With time the disease progresses to involve other cognitive networks such as language. The aphasia in this setting is not primary and therefore the clinical syndrome has a form of an amnestic cognitive impairment (or dementia), in conjunction with progressive aphasia. Aphasia can likewise happen in patients who are primarily affected by other syndromes, such as frontotemporal dementia syndrome, or progressive supranuclear syndrome, or posterior cortical atrophy syndrome. The importance of recognition of nPPAs is mostly with regard to planning of speech and language interventions, as the primary syndrome needs to be taken into account by the speech and language pathologist who plans rehabilitation interventions as discussed later in this chapter.

PROGNOSIS AND TEMPORAL PATTERNS OF PROGRESSION

With progression not only language decline worsens, but also disintegration of additional cognitive domains start to emerge. Therefore designation of PPA-plus (PPA+) is usually used to describe the advanced stages. Aphasia may not be the major cause of distress during the advanced phase. There is some evidence to suggest that progression may happen faster in women [43].

In patients with PPA-S, atrophy usually spreads to the anterior insula, posterior orbitofrontal cortex and contralateral anterior temporal lobe. These changes can lead to the new symptoms of abnormal behaviors and associative agnosias. Combination of agnosia and aphasic syndrome at this time qualifies for the diagnosis of semantic dementia.

Spread of atrophy in PPA-G usually takes course towards dorsolateral prefrontal cortex, motor areas, and basal ganglia and leads additional deficit in executive functions, motor speech, or movement disorders that are characteristic of dysexecutive, speech apraxia, corticobasal, and progressive supranuclear palsy syndrome.

Progression of atrophy in PPA-L can take two courses. Expansion of atrophy through the dorsal language pathway results in a PPA-G syndrome with further worsening resembling that of PPA-G course. In contrast trajectory of atrophy through the ventral pathway results in a syndrome resembling PPA-S and follows the PPA-S route of decline. In a few patients, especially those with Alzheimer disease, the PPA-L pattern persists for many years [24, 38].

CLINICAL APPROACH TO DIAGNOSIS OF PROGRESSIVE APHASIA

A systematic approach to aphasic symptoms can make the clinical diagnosis of aphasia much easier. To determine a specific aphasic syndrome in a in patient with stroke-induced aphasia, this systematic approach usually starts with evaluation of object/picture naming and then assessment of spontaneous speech [44]. As a degenerative disease with different pathophysiology, PPA challenges this approach. In patients with PPA-L, while language output is non-fluent, and the patient has obvious difficulty with word finding and "logopenia," object/picture naming may not be a sensitive test to evaluate language. Also, based on localization of the disease, agrammatism in PPA-G may or may not be associated with non-fluent language output. Impaired syntax has been shown to be associated with abnormality in the arcuate fasciculus, while impaired fluency seems to be associated with abnormality of the aslant tract [45]. A more practical approach [37] is to start the evaluation with following order: word recognition/comprehension→ spontaneous speech (to assess fluency and grammaticality) → Repetition → Object/picture naming → Lexical and semantic fluency, also known as generative naming (Figure 5).

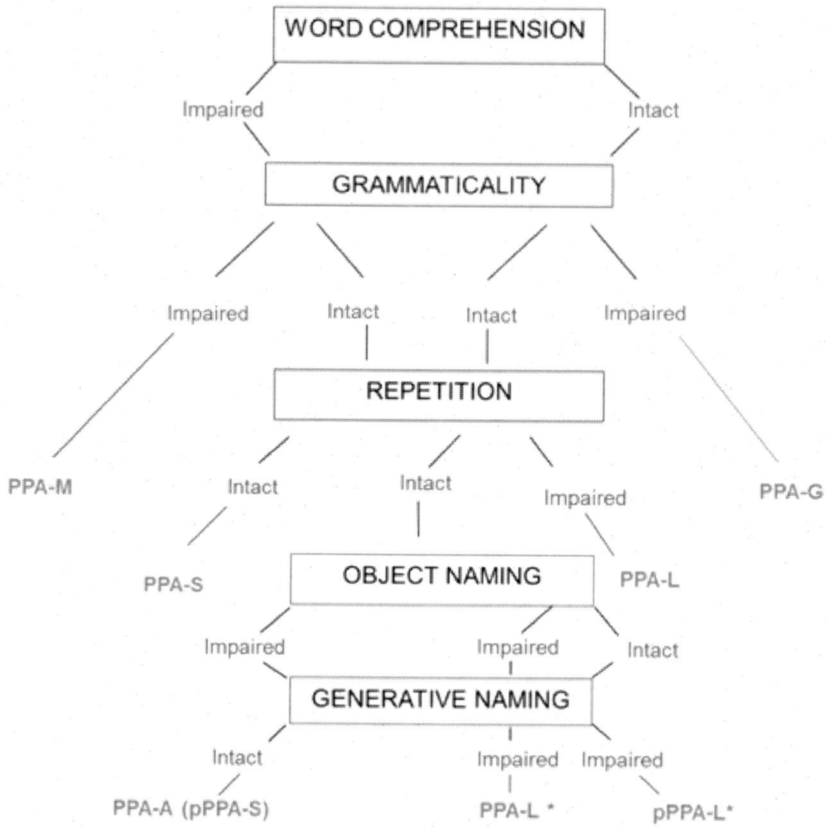

Figure 5. Algorithmic approach to clinical diagnosis of different PPA syndromes. Based on Mesulam et al. (2012) with modifications. PPA-A = Anomic variant of PPA, pPPA-S = prodromal PPA-S. PPA-L* = PPA-L without impaired repetition. pPPA-L = prodromal PPA-L.

Word Comprehension

To evaluate word comprehension in a neurology clinic, the clinician can ask the patient to describe familiar (e.g., elephant), or less familiar (e.g., illumination) words. Also a set of toy animals, tools, fruits, and vegetables can be used to test recognition of these items when their name is provided. Patients with PPA-S, in contrast with PPA-G and PPA-L, have difficulty with describing the words and may not be able to match a given word with the actual object. More detailed evaluation can be performed by a speech-language pathologist (SLP), a neuropsychologist, or for research purposes using the Peabody Picture Vocabulary Test (PPVT) [37, 39, 46].

Spontaneous Speech, Fluency, and Grammaticality

In a neurology clinic, grammaticality can be tested by qualitative evaluation of spontaneous speech, and with direct testing. Spontaneous speech can be evaluated as the clinician converses with the patient about their disease and their current activities and knowledge of news. Cognitively intact individuals have a verbal fluency of 130 ± 20 words per minute (WPM), and their mean length of utterance (MLU) is usually 11.11 ± 0.56 phonemes. In patients with impaired fluency (PPA-G and PPA-L) there is a significant drop in both WPM, and MLU (PPA-G>PPA-L).

Grammaticality of spontaneous speech can be qualitatively evaluated by paying specific attention to usage of verbs, ability to assign words such as subject, object and indirect object to verbs, and usage of verb inflections, all of which are impaired in PPA-G. Also, both patients with PPA-G and PPA-L produce grammatically less complex sentences [47].

A well-researched picture to elicit spontaneous speech is the "Cookie Theft" picture from Boston Diagnostic Aphasia Exam [48]. Nearly all neurologists have this picture as a part of National Institute of Health Stroke Scale (NIHSS) tool kit [49, 50]. Healthy individuals are able to produce 13-24 phrases (called "content units"), while describing the Cookie Theft picture [44, 51]. Individuals with aphasia will have reduced number of correct content units (PPA-S>PPA-L>PPA-G), and impaired MLU (PPA-G>PPA-L>PPA-S).

To directly test the ability to make grammatical sentences the Sentence Production Priming Test (SPPT) of the Northwestern Assessment of Verbs and Sentences (NAVS), can be used in a clinical setting. After presenting a picture of a dog chasing a cat, the patient is asked to produce the following non-canonical sentences after probing the structure [52]:

a. The cat is chased by the dog. (prime: The dog is chased by the cat.)
b. Who is the dog chasing? (prime: Who is the cat chasing?)
c. Pete saw the cat who the dog is chasing. (prime: Pete saw the dog who the cat is chasing.)

In patients with severely diminished verbal output an anagram test can be used. Using this test the clinician presents the patient with single words that are printed on a card, then the clinician asks the patient to form sentences with different syntactic complexity by showing relevant pictures [53].

More detailed evaluation can be performed by an SLP, or neuropsychologist, or for research purposes using the full version of Northwestern Assessment of Verbs and Sentences [52], the full Northwestern Anagram Test [53], and Western Aphasia Battery (WAB) picture description [54].

Repetition

To screen for an impairment in repetition the clinician may use a structurally, or phonologically difficult sentence ("Nelson Rockefeller had a Lincoln Continental," or a sentence with an object relative clause: "Ally saw the cat that the dog was chasing yesterday"). If the patient is not able to repeat these sentences, syntactically less difficult sentences can be used, such as a sentence with subject relative clause "Ally saw the dog that was chasing the dog yesterday," which is more complex than a passive voice ("the cat was being chased by the dog"). If still impaired, this can be follow up by a canonical sentence such as "the dog chased the cat," "the dog barked" or a noun phrase: "the dog," or a single word: "dog."

Impaired repetition is the hallmark of PPA-L syndrome due to abnormal auditory/phonological working memory. Although not a criterion for research diagnosis of PPA-G, patients with PPA-G may also have difficulty with repetition due to impairment of executive aspect of repetition, and processing of closed-class function words such as "if," "but," etc. [30].

Naming

Object/Picture Naming

In a clinic setting, short form of Boston Naming Test (BNT) can be used to evaluate picture naming. It consists of 15 pictures that are organized in order of decreasing frequency. In case the patient is not able to name the picture, each picture is associated with four word options that that patient can choose from [55]. Attention to the patient's paraphasias and their ability to recognize the word from a list, can help the clinician understand the cognitive deficit underlying anomia.

Due to interaction between different networks involved in naming, patients from different subtypes of PPA may have deficit in both pre-semantic and post-semantic levels of word retrieval [56, 57]. However, in patient with PPA-G, paraphasic errors are usually of phonemic type (phoneme substitution) pointing to a post-semantic retrieval deficit. To avoid misdiagnosis of anomia, it is important to rule out motor speech impairments such as apraxia and dysarthrias. Pure motor speech impairments are almost never associated with phonemic paraphasias.

In PPA-L patients, similar to patients with Dementia of the Alzheimer Type (DAT), anomia is due to both pre- and post- semantic deficits [58]. They have difficulty retrieving the word due to impoverished semantic knowledge (lemma level failure), and also due to inability to select the correct form of the word (lexeme level failure) [59]. Therefore phonemic, semantic and circumlocutory paraphasias are evident.

Patients with PPA-S cannot name objects or comprehend the name of the same objects. In this case the naming deficit is described as having a "two-way" deficit. In many cases, they may just say that they do not know what the object is. To avoid misdiagnosis of anomia, it is important to rule out visual agnosia when evaluating picture naming.

Lexical and Semantic Fluency (Generative Naming)

As mentioned above, in milder cases of PPA-G and PPA-L, object/picture naming may not be impaired. In such cases evaluation of lexical and semantic fluency (generative naming), in addition to analysis of spontaneous speech can be helpful. To evaluate lexical (or phonological) fluency, the patient is asked to produce as many words they can in a minute, that start with a certain letter (for example F, A, or S, hence the name FAS test). For semantic fluency, the patient is asked to produce as many words as possible, in a minute that belongs to a certain semantic category such as animals, vegetables, etc. Depending upon age and education, an older adult is able to produce an average of about 14 ± 2 for the lexical and 18 ± 5 for the semantic fluency [60]. Both tests depend on frontal executive, and attention abilities, with semantic fluency requiring access to the semantic knowledge available through the temporal lobe cortex. Therefore semantic fluency is more impaired in PPA-L, and lexical fluency is more impaired in PPA-G. In the presence of a frontal network impairment, these tests may not be as reliable in detecting a language deficit.

Reading and Writing

To evaluate patient's ability to read words and sentences, NIHSS toolkit can be used. NIHSS words and sentences are organized in order of increasing complexity. Before final interpretation of the patient's performance, however, the clinician ought to rule out visual impairment. If the patient is unable to read aloud, written "yes/no" questions can be used. Assessment of reading by having the patient read a command such as "close your eyes" must be interpreted with caution. In this case, the clinician should ensure that praxis is intact [61].

Progressive aphasic patients with involvement of ventral language pathway show signs of surface dyslexia due to involvement of the left temporo-occipital area, fusiform gyrus and the visual word from area. In this case, a patient with PPA-L or PPA-S, has difficulty with reading irregular words such as "yacht," or "choir." Impairment is worse for less frequent word. Unable to read the word, the patient may try to read the word by simply spelling out the word letter by letter, a phenomenon called "letter-by-letter reading."

In patients with PPA-G and PPA-L patient may have more difficulty with reading regular words, as phenomenon called "deep dyslexia." In this case the pathway for grapheme to phoneme conversion is disrupted. The best way to evaluate deep dyslexia is to ask the patient to read a word without a meaning (a pseudoword, such as "larter"), to avoid assistance from the ventral language pathway. In patients with PPA-G written language will have the same errors as oral language with errors in using of grammatical functors, more difficulty with reading verbs and errors with reading grammatical morphemes (e.g., –ed, -ing, etc.) [11].

Impairments in writing usually parallel impairments in reading. To evaluate writing however, the clinician must rule out hand apraxia (apraxic agraphia) and non-apraxic disorders of motor execution.

Imaging and Laboratory Investigations: Role of Biomarkers to Determine Underlying Pathology

Neurodegenerative diseases are the most common underlying cause of PPA. Among neurodegenerative diseases Alzheimer disease (AD) and Frontotemporal lobar degeneration (FTLD) pathologies such as Pick's disease, corticobasal degeneration pathology (CBDp), progressive supranuclear pathology (PSPp), seem to be the most common culprits [62]. The remaining cases have been found to be caused by either rare neurodegenerative disease, such as leukoencephalopathy [63], or more than one neurodegenerative pathology such as combined AD and Lewy body pathologies [64]. Primary rapidly progressive aphasia due to prion disease (Creutzfeldt Jakob disease) has been reported [65]. Also infiltrative left hemisphere white matter tumors, unilateral left hemisphere meningiomas, or progressive vasculitides (e.g., sarcoidosis, or Behcet's disease) can potentially cause a syndrome of primary progressive aphasia.

Among the neurodegenerative causes, Alzheimer pathology accounts for the etiology of PPA in about 60% of PPA-L cases [38, 39]. Other cases are caused by FTLD-Tau (Pick, CBDp, PSPp), or FTLD-TDP A or B pathologies. About 60% of patients with PPA-G are found to have FTLD-tau pathology (Pick, CBDp, PSPp), with the remaining patients having Alzheimer (20%) or FTLD-TDP types A or B (20%) pathology [24, 32]. Almost all cases of PPA-S seem to have FTLD-TDP type C pathology. Due to this overlapping pattern of underlying pathology, except for PPA-S, there is no pathognomonic phenotype for PPA syndromes. Therefore accurate diagnosis of the underlying cause will require biomarker information [24, 38]. Major available biomarkers include imaging, cerebrospinal fluid (CSF) analysis and genetic studies, which will be discussed below. Electroencephalography has not been studied as a biomarker, however, it will be discussed given its common use in clinical neurological work up.

Neuroimaging: Topographical or Progression Biomarkers

Such as other areas of neurology, the next step following formulation of an aphasic syndrome is to determine the anatomical localization of the disease based on the clinical syndrome. Along with meticulous clinical and neuropsychological evaluation neuroimaging findings can increase diagnostic certainty of PPA and help with accurate subtyping, identification of the underlying pathology, and ultimately treatment planning. It is also an important component of research investigating changes in the speech-language network in patients with PPA [66]. Both structural and functional imaging assess the localization of pathology and are therefore called "topographical biomarkers." [67] Changes in brain structural and functional anatomy happen very close to progression of symptoms, and therefore neuroimaging biomarkers are also called "progression biomarkers." All axial images that follow are in radiological orientation, with right side of the image corresponding to the left side of the patient.

Structural Imaging

In a right handed individual, the major gross pathologic hallmark of PPA is asymmetric (typically left greater than right) perisylvian atrophy. Both computed tomography (CT) and magnetic resonance imaging (MRI) scans can be used to evaluate degree of volume loss. Mesulam (1982) reported CT scan evidence of a larger frontal horn and sylvian fissure in the left hemisphere in his first case series. Since then many studies have followed, describing more detailed characteristics of the atrophy in PPA using CT and MRI scans. As compared to brain CT scans, MRI scans have a higher sensitivity for detection of the asymmetric atrophy of PPA. Figure 6 demonstrates CT scan findings of a patient who presented with PPA-G. Sinnatamby and colleagues studied 12 patients with PPA using brain CT and MRI scans and showed a sensitivity of 50% for CT scans as opposed to 83% for MRI scans [68]. Since sensitivity of CT scan is low, its use is typically limited to cases where brain MRI is contraindicated (e.g., in patients with pacemaker).

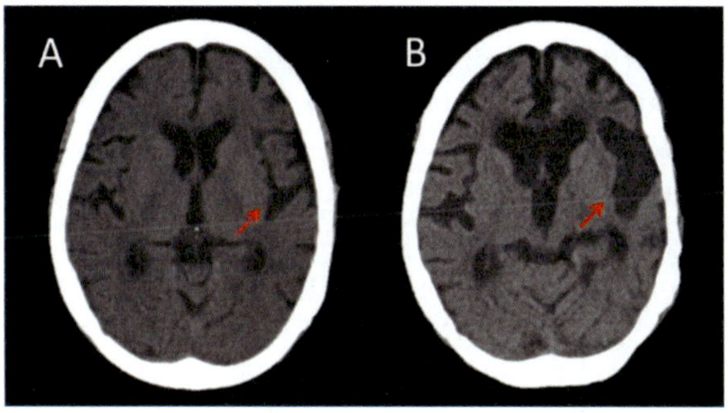

Figure 6. Brain CT scan for a 70 year old woman with PPA, demonstrating left perisylvian atrophy. A) At the time of diagnosis. Red arrow points to the left perisylvian atrophy. B) Scan from 9 years later shows worsening of atrophy in the bifrontal and perisylvian areas (left > right). At this time the patient additional behavioral changes (PPA+ syndrome).

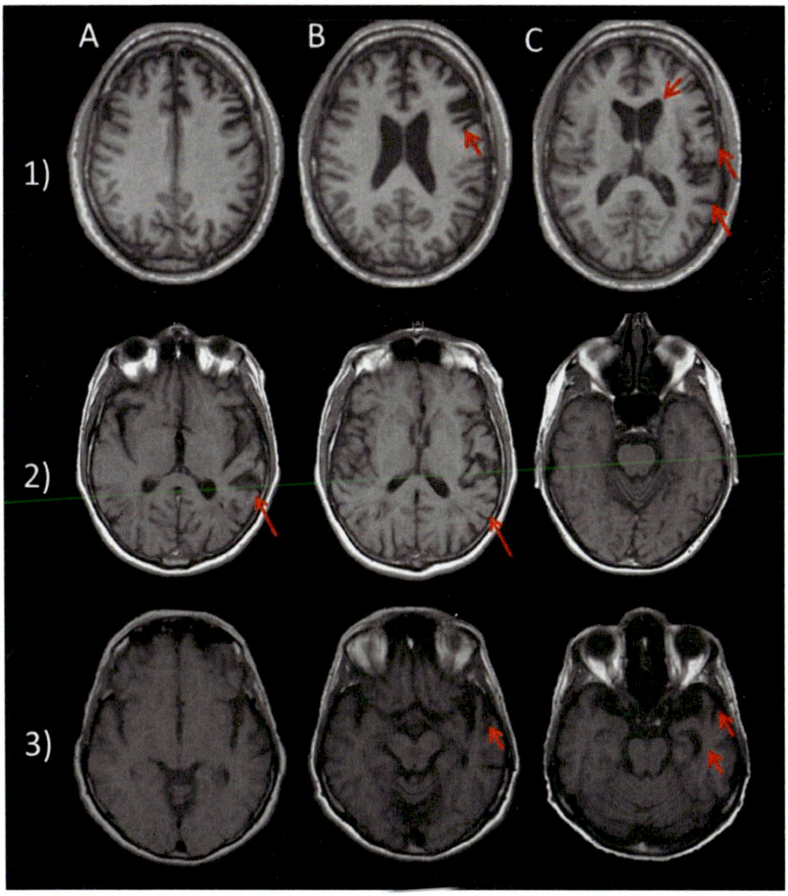

Figure 7. Structural brain MRIs from patients with PPA. Red arrows point to areas of cortical atrophy. 1) PPA-G: red arrows point to atrophy in the left IFG, MFG, and TPJ. Note the ex-vacuo dilatation of the frontal horn of the left lateral ventricle. 2) PPA-L: red arrows point to atrophy in the left STG and supramarginal gyrus. 3) PPA-S: red arrows point to atrophy in the left ATL. Note the severity of atrophy and that the atrophy is more prominent in the anterior aspects of the MTG and ITG. Atrophy has also caused ex-vacuo widening of the temporal horn of the left lateral ventricle.

Thanks to advances in brain volumetric measurements in the 2000s, several research groups have demonstrated that the distribution of atrophy in different subtypes of PPA follows a specific pattern that corresponds to unique patterns of speech-language deficits [41, 46]. The pattern of atrophy in three PPA syndromes are as follows: 1) peak atrophy for PPA-G mostly affects the left inferior frontal gyrus (IFG) and the left temporoparietal junction (TPJ). Atrophy can also be seen in the left premotor cortex; 2) in PPA-L patients, atrophy is more significant in the left TPJ and the left fusiform gyrus (FG). Atrophy can also be seen in left posterior STG and MTG; and 3) PPA-S patients have atrophy in the left anterior temporal lobe (ATL). Figure 7 features structural brain MRIs from patients with PPA. One patient from each PPA subtype and specific areas of atrophy are demonstrated.

Knowledge of patterns of atrophy can increase diagnosis certainty of different PPA subtypes, especially in cases where clinical presentation is less clear, or unclassifiable [69]. Structural MRI also can also be used as a progression biomarker for the progression of disease and to guide the design and evaluating effectiveness of therapeutic interventions. Rogalski and colleagues have demonstrated that, over a period of 2 years, cortical atrophy spreads beyond the initial unique syndromic distributions, with convergence of three major areas of volume loss: IFG, TPJ and lateral temporal cortex [70]. However, as shown in Figure 5, progression of atrophy will favor the left hemisphere [71].

Functional Imaging

SPECT Scan

For a patient with PPA, functional imaging is usually used when structural imaging fails to demonstrate atrophy within the language network [68]. Single-Photon Emission Tomography (SPECT) is based on measurement of regional cerebral blood flow (rCBF) using radiotracers such as Technetium (e.g., 99mTc-hexamethylpropylene amine oxime, or HMPAO).

In PPA, there is a decline in rCBF of the structures within the language network and this pattern can be observed in SPECT images [72-74].

FDG-PET Scan

Positron Emission Tomography (PET) is a functional imaging technique based on measurement of emissions from an injected radiotracer. The most common tracer in clinical practice is Fludeoxyglucose, hence the name FDG-PET (75). FDG is taken in by nerve cells and concentrations of tracer detected by the scanner correlate with metabolic activity of brain tissue. In PPA patients, there is asymmetric reduction of metabolism due to decreased language network metabolism [68, 76-78]. As in structural imaging, each of the three variants of PPA have a unique pattern of decreased metabolism. Location of hypometabolism is within the left parieto-temporal region in PPA-L, within the left ATL region in PPA-S, and within the left frontal lobe in PPA-G [79]. Figure 8 depicts the FDG-PET images from a patient who presented with 2 year history of word finding difficulty. Her word fluency was impaired, especially her lexical fluency, and she had paraphasias in spontaneous speech. Her brain MRI was unremarkable, and therefore an FDG-PET was obtained to objectively determine the localization of brain dysfunction. FDG-PET in her case showed left frontal hypometabolism, a pattern usually seen in PPA-G. Rabinovici and colleagues demonstrated that FDG-PET has an 81% accuracy to diagnose Alzheimer disease, i.e., 81% of patients with an Alzheimer pattern on FDG-PET are found to have underlying AD neuropathology on autopsy [80]. Therefor FDG-PET needs to be combined with other biomarkers such as CSF analysis, amyloid PET, or genetic biomarkers to increase diagnostic certainty of the underlying cause.

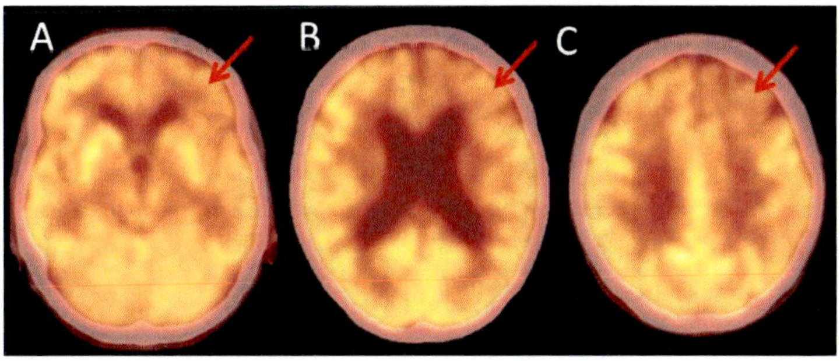

Figure 8. FDG-PET scan of a 73 year old woman who presented with word finding difficulty. Scan shows decreased metabolism in the left IFG and dorsolateral frontal cortex. A pattern seen in PPA-G.

fMRI

Both PET scans and functional MRI (fMRI) can be used to study activity within the language network during linguistic tasks. fMRI relies on changes in blood oxygen level in response to a cognitive task. With the advent of resting state functional imaging, examination of the language network has become possible at rest, i.e., task-free [81]. Compared to PET scan, fMRI is less costly and does not involve injection of a tracer. It therefore has gained popularity over PET scanning for investigation of the physiology of the language network. Currently, fMRI is used to localize "eloquent" cortex for neurosurgical planning [82]. For PPA patients however, it has primarily been used for research purposes with the hope of incorporation into clinical practice in the near future. The purpose of fMRI studies of PPA is, broadly, to examine changes in the speech-language network, to determine compensatory mechanisms through which the brain copes with these changes, and to use the information to plan neuromodulatory treatment and measure effectiveness of therapeutic interventions.

Functional imaging has demonstrated that pathophysiology of language impairment extends beyond the localization of atrophy. Also, unlike patients with stroke-induced aphasia, the region affected by atrophy is not completely dead. Investigating knowledge of homonymous versus synonymous words in a group of PPA-L patients, Sonty and colleagues showed that the atrophied area did in fact show evidence of activation during the task [83]. Their abnormal performance on the language task was therefore found to be due to activation of areas that are abnormally activated (superior parietal sulcus and precentral gyrus), and also due to reduced connectivity of areas that are normally involved in language processing [84]. Wilson et al. showed the same phenomenon of redundant activation [85] in patients with PPA-S and surface dyslexia. Information of this kind can help with planning of treatment with neuromodulatory interventions such as repetitive transcortical magnetic stimulation which will be discussed below.

Although still investigational, there is hope that fMRI may ultimately be used in clinical practice for measurement of treatment effects and predicting network responsivity to speech therapy interventions. For example, we demonstrated that fMRI can unravel the network changes induced by a semantically based intervention that facilitated naming in a logopenic patient. Effects of treatment at the neural level were documented via fMRI, showing recruitment of left dorsolateral prefrontal cortex (DLFPC) during naming tasks (Figure 9) [86].

During the past few years a growing number research has underlined the usefulness of resting state fMRI (rs-fMRI), a task-free from of fMRI, as a potential biomarker to track disease progression in neurodegenerative disease [87, 88]. Comparison of structural and functional imaging as progression biomarkers has shown that depending on different areas of the brain one may precede the other one [89-91]. This has practical implications, as in different stages of the disease the choice of biomarkers may be different. For example, we have shown that in a group of patients with early stages of PPA-G in the absence of significant atrophy on structural brain MRI, rs-fMRI is abnormal (Figure 10), proving it to be a leading indicator of progression and a more appropriate biomarker to measure treatment responsivity in early stages of the disease [92].

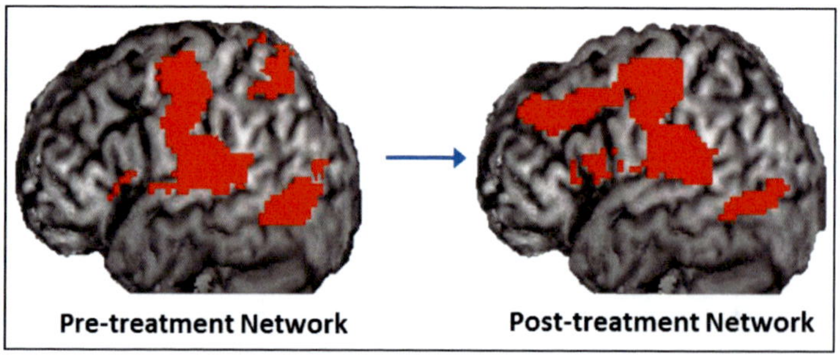

Figure 9. fMRI maps of the main effect of picture naming in a patient with PPA-L before and after receiving semantic based naming treatment. The right picture shows how successful treatment was associated with recruitment of left DLPFC and also Broca's area, both areas are involved in naming.

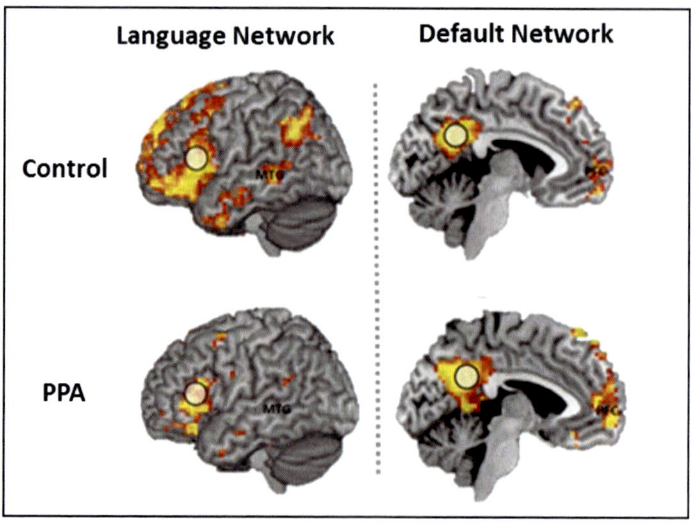

Figure 10. rs-fMRI maps showing resting state functional connectivity of the left IFG seed, the posterior cingulate seen (PCC) with the rest of the brain. While the default networks shows no change in its connectivity with the PCC see, in PPA patients, there is significant decline in the connectivity of IFG seed and the language network.

Figure 11 summarizes use of neuroimaging for topographical detection of site of atrophy in persons with PPA.

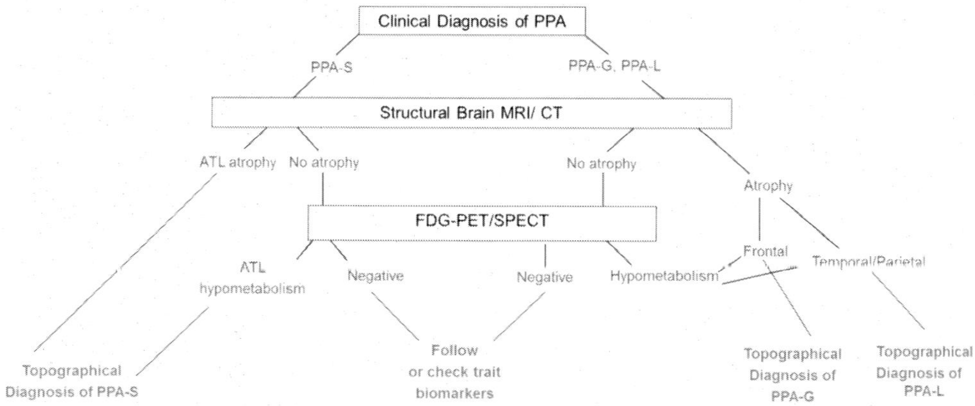

Figure 11. Algorithmic approach to topographical diagnosis of PPA variants using structural (MRI, CT) or functional (PET, SPECT) neuroimaging.

Electroencephalography (EEG): A Possible Physiologic Biomarker

A vast majority of patients with PPA show evidence of asymmetric slowing of the left hemisphere on EEG [93]. Although EEG has never been used as a biomarker in PPA patients, since EEG is commonly used in clinical neurology, knowledge of this asymmetric slowing is important while interpreting EEG data (Figure 12).

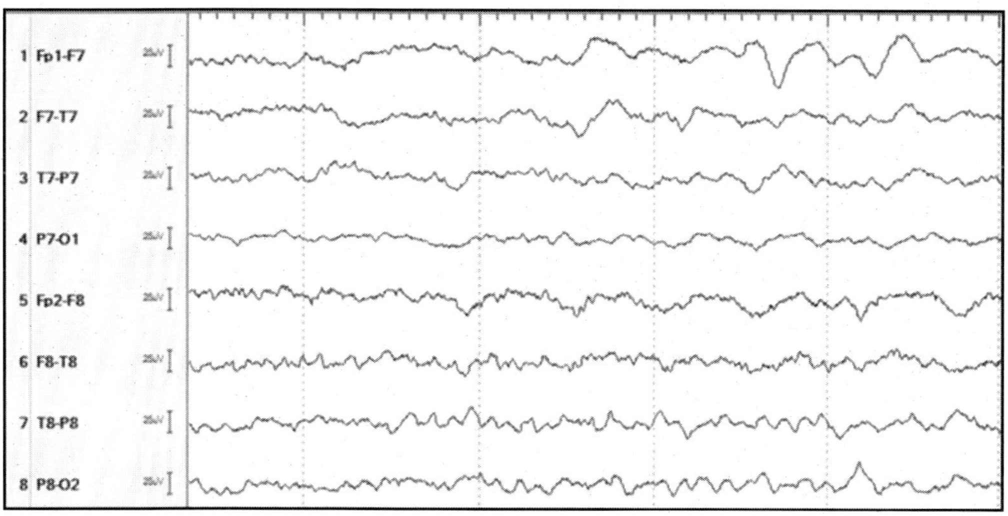

Figure 12. EEG tracing of a 75 year old patient PPA-L+. EEG shows asymmetric slowing of the left hemisphere (leads 1-4) as compared to right hemisphere leads (5-8).

Etiologic or State Biomarkers

Knowledge of the pathologic entity is important for decisions regarding pharmacological treatment of PPA. It also may have prognostic value with regard to the course of the disease and changes in clinical manifestations over time. For example, in most patients with AD pathology, grammar and comprehension remain less affected relative to the progressive impairment in naming [39].

Ligand-Based PET Biomarkers

Currently diagnosis of underlying disease using ligand-based PET scan is only clinically available for Alzheimer disease. About 45% of patients with PPA have underlying Alzheimer pathology or ADp [32]. Therefore it is worthwhile to rule out underlying ADp in all patients. In only one instance, PPA-S with typical left ventropolar ATL atrophy, the underlying pathology is usually FTLD-TDP43 type C and therefore CSF may not be indicated. However, it should be noted that there have been reports of patients with semantic dementia secondary to Alzheimer disease [94].

Amyloid PET scan: A major biochemical breakthrough in 2000's has been the introduction of a tracer that can bind to amyloid plaques in brains of patients with Alzheimer disease. This tracer, which is a neutrally charged benzothiazole derived from thioflavin T, was called the Pittsburgh compound B and the related PET scan was referred to as PiB PET [95]. The PiB tracer, however, has a half-life of about 20 minutes, limiting its feasibility and utility in clinical settings. To improve tracer durability, Wong and colleagues (2010) developed a different compound, Florbetapir, a radiotracer containing the radionuclide Fluorine-18. Florbetapir has a longer half-life (110 minutes) and stays longer in the brain, allowing for more accumulation [96]. It also survives longer, providing increased opportunity for the tracer to be transferred from cyclotron to imaging center. The Food and Drug Administration (FDA) approved Florbetapir PET scanning [97, 98] in 2011 and, since then, it has been clinically available for diagnosis of Alzheimer neuropathology.

Using amyloid PET scans, distribution of amyloid plaques can be demonstrated and Alzheimer disease can be diagnosed as the underlying neuropathology, especially in patients younger than 65 years old. With advanced age, specificity of the amyloid PET scan drops, as normal older adults may have positive scans [99]. Although amyloid PET can determine the presence of AD pathology in PPA, it is unknown whether the distribution of amyloid accumulation follows the distribution of hypometabolism seen on FDG-PET [79]. Leyton and colleagues (2011), in a study of PPA subtypes, showed that 92% of individuals with PPA-L had positive beta-amyloid uptake. In contrast, 11% of PPA-S and 25% of PPA-G individuals had a positive scan [100]. Currently, amyloid PET diagnosis of AD pathology is reported as positive or negative, without sensitivity in measuring amyloid load in different areas of the brain (Figure 13). Future research will focus on quantification of amyloid burden in different brain areas, and, in cases of PPA, within the left hemisphere speech-language network [101]. Amyloid PET has about 92% accuracy for diagnosis of AD pathology [80]. When despite of a clinical diagnosis the result is inconclusive, combination of other biomarkers such as CSF analysis or topographical or genetic biomarkers may increase diagnosis certainty of the underlying cause.

Tau PET scan ([18F] T807 PET scan): Very recently, a new PET ligand, [18F] T807, has been introduced, which binds to Tau pathology in FTLD patients, including patients with PPA.

Preliminary case reports of scans in patients with PPA with known mutations for FTLD-Tau have shown promising results [102]. Further research will reveal whether this ligand is sensitive and specific for diagnosis of tau neuropathology.

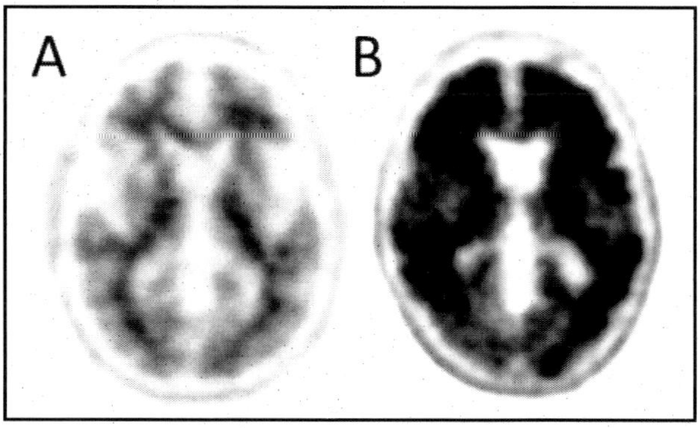

Figure 13. Flobetapir PET scan. A) Normal scan showing Flobetapir distribution in the white matter (black). The border between cortex (white) and subcortical areas (black and gray) can be distinguished. B) Abnormal scan in a 75 year old woman (same patient as in Figure 11) with PPA-L+ demonstrating abnormal activity within the cortical gray matter (black), with loss of the usual gray-white contrast. The findings are consistent with increased beta-amyloid plaque density (positive scan). Note that the scan does not demonstrate the density of the beta-amyloid plaque in different brain regions.

Cerebrospinal Fluid Biomarkers

Cerebrospinal fluid (CSF) provides an excellent source of biomarkers for diseases underlying PPA [62]. Their major contribution to clinical management of patients with PPA is to help with medication selection (see below) and to increase diagnostic certainty for future inclusion of interested individuals in clinical trials.

Currently the only clinically available CSF biomarker is that of Alzheimer disease. Many studies have demonstrated a CSF biochemical profile that is highly associated with an underlying Alzheimer pathology. In Alzheimer disease there is an elevation in CSF levels of phosphorylated tau at its 181 phosphorylation site (p-tau$_{181}$), and a drop in CSF levels of beta-amyloid$_{42}$ peptide [103]. The actual cut off points are different according to different laboratory standards. The combination of tau and beta-amyloid profile is usually presented as the "amyloid/tau index," or ATI. Based on different reports a sensitivity of up to 90-95% and a specificity of 86-95% has been reported for an ATI <0.8 [104, 105]. The lower the ATI the most likely is the presence of Alzheimer pathology. In one study, a low ATI is usually a more robust measure for diagnosis of AD when it is associated with a beta-amyloid$_{42}$ level $\leq$445 pg/ml *and* a p-tau$_{181}$ level >61 pg/ml [106]. An ATI>1.2 has a 95% specificity to rule out Alzheimer disease and differentiate it from FTLD [105].

Panel in Figure 14 demonstrates interpretation of different CSF biomarker profiles based on ATI and p-tau$_{181}$ levels. Once challenging circumstance is when the values are in the "inconclusive" range, or within the borderline zone between different patterns (small broken lines in the panel). Patients in these groups may or may not have Alzheimer disease. In such cases a way to increase diagnostic certainty is to combine CSF results with topographical biomarkers. In case where p-tau_{181} is not elevated enough to make the diagnosis, tau-ligand PET will help with differentiation of AD and FTLD cases. Similarly in cases where beta-$amyloid_{42}$ is not abnormal an amyloid PET scan may be helpful to differentiate AD from FTLD.

Research on CSF biomarkers of FTLDs is still ongoing and these biomarkers are not yet available for clinical use: Reduced ratio of p-tau_{181} to total tau (p/t tau) has been shown to be associated with FTLDs in three cohorts. Reduced p/t ratio is more pronounced for patients with FTLD-TDP than the ones with FTLD-tau, likely due to more rapid neurodegeneration that does not allow phosphorylation of tau [107]. To differentiate FTLD-tau from FTLD-TDP two other biomarkers have shown promise: Fatty Acid Binding Protein 4 (FABP4), and YKL-40 (a marker of inflammation). Both of these biomarkers are elevated in FTLD-tau (108). Other candidate biomarkers for FTLD-TDP disease include tripeptidyl peptidase-1 (TPP1) enzyme (decreased in patients with progranulin mutation), IL-7 cytokine (increased in patients with progranulin mutation), and TDP43 oligomers [107].

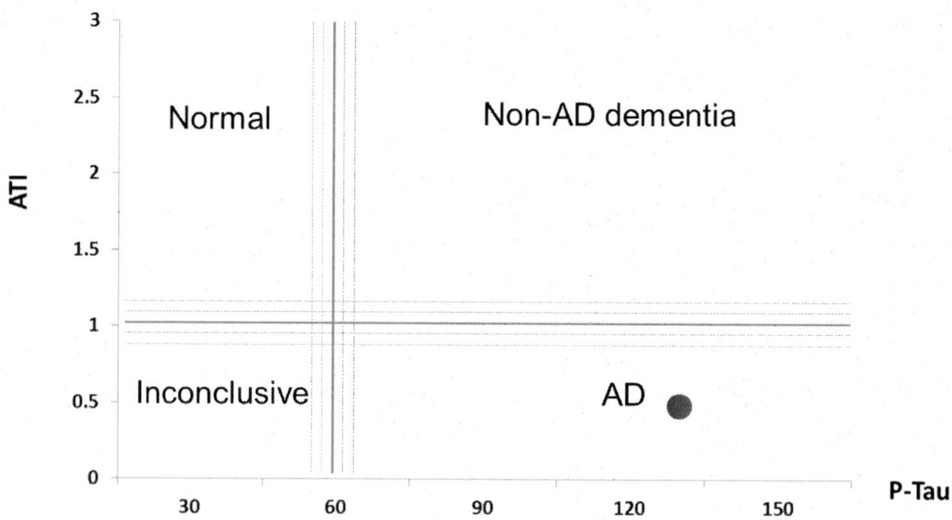

Figure 14. Panel demonstrates interpretation of different CSF biomarker profiles.

GENETIC BIOMARKERS

About half of patients with FTLD have a strong family history of the disease [109]. During the past two decades a number of FTLD related gene mutations have been discovered starting from the MAPT (microtubule-associated protein tau) gene in 1998 [110]. Later the progranulin mutation was found to be the cause of FTLD in a group of patients who had FTD and a linkage to chromosome 17 in the absence of inclusions on neuropathologic examination of their brains [111]. Recent discovery of the C9orf72 mutation has uncovered yet another mutation (a hexanucleotide repeat expansion), which underlies familiar FTLD and motor neuron disease associated with significant psychiatric symptomatology [112].

Between the FTLD related gene mutations and known mutations of familial Alzheimer disease (Presenillin 1 and 1 and amyloid precursor protein, or APP), only progranulin mutation has been shown to be associated with a PPA syndrome, specifically PPA-G [113, 114]. However, it is important to note possession of a PRGN mutation does not necessary guarantee acquiring the PPA syndrome as the mutation can have different phenotypes (phenotypic variability), with other phenotypes being FTD and Parkinson syndromes [115]. Clinical picture in patients with MAPT mutation is that of a semantic dementia. It is important to know however, that other mutation although not associated with a primary progressive aphasic syndrome, may have bvFTD phenotype with additional progressive aphasia which is not primary. In addition to the above mutations, Li et al. (2005) showed an increased incidence of methionine–valine heterozygosity at codon 129 of the prion protein gene *PrP* which has strong association with PPA [116].

APOE ε4 allele is a biomarker that is linked to a genetic risk factor for AD. However, it has been shown that patients with PPA did not have higher incidence of the APOE ε4 allele [117].

From the clinical stand point, unless there is a strong family history of PPA other neurodegenerative syndromes such as FTD or Parkinson, genetic studies of patients with PPA may not have a high yield to determine the underlying cause. Figure 15 summarizes etiologic diagnosis of different PPA syndromes.

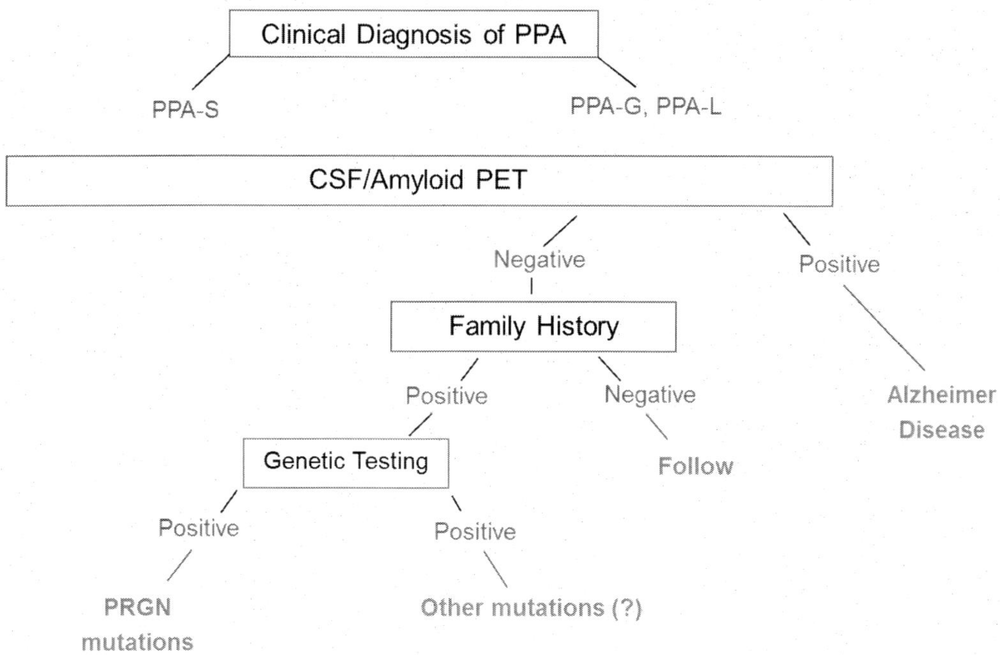

Figure 15. Algorithmic approach to etiologic diagnosis of PPA using CSF and ligand-based PET scan. Only clinically available biomarkers have been included. At this time, CSF profiles suggesting diagnosis of FTLD, and Tau-PET scan are being investigated.

MANAGEMENT OF PROGRESSIVE APHASIAS

PPA is a progressive syndrome. In Figure 16 four levels of intervention to treat PPA are demonstrated. Accumulation of pathology in AD and FTLD can start up to 20 years before symptoms emerge. Therefore an ideal treatment approach would be to treat the underlying cause before it even causes symptoms. With availability of CSF analysis and Amyloid PET, and hopefully Tau PET in a near future, indication for medications and clinical trial enrollments will be not based on diagnosed syndrome, but based on the underlying pathology. In case of PPA cause by underlying Alzheimer disease pathology (PPA-ADp) hope is to detect the pathology well in advance and treat the disease in the preclinical stage. An exciting ongoing clinical trial (the AntiAmyloid treatment of Asymptomatic Alzheimer disease, or A4) at this point tries to answer whether this would be possible. In patients with genetic predisposition (mostly MAPT and GRN mutations) participation in available trials targeting abnormal tau or TDP inclusions is the mainstay of current pharmacological approach to familial PPA.

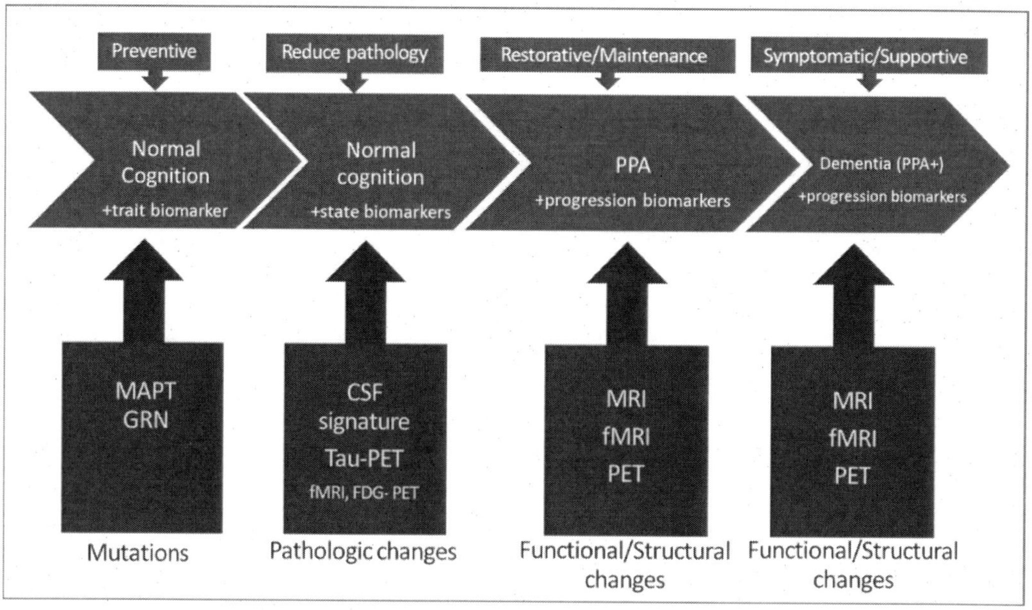

Figure 16. Four levels of intervention for PPA management associated with biomarkers associated with each stage. Schema based in part on a similar approach by Cummings (2014) and Mesulam (2014).

By the time symptoms emerge neurons have started to be affected by the accumulating pathology. During this stage the main principles of PPA management are to 1) slow down the progression of the underlying disease by pharmacological, neuromodulatory, and speech/cognitive interventions, 2) evaluate language function and its effect on activities of daily living on a regular basis, 3) maintain and maximize communication abilities to improve quality of life, 4) make dynamic changes to therapeutic interventions to address symptom changes, 5) family education and life-enriching interventions to adapt to challenges in communication, 6) treatment of depression if it arises. During the most advanced stages of PPA+, the goal of treatments are mostly symptomatic/supportive.

Pharmacological Interventions

There have been few small studies investigating pharmacological intervention in PPA. These studies have examined "restorative" role of candidate drugs, and in one case (steroid) a disease modulation based on inflammatory theory of PPA pathophysiology.

Bromocriptine: A clinical trial of bromocriptin in 6 PPA patients failed to stabilize MLU, however, the patient group had a better MLU compared to the placebo group. Therefore, bromocriptine may have a mild benefit in slowing of language decline in the absence of improving or stabilizing language output [118].

Steroid: Based on autoimmune pathophysiology of PPA brought up by increased association with vasectomy in men, Decker and Heilman [119] administered 60 mg of daily prednisone for 3 months and reported an improvement in naming and verbal fluency. This study, however, was not placebo controlled and needs to be replicated.

Galantamine: Kertesz et al. (2008) investigated effectiveness of galantmine in a group of patients with PPA (N = 22) and behavioral variant frontotemporal dementia (bvFTD, N = 17) in a randomized placebo controlled trial. They found no effect on behavior or language in the total group and a trend of improvement in Clinical Global Impressions of Improvement (CGI-I) in the PPA group. The rational to use galantmine in this study was the fact that aside from being a cholinesterase inhibitor, it also has effect on serotonin and noradrenalin release. Cholinesterase inhibitors such as donepezil, glantamine, or rivastigmine, would be the best candidate medications to use in PPA-ADp. Availability of CSF analysis and to a lesser extent Amyloid PET will allow better selection of patients, not based on theirs syndrome, but based on the underlying pathology of their aphasia.

Memantine: Boxer et al. (2009) in an open-label study of 3 syndromes of FTLD (bvFTD, SD, and PPA-G) showed that over a 26 week period, patients with PPA-G maintained stable in their cognitive and behavioral capacities, although their motor function deteriorated over time. This was in contrast to the SD and bvFTD group who had progressive decline. This study shows some promise for memantine in PPA-G. A follow up placebo control is necessary to replicate these results, and use of "state" biomarkers in future will refine patient inclusion in similar trials. In this study language related outcome measures were not included, which should be considered in future trials.

Omentum transposition surgery (OT): A case report of OT in a 68 year old man with severe PPA-G showed stable symptoms after 36 months of follow up using cognitive and SPECT measures. Shankle et al., state that human omentum is known to have stems cell producing growth factors which may have therapeutic value [120]. Although this study offered an interesting result, its findings have not been replicated since.

Treatment of depression: Progressive language decline in the presence of relatively intact other aspects of cognitive including insight may cause secondary depression in patients with PPA [121]. Different pharmacologic agents have been studies in patients with FTD and can be used in PPA as there syndrome include features of FTD. These agents include trazodone, rivastigmine and selegiline. They can help with depression and agitation but do not have much effect on cognition or language [122].

Neuromodulatory Intervention

Repetitive transcranial magnetic stimulation (rTMS) and transcranial direct current stimulation (tDCS), have been used to improve language function in patients with stroke aphasia with promising results. In these methods magnetic stimulation or direct current are applied to the brain to induce neuromodulation in the remaining network. Since 2006 there have been few studies that have investigated applicability of these method in persons with PPA.

In a case study of a PPA-G patient, Finocchiaro and colleagues demonstrated improvement of verb production in a sentence completion task, after rTMS administration but not after SHAM administration. There was also no effect on memory function proving specificity of their result [123]. This study was followed by a case series of patients with PPA-G (N = 10) and PPA-S (N = 4) by Cotelli et al. [124]. Stimulation of both (50%), left (20%) and right DLPFC (30%) resulted in enhanced action naming in PPA-G but not PPA-S.

Wang and colleagues in 2013 showed improvement in naming, repetition, picture matching and reading after excitatory stimulation of posterior perisylvian area and Broca's area in a case of a person with PPA-G [125].

These studies need to be replicated with higher number of patients. Also, addition of rs-fMRI can guide where and how stimulation should be administered [92].

Speech and Language Interventions

Speech and language interventions is usually performed by a speech-language pathologist who is experienced in working with individuals with PPA. The goal of interventions is to maximize effective communication and improve quality of life. Treatment targets are defined based on individual's communication goals. During early stages of PPA, speech-language interventions are based on brain neuroplasticity, utilizing intact functions of the right hemisphere and left hemisphere non-language networks. In this manner the patient is coached to develop specific compensatory strategies such as self-cueing, and script training for commonplace social scenarios [126].

Early Interventions

In PPA-S and PPA-L variants word finding is the major initial difficulty. Language intervention for each variant, however, is different. In PPA-S, problem with word finding stems from a degraded semantic/conceptual knowledge, and phonological and orthographical skills intact. Language interventions therefore will focus on retraining of concepts. To utilize spared linguistic abilities phonologic cues such as sounds and rhyming is used to help with lexical retrieval [89].

In PPA-L, word retrieval is post-semantic and the patient has decreased phonological abilities. Therefore, utilization of a system of written naming, reading, and searching words' semantic properties underlies retraining interventions [86].

In PPA-G patients word retrieval problem may not be as much as motor and grammatical difficulties. Henry et al. devised a treatment method using structured oral reading as a tool for production of multisyllabic wordsin an individual with mild apraxia of speech. The result of their treatment lasted for a year [127].

Success of speech and language interventions depends on motivation of the patient, intensity of treatment and perseverance with home works. Semantic system needs to be partially intact for treatment to be effective. As PPA is a degenerative condition, no change in language abilities over a long course of years can be considered a positive outcome.

Later Interventions

In later stages of the disease or when language output is significantly impaired alternate modes of communication such as communication book or computer programs or phone applications may be used. With advanced disease, with the addition of executive dysfunction, weakening of memory, or visuospatial abilities, these methods may fail and the focus of intervention will be to enhance communication through education of family members or the patient's care partner.

Psychosocial Interventions and Quality of Life Programs

Clinical management of PPA is not complete without consideration of effect of progressive aphasia and later cognitive on patients their family members. The family needs to be helped as a unit through education (neuro-educational intervention), and planning for future disease progression. Specialized support groups have an important role in with this regard [128]. Patients and families can also receive educational material help and support from international, national, and local organizations, such as the international PPA connection (IMPPACT), Alzheimer association, and association for frontotemporal dementias (aFTD) [126].

Individuals with PPA have been seen to developed outstanding non-linguistic interests and abilities which can enrich their lives significantly. These include emergence of new interest in music, painting, and art work, among others [32, 129]. The patients are highly encouraged to continue such activities alongside their other hobbies and meaningful activities [130].

CONCLUSION

Despite significant progress in determining syndromic variance, neuroimaging characteristics, etiologic biomarker diagnosis, and advances in neuromodulatory and speech-language interventions, there is no pharmacological approach that can significantly slow down the progression of PPA. PPA, therefore remains a devastating syndrome with relentless worsening over time. Current research is now focusing on studying PPA at molecular, neuropathologic, neural network, SLP and psychosocial levels with the final goal to delay the progression of the disease and better improve quality of life in PPA patients.

ACKNOWLEDGMENTS

I hereby would like to thank my mentors and colleagues Drs. Hassan Ashayeri, Jamsheed Lotfi, Nancy Helm-Estabrooks, Cynthia Thompson, Todd Parrish, Marsel Mesulam, Sandra Weintraub, Darren Gitelman, Steve Rapcsak, and Pelagie Beeson for all they taught me in the field of aphasiology and neuroimaging throughout the years. Leisl Jaberg for her help with designing brain figures. Allan Wang for his help with literature search and designing algorithms, and finally Drs. Elizabeth Gerard and Aditi Narechania for their help with deciphering the EEG tracing cited in this chapter.

REFERENCES

[1] Sumerian language. *Encyclopædia Britannica Online 2015* (Retrieved July, 2015).
[2] Zorich Z. Drawing Paleolithic Romania. *Archeology.* 2012;65(1).
[3] Fleagle JG, Assefa Z, Brown FH, Shea JJ. Paleoanthropology of the Kibish Formation, southern Ethiopia: Introduction. *J Hum Evol.* 2008;55(3):360-5.
[4] Yule G. *The study of language.* Fifth edition. ed. Cambridge: New York; 2014. xii, 322 pages p.
[5] Crystal D. The Cambridge encyclopedia of language: New York; 2010.
[6] Prins R, Bastiaanse R. The early history of aphasiology: From the Egyptian surgeons (c. 1700 BC) to Broca (1861). *Aphasiology.* 2006;20(8):762-91.
[7] Catani M, Mesulam M. The arcuate fasciculus and the disconnection theme in language and aphasia: history and current state. *Cortex; A journal devoted to the study of the nervous system and behavior.* 2008;44(8):953-61.
[8] Geschwind N. Disconnexion syndromes in animals and man. *I. Brain.* 1965;88(2):237-94.
[9] Binder J. The Neural Bases of Communication: Evidence From Neuroimaging. *American Speech and Language Association (ASHA);* 2008. p. 1-13.
[10] Hickok G. The functional neuroanatomy of language. *Phys Life Rev.* 2009;6(3):121-43.
[11] Kreutzer JS, Caplan BDJ. *Encyclopedia of clinical neuropsychology:* London; 2011.
[12] Friederici AD, Gierhan SM. The language network. *Curr Opin Neurobiol.* 2013;23(2):250-4.
[13] Wilson SM, Galantucci S, Tartaglia MC, Rising K, Patterson DK, Henry ML, et al. Syntactic processing depends on dorsal language tracts. *Neuron.* 2011;72(2):397-403.
[14] Lukic S, Bonakdarpour B, Ouden Dd, Price C, Thompson C, editors. *Neural mechanisms of verb and sentence production: a lesion-deficit study.* Academy of Aphasia; 2013; Lucerene, Switzerland: Procedia Social and Behavioral Sciences.
[15] Thompson CK, Bonakdarpour B, Fix SC, Blumenfeld HK, Parrish TB, Gitelman DR, et al. Neural correlates of verb argument structure processing. *J Cogn Neurosci.* 2007;19(11):1753-67.
[16] Bonakdarpour B, Thompson C, Fix S. Neural signatures of verb argument structure in agrammatic aphasic and age-matched individuals. *Brain and Language.* 2007;103(1):84-5.

[17]Kielar A, Milman L, Bonakdarpour B, Thompson CK. Neural correlates of covert and overt production of tense and agreement morphology: Evidence from fMRI. *J Neurolinguistics*. 2011;24(2):183-201.
[18]Grodzinsky Y, Friederici AD. Neuroimaging of syntax and syntactic processing. *Current opinion in neurobiology*. 2006;16(2):240-6.
[19]Breier JI, Hasan KM, Zhang W, Men D, Papanicolaou AC. Language dysfunction after stroke and damage to white matter tracts evaluated using diffusion tensor imaging. *AJNR Am J Neuroradiol*. 2008;29(3):483-7.
[20]Mesulam M-M, Thompson CK, Weintraub S, Rogalski EJ. The Wernicke conundrum and the anatomy of langauge comprehension in primary progressive aphasia. *Brain*. 2015;In press.
[21]Hurley RS, Bonakdarpour B, Wang X, Mesulam MM. Asymmetric connectivity between the anterior temporal lobe and the language network. *J Cogn Neurosci*. 2015;27(3):464-73.
[22]Bonakdarpour B, Hurley R, Mesulam M-M. Temporal Pole and the Language Network: Physiologic Evidence from Resting State fMRI. *The 2013 Annual American Neurological Association Metting*; New Orleans, LA2013.
[23]Binder JR, Desai RH, Graves WW, Conant LL. Where is the semantic system? A critical review and meta-analysis of 120 functional neuroimaging studies. *Cerebral cortex*. 2009;19(12):2767-96.
[24]Mesulam M, Rogalski E, Gefen T, Hurley R, Geula C, Weintraub S, et al. Evolving themes in primary progressive aphasia (PPA). *Am J Neurodegener Dis*. 2014;3(Supp 1):4.
[25]Mesulam MM. Slowly progressive aphasia without generalized dementia. *Ann Neurol*. 1982;11(6):592-8.
[26]Weintraub S, Fahey C, Johnson N, Mesulam MM, Gitelman DR, Weitner BB, et al. Vasectomy in men with primary progressive aphasia. *Cogn Behav Neurol*. 2006;19(4):190-3.
[27]Rogalski E, Johnson N, Weintraub S, Mesulam M. Increased frequency of learning disability in patients with primary progressive aphasia and their first-degree relatives. *Arch Neurol*. 2008;65(2):244-8.
[28]Miller ZA, Mandelli ML, Rankin KP, Henry ML, Babiak MC, Frazier DT, et al. Handedness and language learning disability differentially distribute in progressive aphasia variants. *Brain*. 2013;136(Pt 11):3461-73.
[29]Gorno-Tempini ML, Hillis AE, Weintraub S, Kertesz A, Mendez M, Cappa SF, et al. Classification of primary progressive aphasia and its variants. *Neurology*. 2011;76(11):1006-14.
[30]Mesulam MM. Primary progressive aphasia. *Ann Neurol*. 2001;49(4):425-32.
[31]Neary D, Snowden JS, Gustafson L, Passant U, Stuss D, Black S, et al. Frontotemporal lobar degeneration: a consensus on clinical diagnostic criteria. *Neurology*. 1998;51(6):1546-54.
[32]Mesulam MM, Rogalski EJ, Wieneke C, Hurley RS, Geula C, Bigio EH, et al. Primary progressive aphasia and the evolving neurology of the language network. Nature reviews *Neurology*. 2014;10(10):554-69.

[33]Rogalski E, Cobia D, Harrison TM, Wieneke C, Thompson CK, Weintraub S, et al. Anatomy of language impairments in primary progressive aphasia. *J Neurosci.* 2011;31(9):3344-50.

[34]Thompson CK, Lukic S, King MC, Mesulam MM, Weintraub S. Verb and noun deficits in stroke-induced and primary progressive aphasia: The Northwestern Naming Battery. *Aphasiology.* 2012;26(5):632-55.

[35]Henry ML, Beeson PM, Alexander GE, Rapcsak SZ. Written language impairments in primary progressive aphasia: a reflection of damage to central semantic and phonological processes. *J Cogn Neurosci.* 2012;24(2):261-75.

[36]Shim H, Hurley RS, Rogalski E, Mesulam MM. Anatomic, clinical, and neuropsychological correlates of spelling errors in primary progressive aphasia. *Neuropsychologia.* 2012;50(8):1929-35.

[37]Mesulam MM, Wieneke C, Thompson C, Rogalski E, Weintraub S. Quantitative classification of primary progressive aphasia at early and mild impairment stages. *Brain.* 2012;135(Pt 5):1537-53.

[38]Mesulam MM. Primary progressive aphasia and the language network: the 2013 H. Houston Merritt Lecture. *Neurology.* 2013;81(5):456-62.

[39]Mesulam MM, Weintraub S, Rogalski EJ, Wieneke C, Geula C, Bigio EH. Asymmetry and heterogeneity of Alzheimer's and frontotemporal pathology in primary progressive aphasia. *Brain.* 2014;137(Pt 4):1176-92.

[40]Mesulam MM, Weintraub S. Is it time to revisit the classification guidelines for primary progressive aphasia? *Neurology.* 2014;82(13):1108-9.

[41]Gorno-Tempini ML, Dronkers NF, Rankin KP, Ogar JM, Phengrasamy L, Rosen HJ, et al. Cognition and anatomy in three variants of primary progressive aphasia. *Ann Neurol.* 2004;55(3):335-46.

[42]Henry ML, Gorno-Tempini ML. The logopenic variant of primary progressive aphasia. *Curr Opin Neurol.* 2010;23(6):633-7.

[43]Rogalski E, Rademaker A, Weintraub S. Primary progressive aphasia: relationship between gender and severity of language impairment. *Cogn Behav Neurol.* 2007;20(1):38-43.

[44]Helm-Estabrooks N, Albert ML. *Manual of aphasia therapy.* Austin, Tex.: Pro-Ed; 1991. ix, 279 p.p.

[45]Catani M, Mesulam MM, Jakobsen E, Malik F, Martersteck A, Wieneke C, et al. A novel frontal pathway underlies verbal fluency in primary progressive aphasia. *Brain.* 2013;136(Pt 8):2619-28.

[46]Mesulam M, Wieneke C, Rogalski E, Cobia D, Thompson C, Weintraub S. Quantitative template for subtyping primary progressive aphasia. *Arch Neurol.* 2009;66(12):1545-51.

[47]Thompson CK, Cho S, Hsu C-J, Wieneke C, Rademaker A, Weitner BB, et al. Dissociations between fluency and agrammatism in primary progressive aphasia. *Aphasiology.* 2012;26(1):20-43.

[48]Goodglass H, Kaplan E. T*he assessment of aphasia and related disorders.* 2nd ed. Philadelphia: Lea and Febiger; 1983. vii, 102, 31 pages p.

[49]Appelros P, Terent A. Characteristics of the National Institute of Health Stroke Scale: results from a population-based stroke cohort at baseline and after one year. *Cerebrovasc Dis.* 2004;17(1):21-7.

[50]Menn L, Ramsberger G, Helm-Estabrooks N. A linguistic communication measure for aphasic narratives. *Aphasiology.* 1994;8(4):343-59.
[51]Bonakdarpour B, Eftkharzadeh A, Ashayeri H. Melodic intonation therapy in Persian aphasic patients. *Aphasiology.* 2003;17(1):75.
[52]Cho-Reyes S, Thompson CK. Verb and sentence production and comprehension in aphasia: Northwestern Assessment of Verbs and Sentences (NAVS). *Aphasiology.* 2012;26(10):1250-77.
[53]Weintraub S, Mesulam MM, Wieneke C, Rademaker A, Rogalski EJ, Thompson CK. The northwestern anagram test: measuring sentence production in primary progressive aphasia. *Am J Alzheimers Dis Other Demen.* 2009;24(5):408-16.
[54]Kertesz A, Western aphasia battery stimulus b. Raven JC., *Coloured progressive m.* The Western aphasia battery [Visual Material]: San Antonio, TX: PsychCorp; 2007.
[55]Kaplan E, Goodglass H, Weintraub S, Goodglass H. *Boston naming test.* 2nd ed. Philadelphia: Lippincott Williams and Wilkins; 2001.
[56]Hurley RS, Paller KA, Wieneke CA, Weintraub S, Thompson CK, Federmeier KD, et al. Electrophysiology of object naming in primary progressive aphasia. *J Neurosci.* 2009;29(50):15762-9.
[57]Thompson CK, Cho S, Price C, Wieneke C, Bonakdarpour B, Rogalski E, et al. Semantic interference during object naming in agrammatic and logopenic primary progressive aphasia (PPA). *Brain Lang.* 2012;120(3):237-50.
[58]Delazer M, Semenza C, Reiner M, Hofer R, Benke T. Anomia for people names in DAT--evidence for semantic and post-semantic impairments. *Neuropsychologia.* 2003;41(12):1593-8.
[59]Bock K, Levelt WJM. *Language production: Grammatical encoding:* Routledge; 2002.
[60]Mesulam MM. P*rinciples of behavioral and cognitive neurology:* New York; 2000.
[61]Campbell WWJDRN, *Neurologic e. DeJong's the neurologic examination.* 7th ed. Philadelphia, PA: Lippincott Williams and Wilkins; 2013. xii, 819 p. p.
[62]Grossman M. Primary progressive aphasia: clinicopathological correlations. *Nat Rev Neurol.* 2010;6(2):88-97.
[63]Oboudiyat C, Bigio EH, Bonakdarpour B, Baker MC, Rademakers R, Weintraub S, et al. Diffuse leukoencephalopathy with spheroids presenting as primary progressive aphasia. *Neurology.* 2015;85(August 18).
[64]Caselli RJ, Beach TG, Sue LI, Connor DJ, Sabbagh MN. Progressive aphasia with Lewy bodies. *Dement Geriatr Cogn Disord.* 2002;14(2):55-8.
[65]Johnson DY, Dunkelberger DL, Henry M, Haman A, Greicius MD, Wong K, et al. Sporadic Jakob-Creutzfeldt disease presenting as primary progressive aphasia. *JAMA Neurol.* 2013;70(2):254-7.
[66]Bonakdarpour B. Neuroimaging in Primary Progressive Aphasia. *Perspectives in Neurophysiology and Neurogenic Speech and Language Disorders.* 2014;24(4):145-56.
[67]Dubois B, Feldman HH, Jacova C, Hampel H, Molinuevo JL, Blennow K, et al. Advancing research diagnostic criteria for Alzheimer's disease: the IWG-2 criteria. *Lancet Neurol.* 2014;13(6):614-29.
[68]Sinnatamby R, Antoun NA, Freer CE, Miles KA, Hodges JR. Neuroradiological findings in primary progressive aphasia: CT MRI and cerebral perfusion SPECT. *Neuroradiology.* 1996;38(3):232-8.

[69]Wilson SM, Ogar JM, Laluz V, Growdon M, Jang J, Glenn S, et al. Automated MRI-based classification of primary progressive aphasia variants. *Neuroimage.* 2009;47(4):1558-67.

[70]Rogalski E, Cobia D, Harrison TM, Wieneke C, Weintraub S, Mesulam MM. Progression of language decline and cortical atrophy in subtypes of primary progressive aphasia. *Neurology.* 2011;76(21):1804-10.

[71]Rogalski E, Cobia D, Martersteck A, Rademaker A, Wieneke C, Weintraub S, et al. Asymmetry of cortical decline in subtypes of primary progressive aphasia. *Neurology.* 2014;83(13):1184-91.

[72]Gemmell HG, Sharp PF, Besson JA, Crawford JR, Ebmeier KP, Davidson J, et al. Differential diagnosis in dementia using the cerebral blood flow agent 99mTc HM-PAO: a SPECT study. *J Comput Assist Tomogr.* 1987;11(3):398-402.

[73]Kushner M. MRI and 123I-iodoamphetamine SPECT imaging of a patient with slowly progressing. *Adv Func Neuroimaging.* 1989;Winter:17-9.

[74]Neary D, Snowden JS, Shields RA, Burjan AW, Northen B, MacDermott N, et al. Single photon emission tomography using 99mTc-HM-PAO in the investigation of dementia. *J Neurol Neurosurg Psychiatry.* 1987;50(9):1101-9.

[75]Singhal T. Positron emission tomography applications in clinical neurology. *Semin Neurol.* 2012;32(4):421-31.

[76]Chawluk JB, Mesulam MM, Hurtig H, Kushner M, Weintraub S, Saykin A, et al. Slowly progressive aphasia without generalized dementia: studies with positron emission tomography. *Ann Neurol.* 1986;19(1):68-74.

[77]Kempler D, Metter EJ, Riege WH, Jackson CA, Benson DF, Hanson WR. Slowly progressive aphasia: three cases with language, memory, CT and PET data. *J Neurol Neurosurg Psychiatry.* 1990;53(11):987-93.

[78]Tyrrell PJ, Warrington EK, Frackowiak RS, Rossor MN. Heterogeneity in progressive aphasia due to focal cortical atrophy. A clinical and PET study. *Brain.* 1990;113 (Pt 5):1321-36.

[79]Rabinovici GD, Jagust WJ, Furst AJ, Ogar JM, Racine CA, Mormino EC, et al. Abeta amyloid and glucose metabolism in three variants of primary progressive aphasia. *Ann Neurol.* 2008;64(4):388-401.

[80]Rabinovici G, Lehmann M, Rosen H, Ghosh P, Cohn-Sheehy B, Trojanowski J, et al. *Diagnostic Accuracy of Amyloid and FDG PET in Pathologically-Confirmed Dementia Neurology* 2014;S8.005.

[81]Raichle ME, MacLeod AM, Snyder AZ, Powers WJ, Gusnard DA, Shulman GL. A default mode of brain function. *Proc Natl Acad Sci U S A.* 2001;98(2):676-82.

[82]Binder JR. Functional MRI is a valid noninvasive alternative to Wada testing. *Epilepsy Behav.* 2011;20(2):214-22.

[83]Sonty SP, Mesulam MM, Thompson CK, Johnson NA, Weintraub S, Parrish TB, et al. Primary progressive aphasia: PPA and the language network. *Ann Neurol.* 2003;53(1):35-49.

[84]Sonty SP, Mesulam MM, Weintraub S, Johnson NA, Parrish TB, Gitelman DR. Altered effective connectivity within the language network in primary progressive aphasia. *J Neurosci.* 2007;27(6):1334-45.

[85]Wilson SM, Brambati SM, Henry RG, Handwerker DA, Agosta F, Miller BL, et al. The neural basis of surface dyslexia in semantic dementia. *Brain.* 2009;132(Pt 1):71-86.

[86]Beeson PM, King RM, Bonakdarpour B, Henry ML, Cho H, Rapcsak SZ. Positive effects of language treatment for the logopenic variant of primary progressive aphasia. *J Mol Neurosci.* 2011;45(3):724-36.
[87]Damoiseaux JS, Prater KE, Miller BL, Greicius MD. Functional connectivity tracks clinical deterioration in Alzheimer's disease. *Neurobiol Aging.* 2012;33(4):828 e19-30.
[88]Seeley WW, Crawford RK, Zhou J, Miller BL, Greicius MD. Neurodegenerative diseases target large-scale human brain networks. *Neuron.* 2009;62(1):42-52.
[89]Buckner RL, Snyder AZ, Shannon BJ, LaRossa G, Sachs R, Fotenos AF, et al. Molecular, structural, and functional characterization of Alzheimer's disease: evidence for a relationship between default activity, amyloid, and memory. *J Neurosci.* 2005;25(34):7709 17.
[90]Chetelat G, Desgranges B, Landeau B, Mezenge F, Poline JB, de la Sayette V, et al. Direct voxel-based comparison between grey matter hypometabolism and atrophy in Alzheimer's disease. *Brain.* 2008;131(Pt 1):60-71.
[91]Tahmasian M, Pasquini L, Scherr M, Meng C, Forster S, Mulej Bratec S, et al. The lower hippocampus global connectivity, the higher its local metabolism in Alzheimer disease. *Neurology.* 2015;84(19):1956-63.
[92]Bonakdarpour B, Hurley RS, Rogalski E, Mesulam M. Relationship between atrophy and resting state connectivity in Primary Progressive Aphasia. *Am J Neurodegener Dis.* 2014;3(Supp. 1):290.
[93]Mesulam M, Weintraub S. Primary progressive aphasia and kindred disorders. *Handb Clin Neurol.* 2008;89:573-87.
[94]Davies RR, Hodges JR, Kril JJ, Patterson K, Halliday GM, Xuereb JH. The pathological basis of semantic dementia. *Brain.* 2005;128(Pt 9):1984-95.
[95]Klunk WE, Engler H, Nordberg A, Wang Y, Blomqvist G, Holt DP, et al. Imaging brain amyloid in Alzheimer's disease with Pittsburgh Compound-B. *Ann Neurol.* 2004;55(3):306-19.
[96]Wong DF, Rosenberg PB, Zhou Y, Kumar A, Raymont V, Ravert HT, et al. In vivo imaging of amyloid deposition in Alzheimer disease using the radioligand 18F-AV-45 (florbetapir [corrected] F 18). *J Nucl Med.* 2010;51(6):913-20.
[97]Carome M, Wolfe S. Florbetapir-PET imaging and postmortem beta-amyloid pathology. JAMA. 2011;305(18):1857; author reply -8.
[98]Clark CM, Schneider JA, Bedell BJ, Beach TG, Bilker WB, Mintun MA, et al. Use of florbetapir-PET for imaging beta-amyloid pathology. *JAMA.* 2011;305(3):275-83.
[99]Johnson KA, Minoshima S, Bohnen NI, Donohoe KJ, Foster NL, Herscovitch P, et al. Update on appropriate use criteria for amyloid PET imaging: dementia experts, mild cognitive impairment, and education. *J Nucl Med.* 2013;54(7):1011-3.
[100] Leyton CE, Villemagne VL, Savage S, Pike KE, Ballard KJ, Piguet O, et al. Subtypes of progressive aphasia: application of the International Consensus Criteria and validation using beta-amyloid imaging. *Brain.* 2011;134(Pt 10):3030-43.
[101] Martersteck A, Murphy C, Wieneke C, Chen K, Luo J, Thiyyagura P, et al. Is there an asymmetric distribution of in vivo amyloid in primary progressive aphasia? Abstract presented at the 8th Human Amyloid Imaging Conference (January 15–17, 2014), Miami, Florida. 2014.

[102] Dickerson B, Domoto-Reilly K, Hochberg D, Brickhouse M, Stepanovic M, Johnson K. Imaging Tau Pathology In Vivo in FTLD: Initial Experience With 18F T807 PET. *American Academy of Neurology;* Philadelphia2014.

[103] Blennow K, Hampel H. CSF markers for incipient Alzheimer's disease. *Lancet Neurol.* 2003;2(10):605-13.

[104] Tsai A, Malek-Ahmadi M, Kahlon V, Sabbagh MN. Differences in Cerebrospinal Fluid Biomarkers between Clinically Diagnosed Idiopathic Normal Pressure Hydrocephalus and Alzheimer's Disease. *J Alzheimers Dis Parkinsonism.* 2014;4(4).

[105] Tabaraud F, Leman JP, Milor AM, Roussie JM, Barriere G, Tartary M, et al. Alzheimer CSF biomarkers in routine clinical setting. *Acta Neurol Scand.* 2012;125(6):416-23.

[106] Kapaki EN, Paraskevas GP, Tzerakis NG, Sfagos C, Seretis A, Kararizou E, et al. Cerebrospinal fluid tau, phospho-tau181 and beta-amyloid1-42 in idiopathic normal pressure hydrocephalus: a discrimination from Alzheimer's disease. *Eur J Neurol.* 2007;14(2):168-73.

[107] Hu WT. CSF FTLD biomarkders- old foes and new friends. *Am J Neurodegener Dis.* 2014;3(Supp. 1):44.

[108] C. T, N. E, M. K-S, Durieux-Lu C, T. P, J. vS, et al. Identification of novel diagnostic CSF biomarkers for pathological subtypes of FTD with high discriminatory power. *Am J Neurodegener Dis.* 2014;3(Supp. 1):47.

[109] Chow TW, Miller BL, Hayashi VN, Geschwind DH. Inheritance of frontotemporal dementia. *Arch Neurol.* 1999;56(7):817-22.

[110] Hutton M, Lendon CL, Rizzu P, Baker M, Froelich S, Houlden H, et al. Association of missense and 5'-splice-site mutations in tau with the inherited dementia FTDP-17. *Nature.* 1998;393(6686):702-5.

[111] Baker M, Mackenzie IR, Pickering-Brown SM, Gass J, Rademakers R, Lindholm C, et al. Mutations in progranulin cause tau-negative frontotemporal dementia linked to chromosome 17. *Nature.* 2006;442(7105):916-9.

[112] Mahoney CJ, Beck J, Rohrer JD, Lashley T, Mok K, Shakespeare T, et al. Frontotemporal dementia with the C9ORF72 hexanucleotide repeat expansion: clinical, neuroanatomical and neuropathological features. *Brain.* 2012;135(Pt 3):736-50.

[113] Snowden JS, Pickering-Brown SM, Mackenzie IR, Richardson AM, Varma A, Neary D, et al. Progranulin gene mutations associated with frontotemporal dementia and progressive non-fluent aphasia. *Brain.* 2006;129(Pt 11):3091-102.

[114] Mesulam M, Johnson N, Krefft TA, Gass JM, Cannon AD, Adamson JL, et al. Progranulin mutations in primary progressive aphasia: the PPA1 and PPA3 families. *Arch Neurol.* 2007;64(1):43-7.

[115] Kelley BJ, Haidar W, Boeve BF, Baker M, Graff-Radford NR, Krefft T, et al. Prominent phenotypic variability associated with mutations in Progranulin. *Neurobiol Aging.* 2009;30(5):739-51.

[116] Li X, Rowland LP, Mitsumoto H, Przedborski S, Bird TD, Schellenberg GD, et al. Prion protein codon 129 genotype prevalence is altered in primary progressive aphasia. *Ann Neurol.* 2005;58(6):858-64.

[117] Mesulam MM, Johnson N, Grujic Z, Weintraub S. Apolipoprotein E genotypes in primary progressive aphasia. Neurology. 1997;49(1):51-5.

[118] Reed DA, Johnson NA, Thompson C, Weintraub S, Mesulam MM. A clinical trial of bromocriptine for treatment of primary progressive aphasia. *Ann Neurol.* 2004;56(5):750.

[119] Decker DA, Heilman KM. Steroid treatment of primary progressive aphasia. *Arch Neurol.* 2008;65(11):1533-5.

[120] Shankle WR, Hara J, Bjornsen L, Gade GF, Leport PC, Ali MB, et al. Omental therapy for primary progressive aphasia with tau negative histopathology: 3 year study. *Neurol Res.* 2009;31(7):766-9.

[121] Medina J, Weintraub S. Depression in Primary Progressive Aphasia. *J Geriatr Psychiatry Neurol.* 2007;20(3):153-60.

[122] Leger GC, Johnson N. A review on primary progressive aphasia. Neuropsychiatr Dis Treat. 2007;3(6):745-52.

[123] Finocchiaro C, Maimone M, Brighina F, Piccoli T, Giglia G, Fierro B. A case study of Primary Progressive Aphasia: improvement on verbs after rTMS treatment. *Neurocase.* 2006;12(6):317-21.

[124] Cotelli M, Manenti R, Alberici A, Brambilla M, Cosseddu M, Zanetti O, et al. Prefrontal cortex rTMS enhances action naming in progressive non-fluent aphasia. *Eur J Neurol.* 2012;19(11):1404-12.

[125] Wang J, Wu D, Chen Y, Yuan Y, Zhang M. Effects of transcranial direct current stimulation on language improvement and cortical activation in nonfluent variant primary progressive aphasia. *Neurosci Lett.* 2013;549:29-33.

[126] Khayum B, Wieneke C, Rogalski E, Robinson J, O'Hara M. Thinking Outside the Stroke: Treating Primary Progressive Aphasia (PPA). *American Speech and Hearing Association (ASHA) Perspectives on Gerontology.* 2012;17(2):37-49.

[127] Henry ML, Meese MV, Truong S, Babiak MC, Miller BL, Gorno-Tempini ML. Treatment for apraxia of speech in nonfluent variant primary progressive aphasia. *Behavioural neurology.* 2013;26(1-2):77-88.

[128] Morhardt D, Weintraub S, Khayum B, Robinson J, Medina J, O'Hara M, et al. The CARE Pathway Model for Dementia: Psychosocial and Rehabilitative Strategies for Care in Young-Onset Dementias. *The Psychiatric clinics of North America.* 2015;38(2):333-52.

[129] Seeley WW, Matthews BR, Crawford RK, Gorno-Tempini ML, Foti D, Mackenzie IR, et al. Unravelling Bolero: progressive aphasia, transmodal creativity and the right posterior neocortex. *Brain.* 2008;131(Pt 1):39-49.

[130] Brotons M, Koger SM. The impact of music therapy on language functioning in dementia. *Journal of music therapy.* 2000;37(3):183-95.

[131] Thompson CK, Meltzer-Asscher A. Neurocognitive mechanisms of verb argument structure processing. . In: Bachrach A, Roy I, Stockall L, eds. *Structuring the Argument. Multidisciplinary research on verb argument structure*: John Benjamins; 2014.

In: Progressive Cognitive Impairment …
Editor: Gediminas Peter Gliebus
ISBN: 978-1-63485-221-0

Chapter 8

NEUROVISUAL IMPAIRMENT IN NEURODEGENERATIVE DISEASES

Christian Schenk[1], MD, and Alan J. Lerner[2,*], MD
[1] Department of Neurology,
University of Puerto Rico School of Medicine,
San Juan, Puerto Rico
[2] Department of Neurology,
University Hospitals - Case Western School of Medicine,
Cleveland, OH, US

ABSTRACT

The recognition of cortical visual impairment in dementia is challenging, due to the clinical setting where testing of cognitive skills is convoluted by their own decline, confounded by aging, and where the presence of extrapyramidal features are frequently encountered. A lack of common definitions in the study of neurovisual impairment complicates the interpretation of the literature. The clinical spectrum in neurodegenerative dementias, such as in Alzheimer's disease, perceptual impairments and deficits in higher order aspects of spatial orientation and navigation are common and disabling. Cortical visual dysfunction usually manifest through careful behavioral assessments or by using standard neuropsychological measures. New tools and emerging advances in technology are revolutionizing the field of neurovisual evaluation and rehabilitation. The functional implications of visual and spatial dysfunction in the context of other disabling features of these illnesses remain largely unexplored.

INTRODUCTION

Vision plays a central role in human behavior. Changes in visual acuity disturb contrast sensitivity and object recognition from the background, and the ability to function in low light

* Correspondence to: Alan J. Lerner Alan.lerner@uhhospitals.org.

situations. In contrast to changes that commonly take place in the eye, including cataracts, macular degeneration and glaucoma, aspects of visuospatial abilities controlled by the brain change relatively little with age in otherwise healthy adults.

Impairments in the use of vision and space are referred to as visuospatial, visuoperceptual or visuoconstructive deficits, and sometimes called impairments in spatial cognition or spatial behavior. Neurovisual dysfunction in dementia is common and provides important implications for the clinical diagnosis, biomarker discovery and the clinical course of disease. An assessment based on anatomically-focused visual spatial dysfunction can assist the clinician in making an early and accurate diagnosis. A proposed multi-faceted model of visual spatial cognition may help elucidate the specific patterns of visual spatial dysfunction associated with Alzheimer's disease, Parkinson's disease, Lewy Body Dementia, Corticobasal Syndrome, Progressive Supranuclear Palsy, and Frontotemporal Lobar Degeneration.

Elemental perceptual changes influence inputs into visual processing in the cortex. Executive dysfunction is an important mediator of visual and spatial behaviors on neuropsychological tests and in everyday life. Memory is dependent on perception whether visual, auditory or some other modality, and sensory loss leads to memory acquisition failure. Prolonged sensory deprivation may be associated with behavioral changes including agitation, delusions and hallucinations, which are also common in Alzheimer's disease and other dementias. Many phenotypes of visuospatial impairment secondary to neurodegeneration may comprise of partial or complete blindness, failure to notice visual stimuli despite intact vision, difficulty managing one's own body, impairments in managing space immediately around the body and knowing one's way around the city or a building. Functional deficits range from occasionally getting lost to requiring full visual assistance. The literature on the effect of aging has on neurovisual systems is limited [1].

The chapter will begin by describing basic principles of neurovisual systems, followed by some applications of these processes in forms of visuo-constructional apraxias and disorders of analysis and synthesis. Finally we review visuospatial dysfunction in the context of neurodegenerative diseases related to Alzheimer's dementia.

1. The Brain-Visual System

The brain and vision have very exclusive and mutual interactions. More than 25% of the cortex is represented in vision and vision-related processes. In the developing eye, retinal ganglion cells become the source of which the optic nerve sprouts with fibers that in effect become central nervous system axons. Vision is the result of the translation of a sensory input that is processed, associated to a myriad of cognitive processes, including those dependent on awareness and perception, by which reality lies upon. The collection of gathered input provides definition, relativity, and paths for planning and navigation, which aid in making sense of the world. Visual patterns along with auditory processing are the most extensively studied ways of pattern processing in mammals [2, 3].

Visuospatial function is a common neuropsychological category. Similar to attention, "visuospatial" is a term that everyone understands, but difficult to define. Visuospatial processing refers to the spatial perception, recognition, and analysis of visual input. Visual Perceptual skills can be defined as the brain's ability to interpret and process incoming (sensory) information, specifically visual, and generate functional activity as an outcome. Visual perceptual skills are the basic building blocks of all functional activity.

Visuospatial judgment is an example of higher-order visuospatial processing that can involve the analysis of spatial features of visual stimuli such as distances, angles, or basic spatial relations, between stimulus parts or aspects of visual images [4]. Analysis is goal related by definition and often involves a focus on certain spatial features relevant to a particular task or goal. This skillset is essential to human interaction with the environment.

A review of neurovisual literature finds that visual skills in dementia appear as one or a combination of four basic categories: deficits in visuo-perceptive skills, deficits in visuo-spatial skills, deficits in visuo-constructive skills, and deficits in other visual cognitive functions [5].

Table 1. Survey of visual and oculomotor disorders, their etiologies, anatomical localization of the lesion and resulting impairment. Modified from Kerkhof [488]

Deficit	Etiology and localization of lesion	Impairment/Disability
Visual Acuity (near/far)	Primary deficits: bilateral or unilateral postchiasmatic lesion(s); Secondary deficits: eccentric fixation in cerebral hypoxia, visual exploration deficits, disturbed simultaneous perception and spasmodic fixation (Balint/Holmes Syndrome)	Impaired object identification and reading, near work fatigue.
Contrast Sensitivity (spatial, temporal)	Unilateral, bilateral, and diffuse posterior brain lesions; temporal for high spatial and parietal for low spatial frequencies	Blurred vision; recognition of objects, traffic signs, distances or faces impaired at low luminance.
Adaptation (photopic, scotopic)	Posterior thalamic or "posterior" brain lesions, cerebral hypoxia, occasional severe head injury	Blinding/dark or foggy vision; delayed/lost adaptation to different luminance levels; eye strain, impaired depth estimation, reduced acuity, asthenopic disorders
Stereopsis and depth perception	V2 lesions: local stereopsis; temporal lesions: global stereopsis; parietal lesions: 3-D stereo features of objects; right hemispheric preponderance.	Slowed and inaccurate grasping and manipulative movements, impaired depth perception, reduced reading duration.
Convergent fusion	-Vergence movements: midbrain lesion -Sensory fusion: impaired after V2 and/or temporoparietal lesions	Reading difficulties, reduced visual sustained attention in near work conditions, somatic complaints (eye strain)
Homonymous visual field disorders	PCA infarctions, bleedings, cerebral hypoxia, along the whole course of the postchiasmatic visual pathways	Impaired visual search/orientation in 2 D and 3 D Space, reading difficulties, slowed and inaccurate performance in functional visual activities
Visual-spatial perception	**Dorsal visual pathways and basal ganglia after MCA lesions, more frequent and more severe after right cerebral lesions**	**Disturbed perception of geometric relations: subjective visual vertical and horizontal, impaired orientation and localization performance**

Table 1. (Continued)

Deficit	Etiology and localization of lesion	Impairment/Disability
Visual object and face recognition	**Bilateral/sometimes unilateral right PCA lesions or cerebral hypoxia along the ventral visual stream**	**Recognition of objects and faces under unconventional viewing conditions or non-optimal lighting conditions**
Balint/Holmes Syndrome	**Bilateral MCAs of the parietal or frontal branches or bleedings; diffuse lesions in both hemispheres due to cerebral anoxia, encephalitis, trauma, degenerative disease**	**Impairments in visual fixation, reading, grasping, visual search, simultaneous perception, depth and space perception.**
Eye movement disorders		(a) conjugate, tonic imbalance of both eyes to the ipsilesional side; inability to fixate/reach for objects/persons in the contralesional hemispace; hypometric saccades and increase saccadic latencies for saccades to the contralesional hemispace; (b) difficulties following moving objects/vehicles/persons, omissions of critical objects; impaired orientation during self motion of person
(a) Conjugate Eye deviations	(a) large MCA infarctions parietotemporal; more frequent right	
(b) Smooth pursuit	(b) Unilateral superior temporoparietal lesions after MCA infarctions or trauma with brainstem damage	

Visuospatial deficits are commonly encountered in the neurology clinic, either as a result of a focal lesion, or neurodegenerative process like Alzheimer's disease or Dementia with Lewy bodies [6]. As these processes appear to occur automatically and devoid of conscious processing, visuospatial dysfunction might not be evident to the patient or family. A history of becoming lost or disoriented in familiar settings, getting lost while driving, or difficulty recognizing familiar faces may serve as a hint for further evaluation [7].

Sensory perception is notoriously affected by aging through deterioration of hearing and vision, but at the semantic level there is little evidence that meaning categories deteriorate in aging. The subtle decreases in sensory perception with age are mostly in terms of speed and efficiency and recognition may be partial or slow in some cases, even in young subjects [8]. Testing visuoperception in dementia is complicated by age-related ocular impairment, a decline of other cognitive domains and the potential presence of extrapyramidal features.

The ability to navigate is known to require integration of multi-modal sensory information, as well as movement execution and memory capacities, and serves as one of the most complex of brain functions. Discoveries of complex brain structures and processes continues to surprise and awe the scientific community, and it is most recently the neural processes in spatial navigation with a newfound class of neurons (place cells and grid cells) that have led to the 2014 Nobel Prize in Physiology or Medicine [9]. The execution of higher cognitive functions such as navigation opens new avenues of inquiry for understanding cognitive processes like memory, thinking and planning that are also affected in dementia.

Lastly, reports of altered visuospatial abilities in subjects with cerebellar pathology have also been described, with experimental evidence of importance in spatial processing and working memory [10-13]. Processing of visuospatial data by the cerebellum have demonstrated a broad influence in cognitive spatial tasks, such as spatial orientation and line bisection judgment, spatial attention illusory space body perception explorative behavior, mental rotation of objects or faces, visuomotor sequence learning, observational learning and control of movement in space [10, 14-33].

Models of the Visual System, Object Recognition, Attention and Action

Visual neuropsychology is the field of enquiry devoted to elucidating links between the anatomy and physiological functioning of visual cerebro-cortical structures and the visual perceptions and visually-mediated behaviors to which they give rise through experimentation in healthy and brain damaged humans. Altogether these processes target the many ways the brain visually searches, finds, identifies and calculates the "what and where," the "near and far," the "above or below." Due to the complexity that the visual process ensues, many perspectives of theory are to consider: Gestalt psychology, categorical and coordinate spatial relationships, feature integration theory among others [34-42].

Table 2. Syndromes localized to one of the visual cortical areas or Fugal Pathways

Area V1 Anton Syndrome Blindsight Riddoch phenomenon Transient achromatopsia Visual ataxia
Area V2 and V3 Quadrantic homonymous hemianopia
Area V4 Cerebral achromatopsia
Area V5 Akinetopsia
Dorsal Occipitofugal Pathway Balint syndrome "psychic paralysis of gaze" Hemispatial neglect Visual allesthesia Environmental rotation
Ventral Occipitofugal Pathways **Visual-Verbal Disconnection –** Pure Alexia – Color anomia – Object Anomia **Visual-Visual Disconnection –** Prosopagnosia – Object Agnosia **Visual-Limbic Disconnection** – Visual amnesia – Visual hypoemotionality

Source: Girkin and Miller (2001) [489].

From visual neuroscience to cognitive neurology, the prevalent theories that are most applicable to extrastriate clinical syndromes are the Lower and Higher Order Vision, and the Dorsal and Ventral Streams of visual processing [43]. Visuospatial function is part of an experience of perception, a sensory experience that cannot be completely separated from other sensory modalities. Perception has its own fundamentals that depend on what the object is surrounded or what borders it spatially. This process determines how the brain determines color, shape, location or some other quality. The capacity to manipulate 2 dimensional or 3 dimensional figures in the mind falls under spatial visualization or visuospatial ability. Identification of potential causes of visuospatial disorders in dementia include problems with either stimulus salience, motion perception, spatial exploration (scanning and attentional focus) or visual search [44].

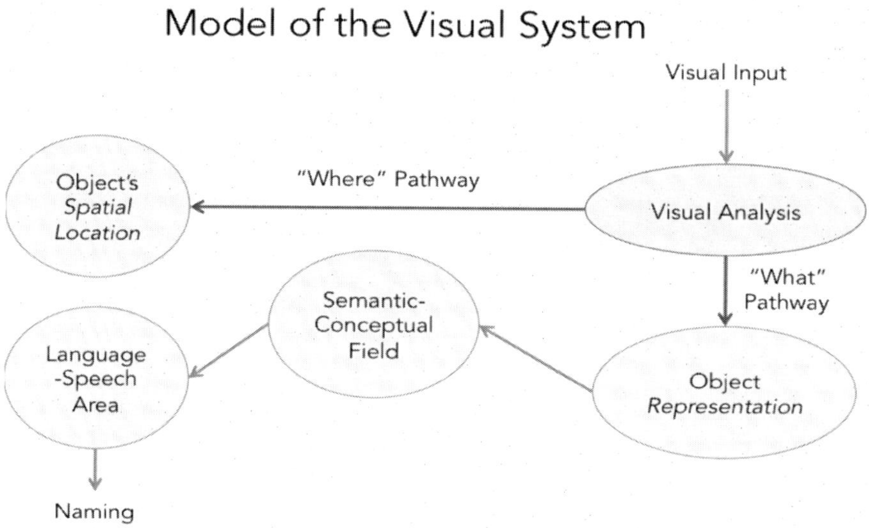

Figure 1. Basic Model of the Visual System.

Ventral and Dorsal Streams: Two-Stream theory of Neural Processing of Vision

The two-streams model of neural processing of vision is a widely accepted and influential hypothesis where humans possess a two part visual system as information exits the occipital lobe: an older dorsal "vision-for action" whose activities guide motor behavior in the absence of awareness and a ventral "vision for perception" stream whose activities lead to a conscious visual experience (Figures 1 and 3) [45]. Although most of what we know about the neurovisual model belongs to data with primates, functional MRI studies and new techniques are promising new ways of exploring the fine-grained neural representation of visual stimuli within the human brain [46].

The dorsal visual-stream is equal with the "where pathway" and is specialized in spatial perception and visual control of action. It is equipped with a quick and "dirty" magno system as a main output. The pathway extends from the dorsal bank of the calcarine fissure into visual association cortices over the superior and lateral surfaces of the posterior hemisphere. Damage to this pathway can alter visuospatial processing, including the control of visually guided eye and hand movements (as in "Balint's syndrome"), impair motion perception (cerebral akinetopsia), or produce simultanagnosia.

The ventral object-recognition stream of vision, or "what" pathway on the other hand, consists of a "slow and detailed" parvo system and anatomically extends from below the calcarine fissure into the visual association cortex in the adjacent medial temporal lobe. Damage to this pathway is associated with impairment in recognition of objects (the agnosias, visual agnosia, prosopagnosia), reading (alexia) and color perception (achromatopsia). The mid- and high-level visual properties supporting object perception in the ventral visual pathway are poorly understood [46]. Object recognition occurs in large part to structures in the inferotemporal cortex (ITC) and facial recognition in the fusiform gyrus. The parahippocampal place area (PPA) responds preferentially to places, such as pictures of houses, while the extrastriate body area (EBA) is specifically involved in the perception of body parts, and finally the middle temporal area (MT) is believed to assist in processing motion.

Fixational eye movements play an important role in perception. Even when attending a single point, gaze is never fixed or at rest. Microscopic movements shift the projection of the stimulus over many receptors on the retina and the observer is never aware of them. Fixation of eye movements and other behavior activity reveal how sensory perception and motor behavior are closely linked and their interaction plays a role in visual perception [47-52]. There is evidence that vestibular function can also influence performance on tests of visuospatial ability [53].

Hemispatial Neglect

Hemispatial neglect is one of the most studied syndromes of cortical visual dysfunction. The term "neglect" is considered by some a misnomer; other proposed or alternative terms include hemi-inattention or hemi-imperception, unilateral spatial agnosia, unilateral visual neglect or fixed hemianopsia.

Hemispatial neglect is defined as the failure to attend, explore, and act upon the contralesional side of space [54]. It is frequently associated with marked anosognosia. When neglect is limited to the body, as in the inability to use information from one side of the body, it is known as unilateral body neglect, personal neglect or hemi-asomatognosia. One theory lies on interhemispheric rivalry, where a contralesional, intact hemisphere undergoes a pathological hyperactivity due to a deficient transcallosal inhibition from the injured hemisphere [55, 56].

One study using repetitive transcranial magnetic stimulation (rTMS) in healthy humans was able to produce two types of neglect: a motor intentional neglect (right frontal rTMS) and sensory-attentional neglect (right parietal rTMS) [57, 58].

In line bisection tasks, patients with left sided unilateral neglect typically bisect horizontal lines significantly to the right of veridical center. Visuospatial neglect has been described predominantly in the azimuthal (horizontal) plane; however, neglect may also be manifested in the altitudinal (vertical) and radial (depth) planes. Normal control subjects generally err to the left of the vericial center when bisecting horizontal lines, a phenomena termed pseudoneglect although the magnitude of bisection errors is much smaller than in neglect patients (Figure 2) [59-64].

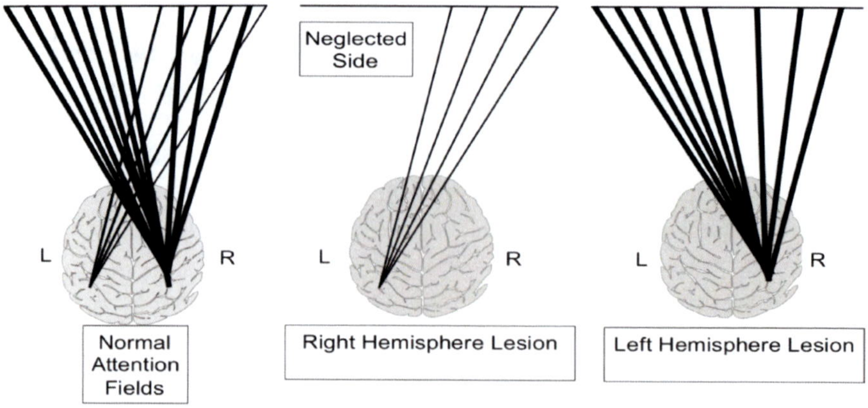

Figure 2. Hemispatial Inattention (neglect) based on laterality of defect. Normal subjects without brain injury have a dominant right-sided parietal visuospatial network.

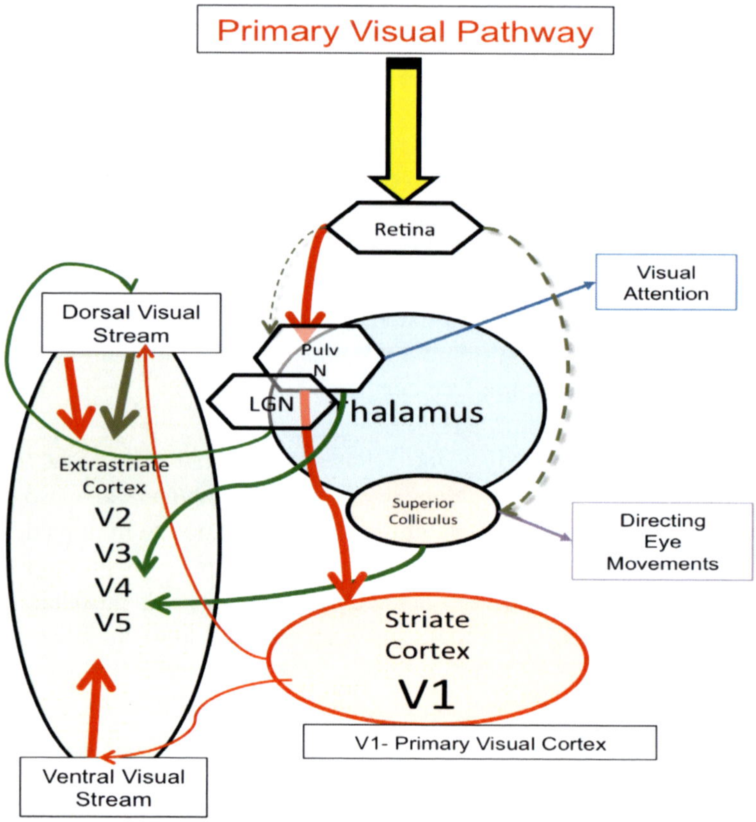

Figure 3. Simplified model of visual processing. The primary visual pathways originates in the retina and travels through the lateral geniculate nucleus of the thalamus and reaches the primary visual (striate) cortex or V1 (Red Arrows). From V1 information travels to the extrastriate cortex along the ventral or dorsal stream. A minority of fibers from the retina deviate (dashed arrows) and reach both the superior colliculus (SC) and the pulvinar nucleus (Pulv N), fibers that bypass V1 and connect directly to the extrastriate visual cortex, as well as the SC and the lateral geniculate nucleus (LGN) where it connects to the extrastriate cortices via the dorsal stream.

Lesions responsible for hemispatial neglect phenomena usually lie within the right posterior parietal lobe, and are classically described in the setting of stroke. In some cases they can also present with hemorrhages to basal ganglia, thalamus and putamen. In neurodegenerative dementias these lesions may also give way to neglect syndromes, and when identified, they become good leads toward specific syndromes, especially in cases of Corticobasal Syndrome or Posterior Cortical Atrophy.

The Agnosias

The agnosias are among the most extensively studied perceptual syndromes despite their rarity in clinical practice. Agnosias are characterized by profound impairment in perceiving, identifying, and/or recognizing stimuli despite adequate sensation and unimpaired language, attention and primary sensation [65, 66]. Visual gnosis or perception was first divided by Lissauer ca. 1890 and are roughly either apperceptive (perceptual) in nature, meaning that there is a failure of visual perception, or associative (semantic), where the person with agnosia reveals a "normal" perception but "stripped of its meaning" (Teuber); it usually involves specific categories such as faces, places or words [67, 68].

Despite the fact that agnosia is relatively rare in focal brain damage, it is striking when it appears, usually in patients with Alzheimer's disease and other cortical dementias. When neuropathology becomes distributed widely across the brain, it is often difficult to determine what is causing it, either anatomically or cognitively, and there is little agreement on the characteristics of neural bases of agnosia.

Visual Agnosia

Agnosias are modality specific, such as tactile agnosia affecting only sense of touch when hearing recognition is intact.

> "I put either pennies, dimes, nickels, quarters, or half dollars in her hand. She named all of them correctly, but when I asked her to open her eyes and name the coins I showed her, she could name only the pennies because of their color. With the other coins she did no better than chance. I tested her visual acuity while she was wearing her glasses, and as her ophthalmologist had said, it was normal.
>
> Source: Heilman [69]

Visual agnosia is identified by a patient's lack of recognition of common objects, colors, words, or faces in drawings, photos or real life. Visual recognition may be determined by a combination of verbal and nonverbal tests. This type of agnosia is typically more severe for small objects than larger ones, and smaller objects are harder to recognize in isolation than when placed in context, like recognizing a pair of scissors on the table but not recognizing them on a bed sheet. During examination with objects such as in the Boston Naming Test, the patient may be asked to copy the picture in question. Further testing may include tests that incorporate Gestalt perception, where the patient needs to integrate pieces of visual information, also known as tests of visual organization: the Hooper Visual Orientation Test, the Benton test of facial recognition, overlapping figures, unusual angles, or when real objects versus non-real objects are presented.

Table 3. Classic Syndromes and Phenomena of Visuospatial Impairment

SYNDROME	Description	Common causes	Comment
Balint's Syndrome; Visual disorientation	Triad: Simultanagnosia, Optic Ataxia, Ocular Apraxia Simultanagnosia: (inability to simultaneously perceive or attend to multiple visual stimuli), Optic Ataxia: (a disorder of visually guided reaching); difficulty in movements that require continual visual guidance such as grasping an object or pouring liquid into a glass. Ocular Apraxia: (an inability to move the eyes voluntarily to a visual target. Fixed angle of gaze that the patient cannot easily shift; perseveration of eye gaze on a single, prominent stimulus;	Hypotension: Sudden and severe hypotension resulting in bilateral borderzone infarction in the occipito-parietal region is reported to be the most frequent cause of complete Balint's syndrome. In Dementia: AD, CBD, CJD	The complete syndrome is rare, and partial syndromes have been reported more frequently. Lack of awareness of the syndrome may lead to misdiagnosis such as blindness, psychosis, or dementia.
Gerstmann's Syndrome	Tetrad: acalculia agraphia finger agnosia left-right disorientation	Stroke Lesion to dominant parietal lobe Left Angular Gyrus Left Middle frontal Gyrus	
Klüver-Bucy syndrome	Visual Agnosia Hypermetamorphosis (strong tendency to react to visual stimulus) Increased oral exploration, placidity Indiscriminate hyper-sexuality Change in dietary habits or behavior Seizures	Bilateral damage to the temporal lobes, medial temporal lobe regions, bilateral Ammon's horn, compression of hippocampi Traumatic Brain Injury with Gliosis Anoxia-ischemic encephalopathy Herpes simplex encephalitis Neurocysticercosis Tubercular meningitis	Neurobehavioral syndrome

In cases where agnosia is suspected, it is important to consider or rule/out motor aphasia and anomic aphasias, where patients may have the name of the object in mind may not be able to verbalize it, but do have the ability to "circumlocute" around the aphasia or give a description of what the object is used for. In the setting of anomic aphasia, subjects can handle objects but cannot come up with the name of the object; agnosic patients will recognize and name the object, improving when presented through another sensory modality [70, 71]. Nonetheless, both phenomena are not all or none in nature, and varying degrees of both may present simultaneously [72].

Scene perception is a complex process in which eye movements are influenced by knowledge structures (top-down control), image features (bottom-up processes) and the interaction between these activities [73]. Simultanagnosia presents as an intermittent failure to see all parts of the environment simultaneously, where certain objects may fall out of view as if they disappear, or conversely, suddenly appear.

Coslett and Saffran describe a patient with the some of the unique experiences encountered by patients with simultagnosia [74]:

> "while walking through the apartment she had lived in for 25 years, 'fell over her dining room table' because she didn't see it as she crossed the room…she reported the converse experience while watching a movie, where a character was having a heated argument, and she 'noted to her surprise and consternation that the character she had been watching was suddenly sent reeling across the room, apparently as a consequence of a punch thrown by a character she had never seen"

When present, it is common to see simultanagnosia as part of Balint's syndrome, hence all patients should be also tested for optic ataxia and optic apraxia. Hemianopia and visual neglect differ from simultanagnosia in where they have deficits only to one side. Simultanagnosia has been noted with stroke of right temporo-occipital areas or bilateral occipitoparietal areas, and in posterior cortical atrophy (PCA). Visual fields may be normal but shrink to "shaft vision" when the patient concentrates on the visual environment [75].

2. Bedside Examination – Testing the Visual Cortical Brain

Following a full examination and evaluation of basic visual sensory function such as visual acuity, visual fields, extraocular movements, additional assessment of secondary cortical visual regions can be sought. This is particularly critical when testing reading capabilities, as homonymous hemianopia disrupts coordination of visuomotor eye movements, which may lead to missing the beginning or end of words. Identification of the extent of visual acuity and other ocular and ophthalmic function in dementia appear to yield inconsistent results when tested out like monocular or binocular vision with full visual fields by confrontation or perimetry.

Tests of visuospatial function include assessment of visual acuity, visual attention, and the ability to read, copy, and make sense of complex visual images. Visuospatial abnormalities may be difficult to isolate as a cognitive feature. Simple tasks used by clinicians to screen patients' abilities include the clock-drawing task (CDT). Since some tests assess only visual orientation and consist of finding objects in space, more in detail tests involve tasks that assess visual perception and the spatial discrimination of position, such as the cancellation tests and the Judgment of Line Orientation test [76]. An even more in-depth assessment would frequently require a consultation with a neuropsychologist.

The Montreal Cognitive Assessment (MoCA) includes a small example of the CDT, and the Mini-Mental Status Exam has a similar profile with the intersecting pentagons test, where visuospatial and constructional abilities are briefly tested. The 12-item Clock Reading Test (CRT) allows a fine-graded assessment of clock-reading ability with a strong focus on visuospatial processing and little executive-processing demand. CRT and CDT are clock-processing tests with different demand profiles and can supplement each other in the neuropsychological evaluation of dementia and visuo-spatial dysfunction [77]. The Visual Cognitive Assessment Test (VCAT) is a visually based testing paradigm of cognitive function that allows easy application to multilingual populations and appears to have good performance in identifying early dysfunction. The VCAT has shown a good sensitivity and specificity for the diagnosis of MCI and mild AD [78].

The following segment points out different deficits and testing modalities commonly used in clinical practice to identify visuocognitive dysfunction:

Testing for Agnosia and Neglect

Testing for Agnosia - Visual agnosia may be tested simply by pointing to a common object, such as a comb and asking the patient to name and describe its use. Asking the patient to describe a complex scene from a photograph tests simultanagnosia; a drawing of a larger letter made up of smaller letters is another testing option, where the global superiority effect dominates for the larger letter.

Testing for Neglect – Classical tests for neglect are based on either cancellation, line bisection, and copying/drawing tasks [79, 80]. When testing extrapersonal visual neglect, it is important to place the patient's body in an unbiased position [81]. This is achieved by placing the patient in a neutral, body-centered, coordinate setting, such as making sure that the patient sits squarely in front of a table, with the trunk parallel to the edge of the desk [82]. Then the patient may bisect a line drawn on a piece of paper. The line or lines should be at least 15cm long and placed in front of the patient.

Line Bisection and Cancellation

Line bisection and line cancellation are two of the tests used most commonly to assess for neglect and because neglect can be induced by a variety of deficits, neither of these tests used alone is as sensitive as both used together (Figure 4) [83].

Instructions: have the patient cross out lines of varying sizes drawn on a sheet of paper, looking at midline bisection of the lines. The task can be performed on parallel lines (bisection) or random lines (cancellation).

Patients with neglect inappropriately bisect the line past the midpoint on the side that is opposite the neglected side. In other words, frequently show omissions and repetitive behavior on cancellation tests. Subjects with homonymous hemianopia usually cross out the line past the midpoint on the same side as their hemianopic defect [84]. The Single Letter Cancellation Test (SLCT) or the Star Cancellation Test are variations of this exercise, where the patient is asked to cross out certain letters or drawings of small stars placed among letters, words, and large stars. Most normal subjects will cross out nearly all stars [85]. The Letter Cancellation Task can also be tested with two letters (Double Letter Cancellation Test - DLCT). An attempt to combine both bisection and cancellation tests is integrated in the Character-line Bisection Task (CLBT) [86].

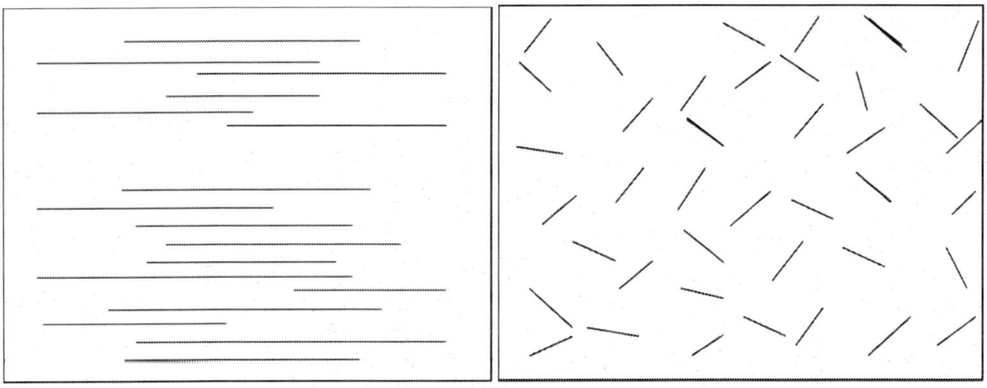

Figures 4. Examples of Line Bisection and Line Cancellation tasks.

Line Extension and Orientation

Line extension task - the subject is presented with half of a line and is asked to complete it towards the left or the right. Because directional motor performance is a major component of this task it should be sensitive enough to reveal premotor aspects in the neglect syndrome. Unilateral neglect preferential or dominant attention depends on dominance of either premotor factors (hypokinesia/hypometria) or perceptual factors. As shown by the landmark task, dominance of premotor factors cause a relative left underextension, most likely due to directional hypokinesia-hypometria [87, 88]. When perceptual factors dominate neglect, we can expect an overextension to the left (right unit drawn shorter than the left).

Line orientation task - the Benton Judgment of Line Orientation (JLO) is perhaps the purist test of spatial perception and is used to test what are called visuoperceptual deficits [89-92]. As with cancellation tests, the task requires very simple stimuli and requires simple responses with minimal movement. Most versions of this test require patients to determine whether lines are the same or different in slope and orientation. Either by match to sample from a multiple choice to best match a particular line, two lines are shown and are asked if they are the same or different. Performance decreases with age, but significantly with brain damage.

Scene Description

Scene Description - ask the patient to describe a scene from a drawing; neglect may be present if the subject limits descriptions to half or a portion of the scene. A good example is the Cookie Theft picture description task from the Boston Diagnostic Aphasia; a scene from a magazine description may also be used. Examination of the Cookie Theft picture is chosen because it is considered an ecologically valid approximation to spontaneous discourse [93]. The Complex Picture Test and the picture description task from the Kentucky Aphasia Test (KAT) are other options for testing [94, 95].

With these simple tests, there are three ways visual neglect may manifest: if the lines are bisected off the midline, a significant percentage of the random lines on one side are not cancelled out, or the numerals on the clock face are clustered to one side. Visual agnosia must be differentiated from object naming problems where in the latter the patient may describe the object after recognizing it, and clues toward a visual agnosia diagnosis may be yielded by the isolation agnosia to the visual sense, and preservation of recognition via other somatosensory means such as touch and feel.

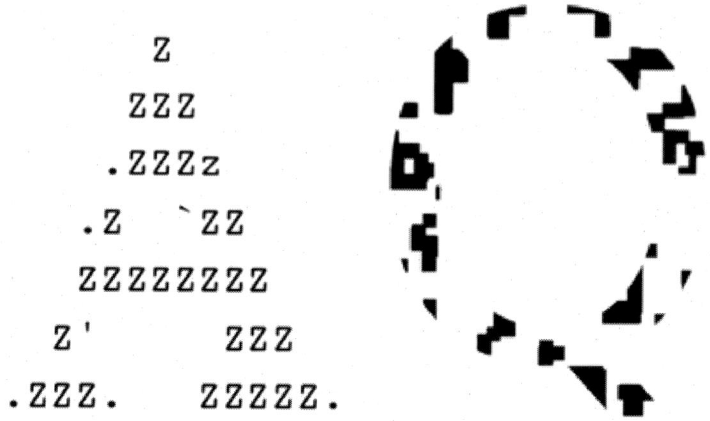

Figure 5. Examples of alternate visuospatial tasks and letter recognition variants.

Large letter composed of small letters (Navon Task). Next is an example of an Incomplete (Degraded 30%) Letter (from the VOSP). Reprinted with permission, Pearson Education Limited.

Visuoconstructive Function

The Clock Drawing Task (CDT) is a standard model, that also has considerable normative data across a wide age range and aging appears to have an effect, with the most common errors occurring in those older than age 70 with incorrect length or proportion of clock hands and incorrect placement of the minute and hand. The CDT can also serve as a screening test given its quick application and provides a more accurate assessment of the visuospatial function and executive function, but is also influenced by other cognitive functions. The test reveals the pattern of frontal and temporal-parietal functioning.

Performance on the CDT has been suggested as a way to differentiate patients with late onset depression (LOD) from early onset depression (EOD). In one study, the LOD group had significantly lower scores on the CDT than patients with EOD and healthy controls [96, 97]. Minute hand functionality in the representation of semantic memory impairment was highly correlated with CDT performance and was significantly different between the EOD and the LOD groups.

In one study, patients with early Alzheimer disease could be discriminated from healthy controls and from participants with mild cognitive impairment, solely by misplacement of the minute hand in the Clock Drawing and Clock Setting [98]. The later stages of Alzheimer disease group showed significantly more impairments in all Clock Test variants. It is assumed that early stage Alzheimer disease deficits in Clock Tests are mainly determined by a reduced access to semantic memory about the appearance and functionality of a clock.

In patients with early stages of AD, access to visual-semantic knowledge appears to be reduced. The fusiform gyrus might be crucial for the visual-semantic retrieval of clock time representation. The minute hand task provokes a stronger activation of areas in the parietal lobes known to be involved in spatial mental imagery, while the semantic task primarily activates regions of the superior temporal lobes associated with verbal conceptual knowledge [100, 101, 102]. Patients with early AD have shown worse performance in both clock tasks in correlation with reduced activation in the occipital lobes and the left fusiform gyrus, and additional activation in the precuneus [103-107]. In advanced AD, degraded knowledge regarding the appearance of a clock can explain the reduced ability to draw a clock face, while in early AD, impaired access to semantic knowledge about the minute hand might explain observed difficulties in drawing, setting, and reading the minute hand (Figure 6) [96]. Deteriorated semantic memory best predicts the performance on the Clock Test. This was concluded by results from a Clock Questionnaire that examined semantic knowledge of the concept of a "Clock" correlated with performance in Clock Drawing, Setting and Reading by control and clinical groups with the ROCF as a control task.

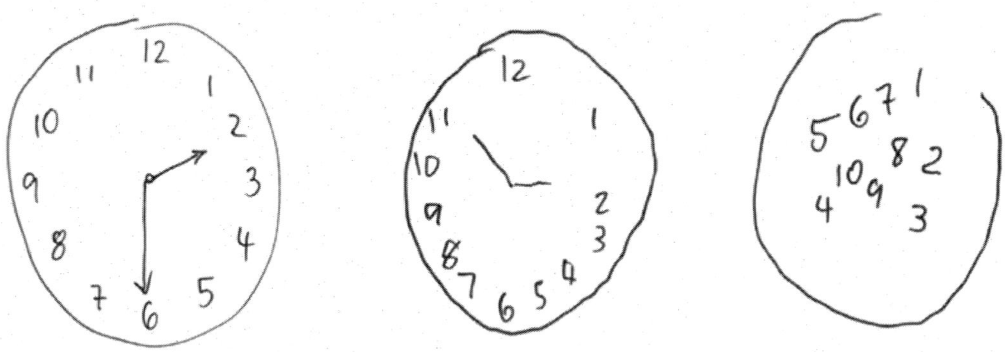

Figure 6. Clock Drawing Task. Samples of clock drawing, showing typical progression of disease by three subjects, where deterioration of pattern processing ability ranges from mild cognitive impairment (MCI) to severe AD. When asked to draw the same clock with the hours showing the time 2:30: in MCI/early AD, the numbers for the hours on the clock are properly drawn, but by the time he/she finished drawing the first part of the clock, the subject forgot what the time details. In late-stage AD, the drawing bears poor resemblance to a clock. Sources: [3, 99].

The 'double-pentagon copy' is included in the Mini Mental State Examination (MMSE) [99, 108, 109, 110]. It is composed of two overlapping pentagons, with the overlapping shape being a rhombus, assessing visual motor ability. Scoring of this subtest in the MMSE relies on a 0/1. The 'double-diamond copy' is part of the Bender-Gestalt Test (Figure 7). It grades the drawing based on sample pictures in a 0-4 score scale, with scores from 0-2 usually reserved for very poor performance such as patients with dementia.

The Rey-Osterreith Complex-Figure Test (ROFC) is one of the most popular tools for assessing construction [111, 112]. The test involves the copying and recall of abstract line drawings. This instrument assesses perceptual organization and visual memory. The figure is well normed for population above 70 years old and has several usable scoring systems, is simple to administer and sufficiently complex to elicit a wide variety of visuospatial deficits. The Extended Complex Figure Test (ECTF) is a variant of the test [113]. The ROCF has multiple scoring systems, among them the Boston Qualitative Scoring System (BQSS) or the Developmental Scoring System (DSS-ROCF), targeted for pediatrics. The test is also known as the Rey-Osterrieth figure, Rey Complex Figure Test (RCTF), the Complex Figure Test (CFT), and Rey Figure (RF) [76].

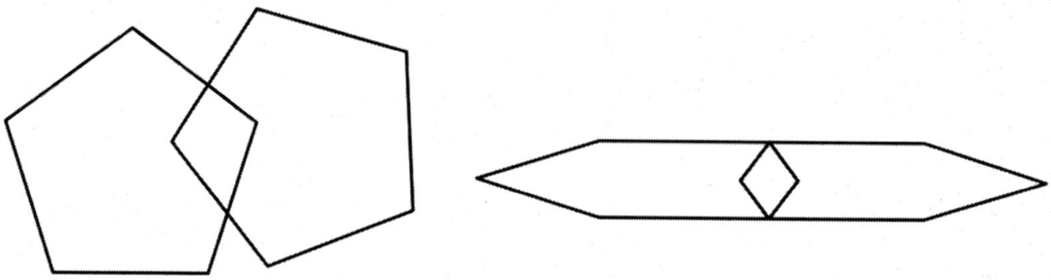

Figure 7. Example of a double pentagon copying model and double diamond.

Standardized Testing

Increasingly, clinicians have come to rely on standardized assessment instruments for diagnosis and management of patients with dementia. Other aspects of dementia such as behavior, function and staging of disease are equally important to capture quantitatively [54]. Standardized testing such as the Block Design subtest of the WAIS-R which measures the spatial/visual orientation, speed of execution, perceptual integration, capacity of planning and organization, among other tests in the neuropsychological laboratory are considerably more detailed than what can be practical and performed at the bedside [85, 114, 115]. The Block Design subtest may be time consuming and shorter alternatives have emerged such as the Design Organization Test (DOT) [116].

An important cognitive battery of visuospatial performance is the Visual Object and Space Perception (VOSP) test [117, 118]. The VOSP consists of a comprehensive group of tests for assessing object or space perception while minimizing the involvement of other cognitive skills. Results are compared to normal controls and with right and left cerebral lesions. Subtests are listed in Table 4.

The VOSP test is divided into two parts of four each, separating ventral and dorsal streams, although in one study did not demonstrate reliability of these two categories as guidelines to detect ventral or dorsal stream dysfunction [119]. Many stimuli for brief testing are included, where testing with fragmented letters is part of the object perception testing stimuli [120, 121]. The silhouette identification task requires subjects to name or identify the silhouette profile of objects and animals viewed from unusual perspectives and it represents both the perceptual and semantic abilities. The recognition of a silhouette as a real (vs. unreal) object or animal is thought to require an intact structural description linked to the right temporal lobe, while naming and other forms of accurate item specific identification require additional semantic processes associated with the left temporal lobe [122].

Table 4. VOSP – Visual Object and Space Perception Battery

Object Perception (Ventral Stream)	
Incomplete Letters	Screening test: subjects name individual letters (1 per card) degraded by 30%
Silhouettes	Subjects identify 15 silhouettes of animals and 15 silhouettes of inanimate objects, presented at unusual angles. Subjects may name, gesture, mimic use, or describe the object (language is minimized)
Object Decision	Subject must select a picture of a real object juxtaposed among 3 nonsense objects. They are not required to name the object, and need only identify which one is real.
Progressive Silhouettes	Cards with shadows of one of two objects, presented at sequentially more recognizable viewpoints. Subjects are shown 10 cards of a gun and 120 cards of a trumpet, with the goal of identifying the object with the fewest number of presented cards.
Space Perception (Dorsal Stream)	
Dot Counting	Counting random assortment of five to nine scattered dots on a card
Position Discrimination	Subjects are shown two cards, each containing a single black dot that is either exactly centered or slightly off-center; subject must specify which card contains the centered dot.
Number Location	Subjects are presented with two cards, one with scattered numbers (from one to nine) and the other with a single dot, corresponding to the position of an individual number. Subjects must indicate which number corresponds to the single dot.
Cube Analysis	Subjects must count stacked blocks (including hidden ones) rendered as drawing on cards. There is one practice item.

Table 5. Visuospatial – Standardized and Battery Testing

Test	Characteristics
The Clock Test (Tuokko, Hadjistravrooulos, Miller, Horton and Beattle, 1995)	Uses the three subsets of Clock Drawing, Clock Setting and Clock Reading. The test is normed in adults 65 and older.
VOT - Hooper Visual Organization Test™ (Hooper, 1958)	A quick assessment of visual integration. Does not require writing or manipulation. Standardized for adults (ages 5 to 91).
Judgment of Line Orientation (JLO) (Benton et al., 1994; 1974, 1983) Benton Line Orientation Task (BLO)	Tests perception and orientation as well as visuospatial judgment. Also a strong visuospatial test, it requires matching the angle and orientation of lines in space. Subjects are asked to match two angled lines to a set of 11 lines that are arranged in a semicircle and separated 18 degrees from each other. Normative data available for ages 7 through 14 and 16 through 74.
Benton Visual Retention Test® BFRT - Benton Facial Recognition Test	Assess visual perception, memory, and visuoconstructive abilities BFRT - There are three parts: (1) matching a frontal view of the target with an identical photograph, (2) matching a frontal view of the target individual with three photos of the target taken from different angles, and (3) matching a frontal view of the target individual with three photos of the target taken under different lighting conditions. No time limits are placed and scores 41 or above are normal. The black and white photos used consist of unfamiliar male and female faces with their hair and clothing shaded out so that subjects must rely on the face.

Table 5. (Continued)

Test	Characteristics
RMF - The Warrington Recognition Memory for Faces	RMF - Subjects are presented with black and white photos of 50 unfamiliar men at a rate of one item every 3 seconds, and are asked to respond 'yes' or 'no' according to whether they find the face pleasant or not pleasant. Immediately following presentation of the target photos, memory for the photos is tested with a forced choice between a target photo identical to that presented earlier and a distracter photo. The number of correct choices determines the score. The maximum score is 50. Means range between 42.4 and 44.3 depending on the age group.
Motor-Free Visual Perception Test – Third Edition (MVPT-3) (Colarusso and Hammill, 2003)	Assess visual perception through spatial relationships, visual closure, visual discrimination, visual memory and figure ground. Originally meant to assess visual perception independent of motor ability in children, however, it has been extensively used and validated in all ages (4-95 y/o).
Rey Complex Figure Test and Recognition Trial (RCFT – Meyers and Meyers, 1995) (Bernstein and Waber, 1994)	Copy, Immediate recall, delayed recall, and recognition. The patient copies the original figure and 3 minutes, as well as 30 minute delays are tested. Validation in adults 18-89.
VOSP – Visual and Object Space and Perception Battery (1991)	Consists of nine tests each designed to assess a particular aspect of object or space perception, while minimizing the involvement of other cognitive sills.
CORVIST - Cortical Vision Screening Test (2001)	Similar to the VOSP. Each of the ten tests focuses on a different aspect of early visual processing by cortical centers. Each is prefaced by a description of its aim, the instructions to the subject, and an indication of its significance.
BIT – Behavioral Inattention Test (initially known as the Rivermead Behavioral Inattention Test). *See also* The Arnadottir OT-ADL Neurobehavioural Evaluation for similar spatial relationship testing.	Short screening battery of tests to assess the presence and the extent of visual neglect on a sample of everyday problems faced by patients with visual inattention*. May be less appropriate for patients with dementia as it was initially targeted for patients with focal brain injuries.
BORB - Birmingham Object Recognition Battery	Measures low-level aspects of visual perception in matching tasks on orientation, size, length, position of objects and a figure-ground task of overlapping figures. Intermediate processes of object recognition are measured in recognition tasks with objects from unfamiliar viewpoints. Object knowledge is tested in an object decision task, a task on functional and associative matching, and a picture-naming task.
"Crossing out" tasks: Albert's Test (lines), Single Letter Cancellation Test (SLCT), Star Cancellation Test, Bells Test.	Hemi-inattention and Neglect Testing, one study found the Bells Test and the Letter-Cancellation Test more likely to detect neglect in patients with spatial neglect than the Line Bisection Test (n=35) [69].
WAIS-III Block design subtest), Cubes Test WAIS-III, or "Wechsler Cubes"	Non-verbal. Wide implementation history.

Test	Characteristics
Raven's Progressive Matrices (Raven et al, 1938)	Visual analysis and synthesis, standardized for adults, non-verbal, long trajectory
Beery VMI - The Beery - Buktenica Developmental Test of Visual-Motor Integration, Fifth Edition (Beery and Beery, 2006)	Measures of visual-motor integration and detects visual-motor deficits predictive of learning difficulties. Requires copying 24 geometric designs that increase in complexity.

The Standardized Road-Map test of Direction Sense of Money was designed to evaluate topographic orientation [123]. It involves important spatial abilities like the capacity to do right–left discriminations, and mental rotation [124, 125]. The test is sensitive to age and gender differences and easily administered [126, 127].

The Corsi Block Tapping Test is further focused on visuo-spatial short-term working memory, where the patient is asked to repeat (or replicate in reverse) the prearranged sequence that the examiner taps on the blocks [128]. The instrument evaluates attention and working memory.

Other examples of domain specific - impairment oriented visuospatial standardized tests include the Benton Facial Recognition Test the Hooper Test of Visual Organization, and the aforementioned Rey-Osterrieth Complex Figure [129-132].

3. Dementia Pathophysiology in Specific Visual and Spatial Deficits

Proteinopathy in Alheimer's Disease

Alzheimer's disease is considered a multi-proteinopathy, with neuropathological correlates of both extracellular amyloid plaques (Neuritic Plaques, NP) and intracellular microtubule associated protein tau (Neurofibrillary Tangles, NFT). Sporadic Alzheimer's disease or idiopathic AD is associated with dysfunctional gene expression in the limbic system and entorhinal cortex of the brain that drives amyloidogenesis, pro-inflammatory signaling, alterations in innate-immunity and related AD-type neuropathology [133, 134, 135].

AD affects several aspects of vision, and visual dysfunction may in turn contribute to performance decrements in other cognitive domains [136]. As the disease progresses, almost every structure of the visual system is affected by Alzheimer's pathology - from the lens and retina to visual association areas, amyloid pathology in the form of beta-amyloid deposits may be found in both the lens of the eye and the retina.

In moderate to late-stages of AD, pro-inflammatory and amyloidogenic pathology spreads through the entorhinal-primary visual sensory cortex-thalamic-retinal axis, which is believed to be responsible in part for the complex visual disturbances, such as spatial and visual agnosia, facial identification problems, perceptual disturbances, and visual hallucinations, associated with end-stages of the AD process.

Although memory loss is typically the first symptom in AD, it is well known that visuospatial deficits are also typical of initial stages and mid-stages of disease, and correlate with clinicopathological patterns described on Thal amyloid phase and Braak NFT staging [140]. In fact, for a long time it was believed that cognitive impairment in AD began with memory impairment as the first symptom followed by attention and later abstract reasoning. While Alzheimer pathology primarily overcomes the hippocampal CA1 and temporal lobe neocortex, it is not clear if the primary visual cortex and the retina are initially spared. Further studies revealed that visuospatial processing or visual function degrade in the earliest stages of AD.

Table 6. Common Neurovisual Deficits in Alzheimer's Disease Patients

Pseudoisochromatic color discrimination tasks.
Object Naming
Facial discrimination
Facial recognition
Low spatial frequency loss (modest increases improve performance)
Spatial processing deficits
Spatially related difficulties (spatial disorientation) likely reflects impaired visuospatial processing in AD Patients

Sources: M. Lehmann et al. (137). DS Geldmacher (138). DA Valenti [139].

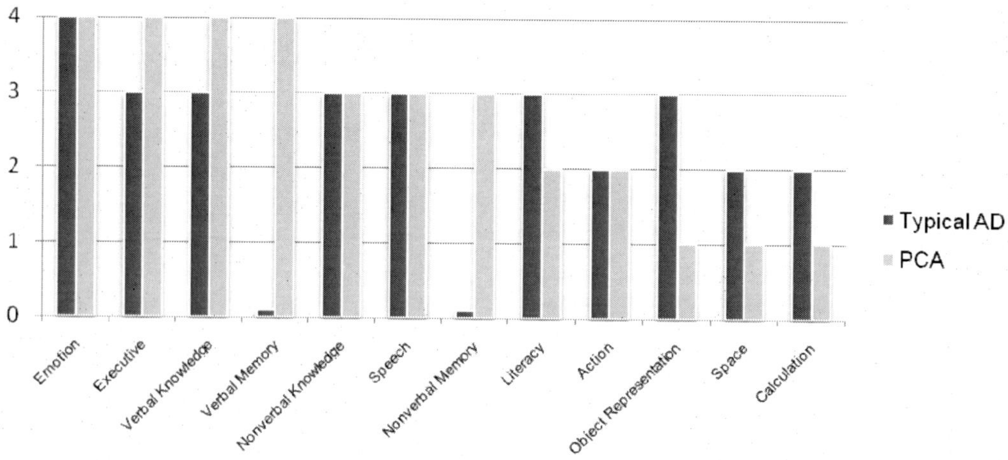

Source: [141].

Figure 8. Core network paradigm of neurodegeneration in AD compared to PCA.

The autopsy findings from the Framingham Heart Study served as evidence that initial pathology of AD may originate in the visual association areas, where more than 50% of non-demented subjects (those without history of memory complaints or cognitively normal) presented with beta amyloid and neurofibrillary tangles in the visual association areas [142, 143]. Some of these patients even had absence of pathology in the hippocampus, thus suggesting that AD may actually start in the visual integration areas, where visual function loss other than visual acuity may become dysfunctional.

In summary, with disease progression, cortical pathology in AD becomes selectively involved in the association areas (sensory and polymodal association cortices in the ventral parietal lobes); these areas most likely lead to many of the visuospatial deficits seen in AD.

Posterior Cortical Atrophy

When the principal symptom in dementia is dominated by visuospatial impairment, the burden of the pathology is usually seen in the parietal and occipital lobes, where very frequently Alzheimer's type pathology is the main culprit. Clinically the syndrome is referred to as posterior cortical atrophy (PCA) or visual variant of Alzheimer's disease, the former being preferred because non-AD dementias are also occasionally seen in patients with prominent visuospatial impairment [144-150]. Patients may display a gradually developing simultanagnosia (Balint Syndrome) and/or manifest early with dominantly and early visuospatial symptoms. The neuropathology is similar, but with neuritic plaques (NP) and neurofibrillary tangles (NFT) in a more posterior cortical regional distribution than the usual patient with AD. Distribution of pathology includes the occipital lobe visual areas V2 and VI (Refer to Section on Posterior Cortical Atrophy) [151, 152].

Classification – Cognitive Domains

Visuo-spatial impairment may be a severe and early feature of degenerative dementias. Symptoms are broadly divisible into dorsal and ventral visual syndromes, which result from focal neurodegeneration in occipito-parietal and occipito-temporal visual association cortices, respectively. Less often, hemineglect or visual field defects result.

DSM-IV refers to agnosia as a feature of AD, which is rarely an initial presentation in early dementia. Milder dysfunction of higher visual and spatial functions was not mentioned in the previous manual and may be due to an area in which standard definitions lacked clarity. The DSM-5 now has descriptions of the general cognitive domains already included in the diagnosis of AD (aphasia, apraxia, agnosia, and impaired executive functioning). Cortical visual assessments are included under the perceptual motor neurocognitive domain [153]. The other five cognitive domains cognitive in the evaluation of neurocognitive disorders are: complex attention, executive function, learning and memory, language and social cognition [154]. NINCDS-ADRDA criteria referred to visual perception and to "praxis" but describe the latter as functions related to visual constructional ability [155].

The available literature on visuospatial dysfunction in AD is broadly dual [156]. One series is focused on visuo-perceptual nature of disorientation, and its association with optic flow perception and visuospatial attention [157-160]. The other series stresses on the cognitive mapping deficits, specifically in using allocentric navigation [161-165].

Changes in the Brain – Alzheimer's Disease

The possibility of identifying individuals most at risk for progression to AD during the preclinical stages is always entertained. The need for sensitive biomarkers in AD is becoming crucial as ever due to the implications that disease begins more than 20 years before the first noticeable symptom emerges. Mounting evidence supports that AD is a syndrome involving neural network disruption before cognitive deficits are detectable. Memory is one of the core deficits involved in the complex interaction of distributed brain networks, but is not the only cognitive domain dependent in these networks.

Advances in the neuroimaging of AD have highlighted dysfunctions in functional connectivity networks (FCNs). Patients with AD experience a brain network breakdown, with disconnections in both structural and functional systems. Certain components of networks have widespread alterations with progression of disease in AD, while others like the medial parietal regions and the subcortical areas are differentially affected depending on the disease stage. Compensatory mechanisms were only seen in the earliest stages of disease, before symptoms set in [166]. During resting state functional MRI (fMRI) studies, regional coherence analysis of signal was found altered in patients with AD and amnestic MCI [167].

Dorsal pathway dysfunctions are thought to underlie visuospatial processing problems in Alzheimer disease (AD). In healthy controls task-induced connectivity decreases between posterior cingulate and middle temporal and occipital visual cortices (ventral visual pathways). Involvement of these areas in visuospatial processing were markedly reduced in AD patients within a small area of the right middle temporal gyrus and superior temporal gyrus when switching from baseline to task condition [168]. These findings are implied to changes in visual processing as well as changes in the DMN connectivity in AD.

When visuospatial processing is examined, the two cortical streams might just be the best-delineated neuronal networks, with abundant data to support it [169-171]. The parietal cortex is in close connection with the medial temporal lobe (MTL) regions of the brain, through the posterior cingulate (retrosplenial cortex), where it also connects with the dorsal and ventral pathways.

Tasks that involve recognition of unusual oriented objects depend strongly on the dorsal visual pathways. Neural correlates in early AD using various task paradigms have also shown a compensation pattern mediated by the ventral pathway for dorsal visual dysfunction, possibly with additional pre-frontal activation [172, 173]. Other studies found the opposite: increased activation or increased deactivation has been interpreted as either dedifferentiation or compensatory mechanisms, while decreased activation or decreased deactivation has been considered as signs of functional loss [174-177]. Functional compensatory mechanisms in early AD appear to be also present in lateral and medial temporal regions [178-181].

Performance with Visuospatial Dysfunction

Patients with AD usually seek an ophthalmic consultation because of disturbances of pattern processing and recognition. Visual deterioration under stress, blurry vision at wide, intermediate or near distances, not fully relieved with glasses, problems with judging depth, eye strain with no apparent cause, reading small print, and restricted depth of focus when reading are some of the main reported symptoms. Depth perception dysfunction may impair tasks such as filling a glass with water. Subjects might also mention that driving a car causes strain or tired eyes, any light sensitivity. Clumsiness, falls, walking into objects, or balance problems are also commonly reported by patients. Individuals with AD frequently show a "closing-in" phenomenon, a tendency to close in on a model while copying it, and considered a form of visuospatial compensation [182-185]. Anatomical correlates of the phenomenon show bilateral orbitofrontal area dysfunction, which may reveal it as an imitation behavior that is commonly observed in frontal lobe damage [186].

Changes involving visual pathways in AD and these also contribute to intellectual deterioration [136]. Visual sensory functions affected in AD include spatial contrast sensitivity, color, stereopsis, temporal resolution and motion [187-209]. Further investigations also evidenced visual attention and "higher" visual (reading, route finding, object localization) and recognition dysfunction [157, 210-216].

Color vision studies in AD have yielded inconsistent results [192, 217-220]. Patients have an unspecific color vision deficiency independent of the severity of the disease. Suggestions of an incomplete achromatopsia in some cases are attributed to lesions in the peristriate and inferotemporal visual cortices. Testing methods vary from study to study, making direct comparisons difficult, and some color vision tests might have been too complicated for patients with AD, leading to unreliable results [217, 221]. As recent studies indicate that problems in naming of colors may result from cognitive decline, conventional color tests should probably not be applied in AD patients [217].

Oculomotor Function in Dementia

Oculomotor dysfunction is well described in neurodegenerative diseases, especially those that involve Parkinsonism. Neurodegeneration in both Parkinson's disease dementia (PDD) and dementia with Lewy bodies (DLB) affect cortical and subcortical networks that are mostly involved in saccade generation [222, 223]. One study showed that patients with PCA were significantly less consistent than typical AD and controls in where they were looking on evaluation of optical scanning during several tasks [73]. When comparing search and non-search tasks, another study found that controls exhibited the lowest between task similar ratings, suggesting they were better able than PCA or AD to respond appropriately to high-level needs by looking at task relevant regions of a scene [224]. Patients with PCA appear to have a significant tendency to fixate upon more low-level salient parts of the scenes than controls [225, 226]. Nevertheless, how these changes impact upon visual information processing remain unclear [227].

Behavioral eye movements in AD (oculomotor function) include impaired oculomotor reaction time, saccade and pursuit generation and target tracking. The most common scanning errors in AD were poor organization of visual search [228]. Patients with AD demonstrate impairments in text and clock reading, with less focused visual exploration strategies correlating with task error rates and dementia severity [229-232]. Ocular Scan Path Analysis in AD has shown perseveration in the oculomotor programming (as well as intrusions) such as returning to previously fixated locations. Eye movement during clock reading displayed impairment in disengagement – probably due to parietal dysfunction in AD [233].

Recent evidence suggests that visuomotor behaviors may be disrupted in the very early stages of Alzheimer's disease. Visuomotor impairments in a group of subjects at increased risk of AD were found to have worse performance as visuomotor task demands increased [234]. Kinematic measures that place demands on visual-spatial and cognitive motor processing may provide an effective behavioral way and potential biomarker to detect subtle early changes associated with risk of AD, with data supporting this notion reporting sensitivity of 81.8% and specificity of 90.9% in differentiating low vs high risk of developing AD. The notion behind this finding lies in that visuomotor impairments may reflect inherent brain alterations that disrupt reciprocal communication between hippocampal, parietal and frontal regions, and thus permits preparing and updating complex reaching movements [235].

Topographic Disorientation

Getting lost is one of the earliest clinical manifestations in AD [236]. Navigation in space is a complex cognitive function that is essential for independence, safety, and quality of life. Episodes of topographical disorientation were reported both in outpatients and patients residing in a community and where almost 90% of patients with AD reported as having their first incident of disorientation in familiar surroundings [237, 238, 239].

Spatial navigation impairment occurs early in the development of AD and can be used for monitoring of disease progression or for evaluation of presymptomatic AD. Spatial disorientation in AD manifests as getting lost in familiar and unfamiliar places. More specific characterization using spatial navigation tests in both real space and virtual environments has shown further impairment in multiple spatial abilities, including allocentric and egocentric navigation strategies, visuo-spatial perception, or selection of relevant information for successful navigation [156]. Patients suffering mild cognitive impairment (MCI), who are at a high risk of developing dementia, show impairment in a subset of these abilities, mainly connected with allocentric and egocentric processing [156]. While spatial disorientation in typical AD patients probably reflects neurodegenerative changes in medial, posterior temporal, parietal, frontal lobes and retrosplenial cortex, the impairment of spatial navigation in MCI seems to be connected mainly to changes in medial temporal and parietal lobes.

Route learning impairment is common in early AD and MCI, and is occasionally also found in elder subjects. Its characteristic appearance is a combination of poor landmark recognition and defective directional guidance, and performance may be predicted by neuropsychological testing [240]. Hippocampal dysfunction may be responsible for any allocentric deficits in older adults, as it is recognized that specifically the right hippocampus plays a critical role in allocentric navigation, particularly when cognitive impairment is present [162].

Deficits in spatial memory, generally defined as the ability to encode, store, and retrieve spatial information in order to build an internal representation of the environment (a 'cognitive map'), is often underestimated in the elderly [241, 242]. Topographical disorientation is an umbrella-term for a set of heterogeneous cognitive deficits, comprising a difficulty, or inability, to find one's way in familiar and unfamiliar environments, learn new routes, recognize places, describe a pathway verbally, and use a map for self-orientation.

Patients with lesions in the nondominant hemisphere, particularly at the junction of the occipito-temporoparietal regions, may manifest predominantly visuospatial dysgnosia, a loss of the sense of "whereness" in the relation of himself to his environment and in the relation of objects to each other. Visuospatial disturbances caused by lesions in the dominant hemisphere may be masked by other gnostic symptoms, whereas patients with more extensive lesions may also exhibit other cognitive disturbances associated with vision [243].

Egocentric, or body-centered, spatial navigation where distance and directions from individuals' body position are used for navigation, is instead parietal lobe dependent and not affected in older adults. Older age may be associated with changes in the medial temporal lobe, which may result in mild spatial navigation deficits, especially in allocentric navigation, whereas egocentric navigation and learning may remain preserved [244-251].

The navigation disability in Alzheimer disease and mild cognitive impairment (MCI) involves a selective impairment of spatial cognition and is associated with atrophy of the right-lateralized navigation network [252]. Among these individuals, deterioration in spatial navigation, manifested by poor hippocampus-dependent allocentric navigation, may occur well before the clinical onset of dementia [176, 253].

Nestor et al. explored topographical disorientation in AD with by developing a virtual navigation test, the Virtual Route Learning Test (VRLT) [254]. The test required participants to learn four routes of increasing complexity following verbal instructions and visual pointers, for later retracing the route in reverse from memory virtually with a joystick. Performance on VRLT demonstrated sensitivity in detecting navigational impairment in very early AD, and specifically discriminated AD patients from patients with Semantic Dementia. The neural basis of performance on VRLT revealed common areas of activation with normal route learning and early neurodegeneration in AD in the retrosplenial, lateral parietal cortices and possibly the hippocampal tail [255].

The Four Mountains Test was found to be fairly specific to the hippocampal topographic memory [253]. When comparing cognitive processes underlying amnestic MCI and frontotemporal lobar degeneration, the authors found a specific impairment in topographical short-term memory that may distinguish AD from FTLD.

Despite the clinical significance of disorientation in Alzheimer's disease, it is not clear which cognitive spatial processes are primarily impaired. Specifically, patients show impairment in translating from an allocentric hippocampal representation to an egocentric parietal one for the purpose of effective spatial orientation and navigation. Serino and Riva suggest that a break in "mental frame syncing," underpinned by damage to the hippocampus and retrosplenial cortex, may be a crucial cognitive marker both for early and differential diagnosis of AD [256]. Identification of these spatial deficits could facilitate the development of early cognitive rehabilitation interventions [248].

Impaired spatial navigation is an early sign of Alzheimer's disease (AD), but this can be difficult to assess in clinical practice. Patients with Alzheimer's disease performed worse in routine recognition tasks or an adaptation of the Morris water maze task [252, 257, 258]. Increased severity of cognitive impairment was associated with worse performance on the Floor Maze Test (FMT), which combines navigation with walking. The FMT was primarily associated with executive dysfunction, and thus may fail to capture impairments in spatial navigation [257].

Visual Search and Attention

Spatial exploration involves a scan and search in order to attend to areas of interest, followed by adjusting the body accordingly for participation or action with the environment. Visual search for a target in an array of distractors relies upon flexible shifts between global and local modes of attentional processing. Visual Attention is usually mixed in almost all types of neuropsychological testing, but is selectively worse in AD where there is poor ability to acquire information in the brief visual stimulus presentations.

Difficulty redirecting focus of attention, narrowing of the functional visual field and the useful field of view are also frequently reported. For example the Nebes and Brady describe an example in mild to moderate AD, where impairment in reorienting attention away from initial stimuli (disengaging) was adversely affected by automatic redirections of attention toward peripherally occurring invalid cues become lost [211, 259]. Activity in primary visual cortex predicts performance in a visual detection task [260]. A qualitative difference in the architecture of visual search between AD and aging may reflect a specific deficit in the disengagement of visual spatial attention, a prolongation of saccade initiation, or inefficiency in planning a search strategy [261]. Visual inattention deficits in visual search tasks appear to depend on the type of stimuli involved and influence in performance on these tests [262].

Visual search is slowed in patients with AD, in part due to an increase in the number and duration of eye fixations made en route to a target [263]. It is thought of this phenomenon as a compensatory adaptation to a narrowing of the zone of focal attention, necessitating more shifts of gaze in order to attend to the global workspace. An increase in the average number and duration of peripheral fixations was seen in older adults and AD patients when compared to younger subjects. Inefficiency of visual search strategies in AD may be due to reduced dynamic ability to adjust the attention zoom ("zoom lens"), coupled with inability to disengage attention from peripheral targets [263].

Depth and Motion Perception

Patients with Alzheimer's disease (AD) commonly have visuospatial deficits such as impaired depth perception (stereopsis) and motion perception [136, 202, 264, 265]. Visual problems such as in spatial orientation and locomotion affected by deficient depth perception in AD can affect quality of life and impair activities of daily living [193]. Known areas of brain activation in response to tasks requiring motion and depth perception include V5 or BA19/37, BA7 in the dorsal parietal cortex and parieto-occipital junction [206]. It is also widely accepted that subjects with AD have more difficulty viewing non-canonical (unusual) views of objects [181].

Posterior Cortical Atrophy

Posterior Cortical Atrophy (PCA) is a type of dementia that presents with a prototypical visuospatial syndrome [145]. Also known as Benson's Syndrome, it is a clinical syndrome of parieto-occipital degeneration.

Nosology for PCA remains inconsistent, but the term "Posterior Cortical Atrophy" is mainly applied to two clinical circumstances [266]:

1. Patients with Alzheimer's disease or preclinical Alzheimer's disease that have manifestations of early and/or dominant symptoms of visual cortical dysfunction combined with neuroimaging that reveals disproportionate selectivity of atrophy to posterior cortices.
2. Patients with clinical manifestations of severe visual cortical dysfunction of unknown etiology with neuroimaging evidence of atrophy of the posterior cortex (may be of different etiologies).

PCA is best classified as a phenomenological presentation of severe visual cortical dysfunction with evidence of atrophy of the posterior cortices evidenced by neuroimaging, and where associated dementia is common [266, 267]. Clinical phenotypes and pathology diagnosis suggest that multiple etiologies contribute to PCA as a syndrome. It is most frequently described as a visual variant of Alzheimer's disease, but about 20% of cases are caused by either Dementia with Lewy Bodies, Corticobasal Degeneration or Prion Disease (including the Heidenhain variant of CJD or HvCJD) [141, 225]. In one-half to two-third of cases, the pathology will show neuritic plaques and neurofibrillary tangles as seen in AD [145].

About 50% of patients with PCA have homonymous hemianopsia, but basic ophthalmoscopic evaluation of vision is usually normal. Anxiety and depression are a common presenting symptom as well, the former being a prominent symptom when compared to AD (268). More commonly disrupting the dorsal visual stream, the PCA syndrome is also described as a disorder of mid-level perception [146]. Patients present visual difficulty with distances and localization, steadiness of static images, problems reading and struggle walking on irregular surfaces. Simultanagnosia appears to be the most common and hence sensitive feature of early PCA [147]. Prominent clinical features also include complex visual disturbances, like those in Balint Syndrome, and deficits lead to multiple impairments in activities of daily living that require visual control. PCA may also feature Gerstmann's syndrome (left-right confusion, dysgraphia, dyscalculia, and finger agnosia), or elements of these syndromes and/or prosopagnosia, central achromatopsia, alexia (inability to read), contralateral hemineglect and visual agnosia [269, 270]. Table 7 lists some features described in the literature that due to the odd and bizarre description that these may sound, they might be tragically, mistaken as a psychiatric symptom.

A systematic review and meta-analysis of neuropsychological and brain morphometry showed that PCA patients exhibited significant decreases in temporal, occipital and parietal gray matter volumes, whereas AD patients showed extensive left temporal atrophy [271]. Compared to healthy controls, PCA exhibits a distribution of brain atrophy similar to AD, in particular atrophy of the left fusiform, left parahippocampal gyrus and left middle temporal gyrus, a shared pattern of wide temporal atrophy. PCA patients exhibit significantly more atrophy in the right occipital gyrus and right posterior lobe when compared to patients with AD, while atrophy in the left parahippocampal gyrus and hippocampus is greater in the AD group [272]. PCA patients exhibit significantly greater impairment in immediate visuospatial memory as well as visuoperceptual and visuospatial abilities than patients with AD, who alternatively showed greater impairment in delayed auditory/verbal memory.

Table 7. Complex Visual Symptoms – Deficits in visuospatial integration in Posterior Cortical Atrophy [137]

- Positive Perceptual Phenomena
- Prolonged Color After-images
- Reverse size phenomena
- Visual crowding
- Perception of movement of static stimuli
- 180° upside-down reversal of vision

Focal atypical presentations of AD such as PCA may be more common than previously thought [141, 273, 274]. Posterior atrophy (PA) appears to be characteristic of AD in patients with typical and atypical clinical presentations (20% and 34% incidence respectively) and is an important factor in the assessment of AD vs Frontotemporal lobar degeneration (FTLD) [137, 272]. Combined with relative sparing of the medial temporal lobe, PA appears to be a hallmark finding for patients with atypical clinical presentations such as PCA [275]. PA appears to be a particular feature of early-onset AD (EOAD), where atrophy of posterior cingulate gyrus, precuneus and parietal lobes was found to be more frequent than in typical AD [276, 277, 278].

In an attempt to grade atrophy of the posterior cortices, including the parietal lobes, the Koedam MRI rating scale was developed, where a PA visual scale is rated from 0-3 in different planes [275]. Compared with other visual rating scales of cortical atrophy, such as the medial temporal lobe atrophy (MTA) or the global cortical atrophy (GCA) visual scales, the initial results of the Koedam MRI rating scale showed good inter-rating agreement ratios and excellent intra-rater agreement ratios [273].

Disabilities in Reading and Writing in Posterior Cortical Atrophy

Problems with reading are frequent and debilitating in PCA, where dyslexia occurs in about 80%–95% of cases [279-281]. Clinical reports describe patients with PCA as having difficulty following text along a printed line, getting lost from one line to the next, seeing words in "false order," and losing their place on a page [279, 282-285]. Dyslexia is likely peripheral in nature, where reading is typical letter by letter, and words written in script with missing or distorted letters may be prominent [279, 280, 285, 286]. This is especially noticeable in musical notation reading. The impairment involves visual analysis of written words with a core defect in recognition of visual-word forms. They may spell words or write cogent sentences, later unable to read them.

Acquired dyslexia may present in patients with PCA where identification of letters within words, even if the words are read correctly, or identifying words flanked by extraneous letters (e.g., "lsoapm") and where reading skills are severely limited [287]. Alzheimers disease produced frequent "blend" errors in a patient described by Saffran, in which letters from one word of a two-word display intruded into the other word [288]. Visual Crowding is an early or prelexical reading deficit, and the extent of visual dysfunction in PCA appears to rely on the proximity (but not identity) of contiguous letters, which significantly influenced the report of a target letter [287].

Written words may be analyzed asymmetrically in space. Erroneous completions of a word based on its stem or ending (eg wish for dish or room for root) suggest misreading or the left or right portion of the word, respectively (neglect dyslexia). Visual paralexias (mistaking k for x or r for p) are common [289]. There may be particular difficulty reading text versus words in isolation, consistent with an interference effect from other similar stimuli in the visual field (attentional dyslexia). Eventually recognition of individual letters may become impossible.

Spatial dysgraphia is an early symptom in PCA [73, 251, 290, 291]. Letter shape selection, formation, placement and sequencing in writing are affected in various stages of the motor output process [292]. Writing dysfunction of the aforementioned kind produce a series of peripheral dysgraphias that may take several different forms. Vascular dementia and CBD presentations of dysgraphia involve an effortful, impoverished, or inconstant letter formation, with or without mixing of upper and lower case letters. In Alzheimer's dementia surface dysgraphia is also frequently found, and non-phonologically plausible errors often increase with disease progression. Surface dysgraphia is a predictable feature in semantic dementia that when compared to AD mechanisms of handwriting are preserved [293].

Surface dysgraphia is the most common spelling impairment in PCA syndromes. Also known as lexical agraphia, it is characterized by impaired spelling of words with exceptional or unpredictable sound-to-spelling correspondences (e.g., cough, yacht), with a tendency to produce phonologically plausible errors (e.g., tomb → TOOM, plane → PLAIN). Spelling of regular words or non-words is well-preserved due to unaffected phoneme-to-grapheme conversion skills. Writing legibility worsens with progression of disease in PCA. Reduplication of letter strokes, poor spacing and placement of letters on the page start to appear, and skewed or undulating lines of script characteristic of spatial dysgraphia are common.

Scene Perception tasks, those that require scanning ocular movement gaze patterns but not a search component, proved that PCA patients were significantly less consistent than typical Alzheimer's disease patients and controls in where they were looking. On searching tasks PCA patients had a significant tendency to fixate upon more low-level salient parts of the scenes than controls irrespective of the viewing task. PCA and AD patients appear to have limitations in their response to high-level needs. Healthy controls respond appropriately by looking at task-relevant regions of a scene than posterior cortical atrophy or typical Alzheimer's disease patients [73].

When compared to AD, PCA shows a younger onset, more focal complex visual symptoms, better verbal fluency and memory impairment is much less prominent memory impairment. If the nature of visual complaints remains elusive, clinically useful signs for the consideration of PCA include unexplained Ishihara color defects and impaired clock drawing, which should prompt special attention to the posterior cortical regions on MRI and consideration of PET- CT imaging to support the diagnosis [294, 295].

PCA Subtypes

While different cortical streams process different types of visual information suggestions of separate parietal (dorsal), occipitotemporal (ventral), and primary visual (striate cortex, caudal) forms of PCA exist [274, 296-301]. Posterior Cortical Atrophy may occur in isolation or as part of a neurodegenerative syndrome. When occurring in isolation, progression usually occurs within five years with development of dementia a typical feature. Recent data suggest some forms of PCA may be part of an extreme phenotypical manifestation of Progranulin (GRN) mutations among other genetic variants in PSEN1, PSEN2, GRN, MAPT, TREM and PRNP [302, 303, 304].

Ryan et al. studied 44 patients with PCA with motor features and their neuroimaging correlates where a total of 30% had asymmetrical left upper limb rigidity and were termed the "PCA-motor" group, limb apraxia was more frequent and asymmetrical in PCA-motor, as was myoclonus and PCA-motor had greater asymmetry of atrophy, involving the right sensorimotor areas. The subgroup with pathology or cerebrospinal fluid all showed evidence of Alzheimer's disease [305].

4. Visuospatial Dysfunction in Other Neurodegenerative Diseases

Parkinsons Disease and Parkinsons Disease Dementia

Cognitive deficits in PD have traditionally been conceptualized as 'subcortical' in nature, but accumulating evidence points to a heterogeneous profile featuring deficits in executive function, attention, processing speed, visuospatial ability, and memory, even during the earliest stages of the disease.

The potential use of exploration strategy measures as a marker of cognitive decline in Parkinson's disease and reveals the efficiency by which fixations and saccades are deployed in the build-up to a cognitive response, rather than merely focusing on the outcome itself. The prolongation of fixation duration, present to a small but significant degree even in cognitively normal subjects with Parkinson's disease, suggests a disease-specific impact on the networks directing visual exploration, although the study also highlights the multi-factorial nature of changes in exploration and the significant impact of cognitive decline on efficiency of visual search.

Some limitations to the study and generalization of visuospatial dysfunction in neurodegeneration appear when studying parkinsonian syndromes, due to the variability of presentation and the considerable overlap exists between PD with dementia (PDD), Lewy body dementia (LBD) and Lewy Body variant of AD.

Parkinson's disease (PD) is characterized mostly by motor and non-motor symptoms. At the time of disease onset, about 25% of PD patients have some degree of cognitive impairment, and about 80% appear to eventually develop dementia [306, 307, 308]. Parkinsons disease dementia (PDD) is considered a late complication of PD, usually after 10 years of disease duration where the prevalence climbs up to 75-90% [308-311]. It is now widely recognized that PDD extends beyond the classical dysexecutive syndrome seen in early PD, and includes additional deficits in recognition memory, attention processes and visual perception as well as visual hallucinations, cognitive fluctuations and as in DLB cases, symptom treatment is very complicated [312-318].

The source of visuospatial dysfunction in PD is unclear [265]. There are subcortical–cortical changes, irregularities of visual scanning and potentially of retinal-level vision in PD [319-323]. Interestingly, unlike Alzheimer's disease, the primary visual cortex can be affected in PD, and neuroimaging studies reporting hypoactivity in cortical areas involved in visual processing in PDD and DLB [233].

Patients with PD without dementia exhibit deficits in multiple domains of visuospatial functioning such as line bisection and Judgment of Line Orientation [320, 321, 324, 325]. Patients become impaired in global/local processing, mental rotation, way finding, visual construction, visuospatial reasoning and angle-size estimation [320, 326, 327, 328]. Problems when attempting to move through narrow spaces such as doorways is a common finding [319, 320, 329].

Judging distance and motion in the street are also commonly reported as reported by a 31-item self-report questionnaire developed by Lee and Harris [319, 329]. Analysis of the PD responses suggested four main factors: motor symptoms of the disease, perception of peripersonal space, retinal changes and type of medication [329].

While independent of executive demands, visual deficits in PD have been linked to freezing of gait. Visual and spatial abilities also have been implied as predictors of the person's ability to drive.

The most common findings of higher visual order dysfunction in PD are noted on tasks requiring preattentive visual processing. Preattentive processing is a process whereby target stimuli are easily detected among distractors that differ by only one feature and fronto-occipito-parietal interactions may be involved in performing these tasks.

In early stages of PD, patients show deficits mainly of Lower Order Vision (LOV), such as reduced color and contrast discrimination. Results from Higher Order Vision (HOV) deficits are less conclusive, especially for facial emotion recognition [330]. PD patients show space perception and object recognition impairments, mostly at advanced stages of the disease [331].

Visuospatial difficulties are more prominent in those whose motor symptoms begin on the left body side (LPD). These patients show a mild type of left-sided visuospatial neglect, whereas those with right onset (RPD) generally do not. In line bisection tasks the LPD tend to deviate to the right of center on horizontal line bisection tasks and downward on vertical line bisection tasks [319, 321, 322, 329, 332-337].

The visual distortion is considered a form of hemispatial-neglect. A bias toward visual exploration of the right side when compared to the left side of space and at perceiving objects on left visual fields as "smaller" than objects to the right [338, 339]. Those with LPD, but not those with RPD or healthy control adults, were found to misjudge the size of virtual doorways through compression, overestimating by 10% the space they would need to pass through the opening [355]. This phenomenon has mainly been attributed to parietal dysfunction [322]. At a perceptual level, LPD do not have a systematically biased way of representing space in the left hemifield that differs from healthy individuals. Nor do they perceive stimuli on the left as less salient than stimuli on the right, suggesting that the neglect-like syndrome instead presumably arises from dysfunction of higher order attention [335].

Typically, patients with Parkinson's disease will have a period of no or very little decline followed by an inflexion point, after which a much more rapid decline occurs; the time to this inflexion point varies greatly between patients [340]. Declines in visuospatial and verbal memory are more rapid in patients with Parkinson's disease who have dementia than in people with Alzheimer's disease; overall decline in Parkinson's disease is less rapid than or similar to that of Alzheimer's disease [341, 342].

Bohnen and colleagues' longitudinal study has provided insights into early metabolic features of dementia in Parkinson's disease, where they reported early metabolic changes in the visual association cortex and posterior cingulate cortex, that could be used as possible useful biomarkers of incident dementia in Parkinson's disease [343]. Subjects who developed dementia had reduced activity in subcortical and cortical areas compared with those with Parkinson's disease whose cognitive function did not decline for 2 years.

The Movement Disorder Society's criteria are practical and timesaving. Level II criteria more frequently classify subjects with PDD than does traditional neuropsychological testing. Whereas Level II criteria may overclassify subjects as having PDD, these are very accurate in ruling out dementia [344]. Level II criteria testing recommended for visuoconstructive, visuospatial and visuoperceptive tests in PD are similar to neurovisual testing in AD. The patient may be tested in a combination of the Clock Drawing Task, Benton Line Orientation

Test, Cube Analysis (VOSP), Benton face recognition test, and Fragmented letters (VOSP) [345].

Finally, visual field impairment in PD has not been well studied, but data points to loss of contrast sensitivity of visual stimuli, delays in visual evoked potentials, delayed pattern electroretinogram latency, and reduced amplitude in the pattern electrooculogram (EOG) are reported. Basic visual sensory function is reduced and may be due to a reduction of dopamine in the retina [193].

Dementia with Lewy Bodies

Visuospatial and visuoconstructive disabilities in DLB are disproportionately severe, especially when compared to performance with AD patients. Radionuclear studies have demonstrated that glucose metabolism and blood flow are significantly decreased in the occipital lobes, including the primary visual cortex and visual association cortex, in DLB as compared with AD. Visual perceptive deficits in DLB are also disproportionately severe and play a crucial role in the development of visual hallucinations, delusional misidentification syndromes, visual agnosias and visuoconstructive disability that is characteristic of the disease [122, 321, 346, 349, 350]. When hallucinations are present, the clinical picture becomes especially deficient in performance at visuospatial tasks [321, 351].

Visuospatial deficits appear to predict the rate of cognitive decline in autopsy-verified DLB [387]. There is evidence that the New Qualitative Scoring MMSE Pentagon Test (QSPT) is a sensitive measure of visuo-constructive abilities, which is able to differentiate DLB from AD at disease onset and as the diseases progress [352, 353]. Both the Standard Mini Mental Status Exam (MMSE) and the Montreal Cognitive Assessment (MoCA) tests appear to be poor screening tools of visuospatial impairment in Parkinson's Disease Dementia (PDD) [354, 355, 356].

Clinical history plus a brief assessment of visuospatial function may be of the greatest value in correctly identifying DLB early during the course of disease. Although not a core feature, visuospatial/constructional impairment was observed in most of the DLB cases (74%) [357]. The best model for differentiating DLB from Alzheimer's disease in the earliest stages of disease includes visual hallucinations and visuospatial/constructional dysfunction, but not spontaneous extrapyramidal symptoms (EPS) as predictors [358].

Visuoconstructional tasks, in combination with other tests can differentiate DLB from normal aging and from AD with sensitivity in excess of 80% and specificity in excess of 90%, and poor performance on visuoperceptual and constructional tasks may indicate the need for more careful monitoring for development of hallucinations [359, 360]. Visual dysfunction of a DLB group free of hallucinations in contrast, did not differ much when compared to groups with corticobasal syndrome [361].

On brief screening tasks, such as pentagon-copying, reports show that patients with DLB or DLB and PDD tend to reveal greater impairment compared to AD [309, 357, 362, 363]. Copying impairments in PDD and DLB were specifically related to disturbances in praxis and perceptual processing. Impairments on visuoconstructional tasks probably do not simply reflect the motor demands of the tasks and the motor impairment of PDD and DLB, since DLB and PDD are also more impaired than AD on the matching portion of the Benton Visual Retention Test [364]. DLB patients also are more impaired than AD patients on other tasks without significant motor demands. Specifically, on the VOSP battery, DLB patients were more impaired than AD patients on three of five subtests (cubes, letters, and object decisions) [122]. DLB patients showed particularly striking deficits in visuospatial and visuoperceptual abilities despite showing even better skills on verbal memory tests or semantic memory relative to AD groups. Patients with hallucinations and DLB usually perform worse than those without hallucinations, for example in the figure-ground segregation tests or the Benton Judgment of Line Orientation [365, 366, 367].

Studies performed with metabolic or blood flow radioligands on DLB patients have classically shown decreased uptake in the occipital lobes, including the primary visual cortex and visual association cortex [368, 369]. The physiopathology underlying visual hallucinations in DLB is not well understood. Causative models for complex visual hallucinations have suggested that the origin of this deficit may be related to a range of pathological alterations affecting both the dorsal and ventral visual streams.

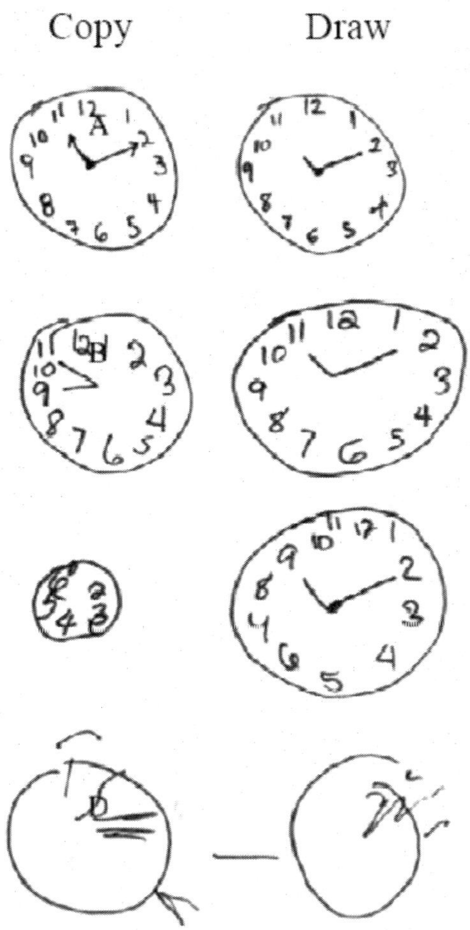

Figure 10. Typical drawings on the CDT produced by (A) controls, (B) patients with PD, (C) patients with AD, and D) patients with LBD. The CDT scores were better in general in the "copy" than the "draw" parts of the test, unlike the DLB group where the "copy" parts of the test were in general the same than that for the "draw" part. Modified from Gnanalingham [358].

DLB patients are also characterized by marked cortical thinning in posterior regions of the brain when compared with AD patients and age-matched healthy controls. Hallucination severity in DLB is correlated with reduced activation in bilateral medial occipital lobes, although it is unconfirmed whether this is the result of deficits in top-down or bottom-up visual processing pathways [370].

Other structural abnormalities indicate that the cuneus, and higher visual areas appear to also be related to visual hallucinations in DLB, and findings are consistent with many other findings not only in neuroimaging, but also neuropathological and electrophysiological studies [351, 368, 371-383]. The presence of Lewy Body pathology links DLB and PD. Despite that in patients with PD the neuropathology appears to be mostly limited to subcortical structures, visuospatial dysfunction remains a frequent associated impairment [384-388]. Multiple visual and spatial impairments and correlations have been found with side-of-disease or laterality of symptom onset and gender. A reduction in gray matter of the posterior cortices is linked to impaired visuospatial and visuoperceptual performance measures [389, 390]. In this view, Parkinsons Disease and driving capacity remains a subject of intense research [391-395].

Atypical Parkinsonian Disorders

Corticobasal Ganglionic Degeneration (CBD) is a disorder that typically presents between 60-80 years of age, with prominent symptoms such as focal rigidity, dystonia, apraxia, pronounced asymmetry of symptoms, parkinsonism, and cortical sensory deficits as core features of this disorder. Dementia occurs as a late feature of the disease. Neuroimaging usually shows an asymmetric cortical atrophy in 50-96% of cases [396]. Neuropathology reveals specific atrophy of the frontoparietal lobes, tau-positive neuronal inclusions, ballooned neurons, and astrocytic plaques [397].

Although few studies have characterized the visual cortical processing deficits in CBD, the most common apparent pattern of visual cortical symptoms is visuospatial dysfunction, which is consistent with the prominent pathological cortical changes noted in the parietal lobes [398, 399, 400]. The most characteristic neuropsychological feature of CBD is limb apraxia, usually asymmetric ideomotor and limb-kinetic in nature [401]. Episodic memory is generally spared or mildly impaired compared to AD. Other cognitive features include constructional and visuospatial difficulties, acalculia, frontal dysfunction and non-fluent aphasia [144, 402]. Temporal and parietal hypoperfusion on SPECT, usually asymmetric, occurs contralateral to clinically evident apraxia. There is limited data on whether manipulation of visual inputs have an impact on the expression of ideomotor apraxia.

Patients with corticobasal ganglionic degeneration often develop symptomatic involvement of contiguous sensorimotor cortices causing mixed perceptual-motor syndromes. Characterization of the visual processing awaits further study, but typically the other features of CBD make the cause of the visual cortical deficits more apparent. Some cases of CBD present initially with posterior visual cortical dysfunction, and it is one of the etiologies to suspect in Posterior Cortical Atrophy (PCA) [267]. Progressive supranuclear palsy is closely related to CBD, but prominent deficits are primarily linked to oculomotor, postural and executive function [403].

When comparing CBD with AD, in patients with CBS a failure in specific subsets of the VOSP is associated with greater odds of underlying AD as an etiology. There may be preferential involvement of the dorsal stream in CBS-AD. Some subtests of the VOSP accurately distinguish patients with CBS-AD from those without AD pathology (e.g., Cube Analysis sensitivity 100%, specificity 77%) [121]. CBD patients show more impaired praxis than those with AD and do poorly at measures of phonemic fluency (number of D words produced in 1 min). They also scored significantly better on verbal memory (California Verbal Learning Test-Short Form), and show a trend in the predicted direction on visual memory (modified Rey figure).

Other Neurodegenerative Forms of Dementia

Neither vascular dementia nor any of the atypical neurodegenerative syndromes have extensive literature on visual and spatial impairment. As with many cognitive domains, those tasks dependent on executive function also affect performance on visuoconstructive tasks [404]. Qualitative analysis of error patterns in AD vs VaD where the vascular group (or subcortical dementia groups) made more spatial and planning errors than the AD group [103, 405, 406, 407].

Logopenic aphasia (LPA) usually presents with dysfunction in the left temporoparietal areas (posterior superior temporal and inferior parietal). Since these same areas mentioned overlap with atrophy of core structures for aphasia and attentional syndromes, it may be prudent to screen LPA patients for spatial neglect and extinction [408].

Frontotemporal dementia is characterized by preservation of visuospatial abilities and is frequently used as a hallmark finding when examining borderline cases of FTD vs AD. Language performance on the other hand is and progresses worse in FTD relative to AD [409, 410]. When comparing clock drawing in similar groups, the AD group committed more spatial errors and more stimulus-bound responses, conceptual deficits and planning errors than the FTD group.

Some data on patients with Amyotrophic Lateral Sclerosis (ALS) also demonstrate problems in visuoperceptual tasks and visuospatial reasoning as an associated cognitive deficit. Reports of marked visuomotor impairment on visual search tasks are also reported on patients with Huntington's disease, where deficits in spatial learning and memory are prominent cognitive features [411-414]. When examining visuospatial bias, Ho et al. found that patients' trinucleotide (CAG) repeat length correlated with an increasing leftward bias on line bisection task when compared to controls (increased pseudo-neglect) [415]. MRI correlated this deficit with reduced density in the angular gyrus (BA39) bilaterally.

Following a neurological event such as a traumatic brain injury (TBI), cerebrovascular accident (CVA), multiple sclerosis (MS), among other insults, imbalances in vision can affect balance, posture, ambulation, reading, attention, concentration and cognitive function in general [416]. Imbalances between focal and ambient visual processes include rare syndromes like Post Trauma Vision Syndrome (PTVS) and Visual Midline Shift Syndrome (VMSS) [417, 418, 419].

Following a cerebrovascular accident (CVA), individuals initially tend to lean toward the side of the hemiparesis, that when present chronically the condition is also known as Pusher

Syndrome [420, 421, 422]. This type of body-orientation-perception syndrome appears to be unrelated to vestibular function, and more akin to a sensorimotor mismatch for example.

Detailed assessment of visual function in patients with stroke can help to clarify the risk of various types of visual impairment. Moreover, as visual function assessment in patients with stroke is difficult, knowledge of the correlation of visual impairments with different neurological dysfunctions observed in stroke and lesion side will help predict vision problems and inform optimal corrective measures in treating patients with stroke.

Creutzfeldt-Jakob Disease

Creutzfeldt-Jakob disease (CJD) is the most important form of transmissible spongiform encephalopathy in humans, with at least four different varieties of this disease. Two variants of vCJD have been described, a visual or Heidenhain variant (HvCJD) and a cerebellar-ataxic variant [423-430]. Acquisition and deposition of prion protein (PrP) is the main pathophysiological mechanism. In CJD, visual symptoms as disease presentation are documented in about 10% of cases, and expand to approximately 50% during the course of the disease. Visual symptoms range from diplopia, supranuclear palsies, complex visual disturbances, homonymous visual field defects, hallucinations and cortical blindness. Saccadic and smooth pursuit movements appear to be rarely affected [431].

Posterior Cortical Atrophy as previously mentioned, may be a presentation in both AD and CJD. Even in patients with more typical patterns of dementia, the degree of visuo-spatial impairment may hinder driving skills, and the issue of driving should be addressed early in the clinical course [432].

A variety of visual symptoms in CJD appear to be associated with the development of posterior cortical atrophy especially when it affects the visual cortex. Studies have suggested that there is vacuolation in lamina IV of the primary visual area (V1) with preservation of the Band of Gennari and extensive PrP deposition in all cortical laminae, especially in vCJD [433]. Patients may develop difficulties in identifying objects, depth perception, symptoms of Balint Syndrome and prosopagnosia, as well as alexia. Dissociation of visual processing from more complex language functions, visual hallucinations and visuospatial recognition problems may also occur. Hallucinatory behavior is especially common in vCJD. Cortical blindness occurs in about 25-50% of cases of vCJD and may reflect the extensive pathology that develops in the visual cortex [431, 432].

5. Functional Impairment and Rehabilitation

The clinical pictures of the neurodegenerative diseases are dominated by functional impairment. One reason for the lack of broad understanding of the visuospatial impairments in these conditions may be an underappreciation of the role of low vision as a contributor to the disability, by the clinician, family, or patient. Problems with gait or visually guided behaviors are often attributed directly to the apraxia or to extrapyramidal motor dysfunction.

Healthy elderly patients appear to under-report their actual degrees of visual disability. An increased risk of falls and higher dependence in ADL's are some of the factors associated with reduced visual function in both community dwelling and nursing home samples. A study by Fukui and Lee showed how their results on global cognitive testing (Revised Hasegawa Dementia Scale) correlated with the performance on instrumental ADL's, while figure copying with basic ADL's, and Clock Reading Test contributed significantly to both Basic and Instrumental ADL's [103, 434].

In hemispatial neglect after stroke, conventional tests of neglect were not good predictors of everyday difficulties. The Catherine Bergego Scale (CBS) was conceived in order to provide a general idea of the presence and extent of neglect on a sample of real everyday-life activities [435, 436]. A functional scale consisting of 10 items related to neglect in everyday life. Assessment occurs via direct observation of spontaneous (i.e., self-initiated) behaviors, such as brushing hair on both left and right sides and remembering to take care of the left limb that may be weaker and hanging outside the wheelchair. By comparing the therapist's observations and the patient's self-report, an anosognosia score can be calculated. Of the existing 28 standardized assessments, the CBS is the only one assessing performance in personal (body parts or on the body surface), peri-personal (within arm's reach) and extra-personal spaces (beyond arm's reach), as well as in perceptual, representational, and motor domains [437]. A revised modified version of the CBS, the Kessler Foundation Neglect Assessment Process (KF-NAP) was measured against the Barthel Index (BI) and the Functional Impairment Measure (FIM), where the KF-NAP uniquely quantifies symptoms of spatial neglect by measuring functional difficulties that are not captured by the FIM or BI [438, 439].

Wandering and Getting Lost

Prevention is key to help lower the chances of wandering in dementia. Strategies such as carrying out daily activities or having a daily routine, camouflaging doors and door knobs, keeping car keys out of sight and having a plan in place beforehand, so caregivers know what to do in case of an emergency are essential. Knowledge of places where person might wander, might provide leads when they become lost; this could include past jobs, former homes, places of worship or a restaurant.. If the person is right or left handed also provides a clue, as wandering generally follows the direction of the dominant hand.

There continues to be limited agreement on what are the most valuable of rehabilitation techniques or what are the mechanisms underlying any of the ameliorating effects seen in some studies. Many dementia conditions present with heterogeneous forms of neglect more frequently as a norm than they are the exception [440]. Restorative therapy may rely in sensory stimulation, visual scanning practice and functional tasks such as map reading. Compensatory strategies might incorporate the use of written notes to remind patients to do important tasks and rearranging the environment to facilitate movement, as we will discuss next.

Compensatory and Rehabilitation Strategies

Occupational therapists treat visual spatial disorders with the goal of improving the patient's ability to accomplish daily activities. Rehabilitation aims to compensate for these deficits in order to regain quality of life for patients. The nature of these deficits and their impact on activities of daily living can be quite varied and require specific rehabilitation approaches. The most important domains that may be involved are near tasks, especially reading, distance tasks relating to orientation and mobility, and social requirements related to communication [441].

In visual neglect and visual inattention it seems logical to compensate for their deficits by constant verbal or visual cues to "look to the left." The reality is that this approach usually fails miserably. It is usually other coping mechanisms that may not be as intuitive, the ones that will help restore a lost part of the world. Special glasses with prisms or caloric stimulation to the ear canal appear to work in standard tasks of neglect but their transfer or usefulness in activities of daily living is usually not accomplished. These and other non-pharmacological approaches have yielded that enhanced stimulus strength improves visual cognition in aging and AD [442]. When topographical disorientation is an issue, a specific set of landmarks such as pictures, icons, or written signs can be designed to facilitate getting about [443].

Pharmacological study results available in the setting of neglect is rather small, and the observed responses vary. Most of the agents target the dopaminergic system, where levodopa, bromocriptine and apomorphine showed positive effects on hemispatial neglect. The dopaminergic network related to improvement in neglect is not well understood, although a hypothesis is that dopaminergic circuits principally mediate the premotor components of spatial exploration behavior [444, 445, 446]. Some authors suggest that these circuits are purely motor, whereas others maintain that dopaminergic circuits also mediate perceptive aspects [447, 448, 449]. Dopamine agonist therapy has been found to reduce neglect but only minimal and equivocal research is available to support the usefulness of this pharmacotherapy [450].

Improvements in perceptual-motor aspects of neglect were found in four patients with Parkinsons disease where stimulation with apomorphine helped them point to objects in their left space when compared to placebo. The results showed improvements in perceptual-motor aspects but not in the perceptual aspect of neglect [451]. Any evidence linking amphetamines as therapy for improvement in neglect remains in preclinical stages [452]. Finally, cholinesterase inhibitor dose required in some behavioral symptoms in dementia with Lewy bodies may be higher, and there is evidence that both acetylcholinesterase inhibitors and uncompetitive NMDA receptor antagonists may improve visuospatial function among persons with neurodegenerative dementias [65, 453].

Motivation could potentially influence neglect in relation to dysfunction of attention [454-461] There is very preliminary evidence suggesting that some motivational stimulation may act as a surrogate for dopaminergic pharmacological therapy. More studies addressing clinical tasks and employing motivational processes in the context of rehabilitation are needed [462, 463].

When examining systematic reviews on neurovisual rehabilitation and treatment strategies, the most common phenomenon studies are focused on hemi-inattention [454, 464]. The goal is set to reducing the disabling effects of neglect and increasing independence. Unfortunately, no rehabilitation approach can be supported when based on the evidence available from Randomized Controlled Trials [465].

Table 8. Rehabilitation strategies in Neurovisual Disorders

Eye Patching [466]
Prism Adaptation [467, 473]
Vestibular Stimulation [474]
Galvanic Vestibular Stimulation [475, 476, 477]
Transcutaneous electrical nerve stimulation [478-482]
Optokinetic Stimulation [483, 484]
Transcranial Magnetic Stimulation (TMS) and transcranial Direct Current Stimulation (tDCS) [511-515]
Noradrenergic stimulation [485]
Videogame based neglect rehabilitation [486]

Prism adaptation is currently the most explored and studied rehabilitation technique for neglect [470, 471]. The effect extends to walking trajectories and when applied to the upper right limb, in some cases it even improved the walking trajectory for up to 15 months after treatment [468]. Repetitive transcranial magnetic stimulation (rTMS) aimed at reducing the activity of the left healthy hemisphere. Six patients suffering from visual extinction underwent low frequency TMS over the left parietal lobe where their performance in an attentional tracking task significantly improved in the contralesional visual field immediately after stimulation protocols. Performance remained unaltered in the ipsilesional field. TMS was also used in the recovery of visual extinction based on the interhemispheric inhibition hypothesis with positive results [487].

CONCLUSION

Visuospatial deficits are common in many neurodegenerative diseases. The progressive nature of these phenomena along with no solid proof of treatment modalities, and the relative invisibility of the symptoms to the outsider, makes it one of the hardest deficits to diagnose, let alone to treat. The field in visuospatial function is expanding rapidly by both understanding the pathology of these disease states and widening the research field for brain stimulation, assistive and technological, as well as pharmacological treatments. Awareness of the nature of neuropsychiatric impairments in dementia is increasing and is currently best dealt with social and behavioral interventions while lessening the risk of polypharmacy that may lead to confusion and falls. Improving guidance and referral for other needs affected by declines in visual function may be warranted, such as home modification or personal management.

REFERENCES

[1] Jenkins L, Myerson J, Joerding JA, Hale S. Converging evidence that visuospatial cognition is more age-sensitive than verbal cognition. *Psychology and Aging*. 2000.

[2] Sweeny TD, Grabowecky M, Suzuki S. Awareness Becomes Necessary Between Adaptive Pattern Coding of Open and Closed Curvatures. *Psychological Science*. 2011 Jul 20;22(7):943–50.

[3] Mattson MP. Superior pattern processing is the essence of the evolved human brain. *Frontiers in Neuroscience.* 2014;8:265.

[4] de Graaf TA, Roebroeck A, Goebel R, Sack AT. Brain network dynamics underlying visuospatial judgment: an FMRI connectivity study. *J Cogn Neurosci.* 2010 Sep;22(9):2012–26.

[5] Li X, Rastogi P, Gibbons JA, Chaudhury S. Visuo-cognitive skill deficits in Alzheimer's disease and Lewy body disease: A comparative analysis. *Ann Indian Acad Neurol.* 2014 Jan;17(1):12–8.

[6] Schoenberg MR, Scott JG. Deficits in Visuospatial/Visuoconstructional Skills and Motor Praxis. The Little Black Book of Neuropsychology. *Springer Verlag;* 2011. p. 986.

[7] Mendez MF, Mendez MA, Martin R, Smyth KA, Whitehouse PJ. Complex visual disturbances in Alzheimer's disease. *Neurology.* 1990;40:439–43.

[8] Cerella J, Birren JE, Schaie KW. Aging and information-processing rate. In: Birren JE, Schaie KW, editors. Handbook of the psychology of aging. 3rd ed. San Diego: Associated Press; 1990.

[9] Moser M-B, Rowland DC, Moser EI. Place cells, grid cells, and memory. *Cold Spring Harb Perspect Biol.* 2015 Feb;7(2):a021808.

[10] Molinari M, Leggio MG. Cerebellar information processing and visuospatial functions. *The Cerebellum.* 2007;6(3):214–20.

[11] Molinari M, Chiricozzi FR, Clausi S, Tedesco AM, De Lisa M, Leggio MG. Cerebellum and Detection of Sequences, from Perception to Cognition. *Cerebellum.* 2008 Oct 22;7(4):611–5.

[12] Lalonde R. Visuospatial abilities. International Review of Neurobiology. *Elsevier;* 1997;41:191–215.

[13] Thürling M, Hautzel H, Küper M, Stefanescu MR, Maderwald S, Ladd ME, et al. Involvement of the cerebellar cortex and nuclei in verbal and visuospatial working memory: A 7T fMRI study. Neuroimage. *Elsevier Inc;* 2012 Sep 1;62(3):1537–50.

[14] Fink GR, Marshall JC, Shah NJ, Weiss PH, Halligan PW, Grosse-Ruyken M, et al. Line bisection judgments implicate right parietal cortex and cerebellum as assessed by fMRI. Neurology. 2000 Mar 28;54(6):1324–31.

[15] Lee TMC, Liu H-L, Hung KN, Pu J, Ng Y-B, Mak AKY, et al. The cerebellum's involvement in the judgment of spatial orientation: a functional magnetic resonance imaging study. *Neuropsychologia.* 2005;43(13):1870–7.

[16] Stoodley CJ, Schmahmann JD. Functional topography in the human cerebellum: A meta-analysis of neuroimaging studies. *Human Brain Mapping Journal.* 2009 Jan 15;44(2):489–501.

[17] Stoodley CJ, Valera EM, Schmahmann JD. Functional topography of the cerebellum for motor and cognitive tasks: An fMRI study. *Human Brain Mapping Journal.* 2012 Jan 16;59(2):1560–70.

[18] Hildebrandt H, Spang K, Ebke M. Visuospatial hemi-inattention following cerebellar/brain stem bleeding. *Neurocase.* 2002;8(4).

[19] Silveri MC, Misciagna S, Terrezza G. Right side neglect in right cerebellar lesion. *Journal of Neurology, Neurosurgery and Psychiatry.* 2001 Jul;71(1):114–7.

[20] Schutter DJLG, Kammers M, Enter D, van Honk J. A case of illusory own-body perceptions after transcranial magnetic stimulation of the cerebellum. *The Cerebellum.* 2006 Sep 1;5(3):238–40.

[21] Kinsey K, Anderson SJ, Hadjipapas A, Nevado A, Hillebrand A, Holliday IE. Cortical oscillatory activity associated with the perception of illusory and real visual contours. *Int J Psychophysiol.* 2009 Sep;73(3):265–72.

[22] Azanon E, Haggard P. Somatosensory processing and body representation. *CORTEX.* 2009 Oct 1;45(9):1078–84.

[23] Deluca C, Golzar A, Santandrea E, Gerfo Lo E, Eštočinová J, Moretto G, et al. The cerebellum and visual perceptual learning: evidence from a motion extrapolation task. *CORTEX.* 2014 Sep;58:52–71.

[24] Pierce K, Courchesne E. Evidence for a cerebellar role in reduced exploration and stereotyped behavior in autism. *BPS.* 2001 Apr 15;49(8):655–64.

[25] Kawa R, Pisula E. Locomotor activity, object exploration and space preference in children with autism and Down syndrome. *Acta Neurobiol Exp* (Wars). 2010;70(2):131–40.

[26] Adduri CA, Marotta JJ. Mental rotation of faces in healthy aging and Alzheimer's disease. *PLoS ONE.* 2009.

[27] Tagaris GA, Richter W, Kim SG, Pellizzer G, Andersen P, Ugurbil K, et al. Functional magnetic resonance imaging of mental rotation and memory scanning: a multidimensional scaling analysis of brain activation patterns. *Brain Res Brain Res Rev.* 1998 May;26(2-3):106–12.

[28] Molinari M, Petrosini L, Misciagna S, Leggio MG. Visuospatial abilities in cerebellar disorders. *Journal of Neurology, Neurosurgery and Psychiatry.* 2004 Feb;75(2):235–40.

[29] Werner S, Schorn CF, Bock O, Theysohn N, Timmann D. Neural correlates of adaptation to gradual and to sudden visuomotor distortions in humans. *Exp Brain Res.* 2014 Jan 22;232(4):1145–56.

[30] Molinari M, Leggio MG, Solida A, Ciorra R, Misciagna S, Silveri MC, et al. Cerebellum and procedural learning: evidence from focal cerebellar lesions. *Brain.* 1997 Oct;120 (Pt 10):1753–62.

[31] Petrosini L, Graziano A, Mandolesi L, Neri P, Molinari M, Leggio MG. Watch how to do it! New advances in learning by observation. *Brain Res Brain Res Rev.* 2003 Jun;42(3):252–64.

[32] Jackson PL, Meltzoff AN, Decety J. Neural circuits involved in imitation and perspective-taking. *Neuroimage.* 2006 May;31(1):429–39.

[33] Nitschke MF, Arp T, Stavrou G, Erdmann C. The cerebellum in the cerebro-cerebellar network for the control of eye and hand movements—an fMRI study. *Prog Brain Res.* 2005;148:151.

[34] Brooks A, van der Zwan R, Mercier M, Blanke O. Visual neuropsychology. *Encyclopedia of Neuroscience;* 2009. pp. 4318–22.

[35] van der Ham IJM, Duijndam MJA, Raemaekers M, van Wezel RJA, Oleksiak A, Postma A. Retinotopic Mapping of Categorical and Coordinate Spatial Relation Processing in Early Visual Cortex. Hamed SB, editor. *PLoS ONE.* 2012 Jun 19;7(6):e38644.

[36] Baumann O, Chan E, Mattingley JB. Distinct neural networks underlie encoding of categorical versus coordinate spatial relations during active navigation. *Human Brain Mapping Journal.* 2012 Apr 15;60(3):1630–7.

[37] Saneyoshi A, Michimata C. Categorical and coordinate processing in object recognition depends on different spatial frequencies. *Cogn Process.* 2014 Sep 19;16(1):27–33.

[38] Treisman AM, Gelade G. A feature-integration theory of attention. *Cogn Psychol.* 1980 Jan;12(1):97–136.

[39] Müller HJ, Krummenacher J. Visual search and selective attention. *Visual Cognition.* 2006 Aug;14(4-8):389–410.

[40] Weidner R, Krummenacher J, Reimann B, Müller HJ, Fink GR. Sources of top-down control in visual search. *J Cogn Neurosci.* 2009 Nov;21(11):2100–13.

[41] Chan LKH, Hayward WG. Feature integration theory revisited: Dissociating feature detection and attentional guidance in visual search. *Journal of Experimental Psychology: Human Perception and Performance*. 2009;35(1):119–32.

[42] Green M. Visual search, visual streams, and visual architectures. *Percept Psychophys.* 1991 Oct;50(4):388–403.

[43] Farah MJ. The Cognitive Neuroscience of Vision. *Wiley-Blackwell;* 2000.

[44] Cronin-Golomb A. Visuospatial Function in Alzheimer's Disease and Related Disorders. In: Cronin-Golomb A, editor. *The Handbook of Alzheimers Disease and Other Dementias.* 1st ed. Blackwell Publishing; 2011. pp. 457–82.

[45] Milner D, Goodale M. The Visual Brain in Action. 2nd ed. Oxford University Press; 2006.

[46] Leeds DD, Pyles JA, Tarr MJ. Exploration of complex visual feature spaces for object perception. *Frontiers in computational neuroscience.* 2014;8.

[47] Rucci M, Victor JD. The unsteady eye: an information- processing stage, not a bug. *Trends in Neurosciences.* 2015 Apr 1;38(4):195–206.

[48] Spering M, Carrasco M. Acting without seeing: eye movements reveal visual processing without awareness. *Trends in Neurosciences.* 2015 Apr 1;38(4):247–58.

[49] Gur M. Space reconstruction by primary visual cortex activity: a parallel, non-computational mechanism of object representation. *Trends in Neurosciences.* 2015 Apr 1;38(4):207–16.

[50] Jensen O, Bonnefond M, Marshall TR, Tiesinga P. Oscillatory mechanisms of feedforward and feedback visual processing. *Trends in Neurosciences.* 2015 Apr 1;38(4):192–4.

[51] Engbert R. Microsaccades: a microcosm for research on oculomotor control, attention, and visual perception. *Progress in Brain Research. Elsevier;* 2006. pp. 177–92.

[52] Gonçalves de Freitas Pereira ML, Zuben de Arruda Camargo von M, Aprahamian I, Vicente Forlenza O. Eye movement analysis and cognitive processing: detecting indicators of conversion to Alzheimer's disease. *Neuropsychiatric Disease and Treatment* [Internet]. 2014;10:1273–85.

[53] Bigelow RT, Semenov YR, Trevino C, Ferrucci L, Resnick SM, Simonsick EM, et al. Association Between Visuospatial Ability and Vestibular Function in the Baltimore Longitudinal Study of Aging. *Journal of the American Geriatrics Society.* 2015 Sep;63(9):1837–44.

[54] Martha J. Farah and Russel A. Epstein. Disorders of Visual-spatial Perception and Cognition. Clinical Neuropsychology. Kenneth M. Heilman and Edward Valenstein (eds). *Oxford University Press*; 2011. Chapter 7. p.152-166.

[55] Cazzoli D, Müri RM, Hess CW, Nyffeler T. Treatment of hemispatial neglect by means of rTMS--a review. *Restor Neurol Neurosci.* 2010;28(4):499–510.

[56] Fellrath J, Blanche-Durbec V, Schnider A, Jacquemoud A-S, Ptak R. Visual search in spatial neglect studied with a preview paradigm. *Frontiers in Human Neuroscience.* 2012;6:93.

[57] Ghacibeh GA, Shenker JI, Winter KH, Triggs WJ, Heilman KM. Dissociation of neglect subtypes with transcranial magnetic stimulation. *Neurology.* 2007 Sep 11;69(11):1122–7.

[58] Sack AT, Sperling JM, Prvulovic D, Formisano E. Tracking the mind's image in the brain II: transcranial magnetic stimulation reveals parietal asymmetry in visuospatial imagery. *Neuron.* 2002. Jul 3;35(1):195-204.

[59] McCourt ME, Jewell G. Visuospatial attention in line bisection: stimulus modulation of pseudoneglect. *Neuropsychologia.* 1999 Jun;37(7):843–55.

[60] Porac C, Searleman A, Karagiannakis K. Pseudoneglect: Evidence for both perceptual and attentional factors. *Brain and Cognition.* 2006 Aug;61(3):305–11.

[61] Bowers D, Heilman KM. Pseudoneglect: effects of hemispace on a tactile line bisection task. *Neuropsychologia.* 1980;18(4-5):491–8.

[62] Ribolsi M, Di Lorenzo G, Lisi G, Niolu C, Siracusano A. A critical review and meta-analysis of the perceptual pseudoneglect across psychiatric disorders: Is there a continuum? *Cogn Process.* 2014 Nov 7;16(1):17–25.

[63] Jewell G, McCourt ME. Pseudoneglect: a review and meta-analysis of performance factors in line bisection tasks. *Neuropsychologia.* 1999 Nov 11;38(1):93–110.

[64] Benwell CSY, Thut G, Grant A, Harvey M. A rightward shift in the visuospatial attention vector with healthy aging. *Frontiers in aging neuroscience.* 2014;6:113.

[65] Arciniegas DB, Anderson CA, Filley CM. Behavioral Neurology and Neuropsychiatry. *Cambridge University Press*; 2013. pp. 529-530.

[66] Moore D, Puri BK. Textbook of Clinical Neuropsychiatry and Behavioral Neuroscience 3E, 3rd ed. *CRC Press;* 2012. pp. 36-37.

[67] Lissauer H. Ein Fall von Seelenblindheit nebst einem beitrage zue Theoric derselben. *Archiv fur Psychiatrie und Nervenkrankheiten.* 1890 Jun 29;21:222–70.

[68] Teuber HL. Alteration of perception and memory in man. In: Weiskrantz L, editor. Analysis of Behavioral Change. New York: *Harper and Row;* 1968. pp. 274–328.

[69] Heilman KM. Matter of Mind: A Neurologist's View of Brain-Behavior Relationships. *Oxford University Press*, USA; 2002. p. 180-183.

[70] Spreen O, Benton AL, Van Allen MW. Dissociation of visual and tactile naming in amnesic aphasia. *Neurology.* 1966. 16; 807.

[71] Goodglass H, Barton MI, Kaplan EF. Sensory modality and object-naming in aphasia. *J Speech Hear Res.* 1968 Sep;11(3):488–96.

[72] De Renzi E, Saetti MC. Associative agnosia and optic aphasia: qualitative or quantitative difference? *CORTEX.* 1997;33(1):115–30.

[73] Shakespeare TJ, Pertzov Y, Yong KXX, Nicholas J, Crutch SJ. Reduced modulation of scanpaths in response to task demands in posterior cortical atrophy. *Neuropsychologia.* 2015 Feb;68:190–200.

[74] Coslett HB, Saffran E. To see but not two see. *Brain.* 1991;114:1523–45.

[75] Farah MJ. Visual Agnosia. *MIT Press;* 2004.

[76] Strauss E. A Compendium of Neuropsychological Tests. Oxford University Press, USA; 2006.

[77] Schmidtke K, Olbrich S. The Clock Reading Test: validation of an instrument for the diagnosis of dementia and disorders of visuo-spatial cognition. *International Psychogeriatrics.* 2007 Apr;19(2):307–21.

[78] Kandiah N, Zhang A, Bautista DC, Silva E, Ting SKS, Ng A, et al. Early detection of dementia in multilingual populations: Visual Cognitive Assessment Test (VCAT). *Journal of Neurology, Neurosurgery and Psychiatry.* 2015 Feb 17.

[79] Brucki SMD, Nitrini R. Cancellation task in very low educated people. *Archives of Clinical Neuropsychology.* 2008 Mar;23(2):139–47.

[80] Mesulam MM. Principles of Behavioral and Cognitive Neurology, 2nd Edition. 2nd ed. *Oxford University Press,* USA; 2000.

[81] Mennemeier M, Chatterjee A, Heilman KM. A comparison of the influences of body and environment centred reference frames on neglect. *Brain.* 1994 Oct;117 (Pt 5):1013–21.

[82] Cubelli R, Sala Della S, Spinazzola L. Left of what? The role of egocentric coordinates in neglect. *J Neurol.* 1997. Oct;63(4):483-9.

[83] Albert ML. A simple test of visual neglect. *Neurology.* 1973 Jun;23(6):658–64.

[84] Barrett AM, Peterlin BL, Heilman KM. Ipsilateral neglect versus hemianopic compensation. *Neurology.* 2003 Jul 8;61(1):120–3.

[85] Lezak MD, Howieson DB, Bigler ED, Tranel D. Neuropsychological Assessment. 5 ed. *Oxford University Press*, USA; 2012. p. 377-383.

[86] Lee BH, Kang SJ, Park JM, Son Y, Lee KH, Adair JC, et al. The Character-line Bisection Task: a new test for hemispatial neglect. *Neuropsychologia.* 2004 Jan;42(12):1715–24.

[87] Milner AD, Harvey M, Roberts SC, Forster S. Line bisection errors in visual neglect: misguided action or size distortion? *Neuropsychologia.* 1993 Aug 2;31(1):39–49.

[88] Geminiani G, Camaschella E, Mariani C, Alberoni M, Farina E. Direction and position factors in performance of line extension task by unilateral neglect subjects. *Neuropsychologia.* 2002;40(11):1834–40.

[89] Qualls CE, Bliwise NG, Stringer AY. Short forms of the Benton Judgment of Line Orientation Test: development and psychometric properties. *Archives of Clinical Neuropsychology.* 2000 Feb;15(2):159–63.

[90] Woodard JL, Benedict RH, Salthouse TA, Toth JP, Zgaljardic DJ, Hancock HE. Normative data for equivalent, parallel forms of the Judgment of Line Orientation Test. *J Clin Exp Neuropsychol.* 1998 Aug;20(4):457–62.

[91] Benton A, Hamsher K, Varney NR, Spreen O. Contributions to Neuropsychological Assessment. New York: Oxford; 1983.

[92] Benton A, Tranel D. Visuoperceptual, visuospatial, and visuoconstructive disorders. In: Heilman KM, Valenstein E, editors. Clinical neuropsychology. *Oxford University Press*; 1993.

[93] Williams C, Thwaites A, Buttery P, Geertzen J. The Cambridge Cookie-Theft Corpus: A Corpus of Directed and Spontaneous Speech of Brain-Damaged Patients and Healthy Individuals. *LREC.* 2010.

[94] Rothenberg KG, Piądło R, Nagaraj UD, Friedland RP. The complex picture test in dementia. *Dement Geriatr Cogn Dis Extra.* 2012 Jan;2(1):411–7.

[95] Marshall RC, Wright HH. Developing a Clinician-Friendly Aphasia Test. *American Journal of Speech-Language Pathology.* 2007 Oct 23;16:295–315.

[96] Klein L, Saur R, Müller S, Leyhe T. Comparison of Clock Test Deficits Between Elderly Patients With Early and Late Onset Depression. *J Geriatr Psychiatry Neurol.* 2015 Jun 4;1(8).

[97] Matsuoka T, Narumoto J, Shibata K, Okamura A, Nakamura K, Nakamae T, et al. Neural correlates of performance on the different scoring systems of the clock drawing test. *Neuroscience Letters.* 2011 Jan 10;487(3):421–5.

[98] Quental N, Brucki S. Visuospatial function in early Alzheimer's disease. *Dementia and Neuropsychologia.* 2009;3(3):234–40.

[99] Leyhe T, Saur R, Eschweiler GW, Milian M. Clock Test Deficits Are Associated With Semantic Memory Impairment in Alzheimer Disease. *J Geriatr Psychiatry Neurol.* 2009 Nov 17;22(4):235–45.

[100] Formisano E, Linden DEJ, Di Salle F, Trojano L, Esposito F, Sack AT, et al. Tracking the mind's image in the brain I: time-resolved fMRI during visuospatial mental imagery. *Neuron.* 2002 Jul 3;35(1):185–94.

[101] Leyhe T, Erb M, Milian M, Eschweiler GW, Ethofer T, Grodd W, et al. Changes in Cortical Activation during Retrieval of Clock Time Representations in Patients with Mild Cognitive Impairment and Early Alzheimer's Disease. *Dementia and Geriatric Cognitive Disorders.* 2009;27(2):117–32.

[102] Jefferies E. The neural basis of semantic cognition: Converging evidence from neuropsychology, neuroimaging and TMS. *CORTEX.* 2013 Mar 1;49(3):611–25.

[103] Fukui T, Lee E, Kitamura M, Hosoda H, Bokui C, Ikusu K, et al. Visuospatial dysfunction may be a key in the differentiation between Alzheimer's disease and subcortical cognitive impairment in moderate to severe stages. *Dementia and Geriatric Cognitive Disorders.* 2009;28(4):288–94.

[104] Sperling RA, Dickerson BC, Pihlajamäki M, Vannini P, LaViolette PS, Vitolo OV, et al. Functional alterations in memory networks in early Alzheimer's disease. *Neuromolecular Med.* 2010 Mar;12(1):27–43.

[105] Boccia M, Acierno M, Piccardi L. Neuroanatomy of Alzheimer's Disease and Late Life Depression: A Coordinate-Based Meta-Analysis of MRI Studies. *Journal of Alzheimer's Disease.* 2015 Apr 13.

[106] Morbelli S, Drzezga A, Perneczky R, Frisoni GB, Caroli A, van Berckel BNM, et al. Resting metabolic connectivity in prodromal Alzheimer's disease. A European Alzheimer Disease Consortium (EADC) project. *Neurobiology of Aging.* 2012 Nov;33(11):2533–50.

[107] Lebedeva A, Westman E, Lebedev AV, Li X, Winblad B, Simmons A, et al. Structural brain changes associated with depressive symptoms in the elderly with Alzheimer's disease. *Journal of Neurology, Neurosurgery and Psychiatry.* 2014 Aug;85(8):930–5.

[108] Folstein MF, Folstein SE, McHugh PR. "Mini-mental state." A practical method for grading the cognitive state of patients for the clinician. *Journal of psychiatric research.* 1975 Nov;12(3):189–98.

[109] Folstein MF, Robins LN, Helzer JE. The Mini-Mental State Examination. *Arch Gen Psychiatry.* 1983 Jul 6;40:812.

[110] Fountoulakis KN, Siamouli M, Panagiotidis PT, Magiria S, Kantartzis S, Terzoglou VA, et al. The standardised copy of pentagons test. *Ann Gen Psychiatry.* BioMed Central Ltd; 2011 Apr 11;10(1):13.

[111] Rey A. Reativo delle figure complesse A e B. Florence*: Organizzazioni Speciali;* 1983.

[112] Osterrieth PA. Le test de copie d"une figure complexe; contribution à l"étude de la perception et de la mémoire. *Archives de psychologie.* 1944.

[113] Fastenau PS. Development and preliminary standardization of the "extended complex figure test" (ECFT). *J Clin Exp Neuropsychol.* 1996 Feb;18(1):63–76.

[114] Wechsler D. WAIS-R, Wechsler Adult Intelligence Scale-Revised, Manual. 1981.

[115] Groth-Marnat G, Teal M. Block design as a measure of everyday spatial ability: a study of ecological validity. *Perceptual and Motor Skills.* 2000 Apr;90(2):522–6.

[116] Burggraaf R, Frens MA, Hooge ITC, van der Geest JN. A Quick Assessment of Visuospatial Abilities in Adolescents Using the Design Organization Test (DOT). *Appl Neuropsychol Child.* 2014 Dec 31:1–6.

[117] Warrington EK, James M. The visual object and space perception battery. Bury St Edmunds, England: Thames Valley Test Company; 1991.

[118] Herrera-Guzmán I, Peña-Casanova J, Lara JP, Gudayol-Ferré E, Böhm P. Influence of age, sex, and education on the Visual Object and Space Perception Battery (VOSP) in a healthy normal elderly population. *Clin Neuropsychol.* 2004 Aug;18(3):385–94.

[119] Videaud H, Torny F, Prado-Jean A, Couratier P. Use of the Visual Object and Space Perception (VOSP) test battery in two cases of posterior cortical atrophy. *Neurocase.* 2008;15(1):32–6.

[120] Quental NBM, Brucki SMD, Bueno OFA. Visuospatial Function in Early Alzheimer's Disease—The Use of the Visual Object and Space Perception (VOSP) Battery. Laks J, editor. *PLoS ONE.* 2013 Jul 16;8(7):e68398.

[121] Boyd CD, Tierney M, Wassermann EM, Spina S, Oblak AL, Ghetti B, et al. Visuoperception test predicts pathologic diagnosis of Alzheimer disease in corticobasal syndrome. *Neurology.* 2014 Aug 5;83(6):510–9.

[122] Calderón J, Perry RJ, Erzinclioglu SW, Berrios GE, Dening TR, Hodges JR. Perception, attention, and working memory are disproportionately impaired in dementia with Lewy bodies compared with Alzheimer's disease. *Journal of Neurology, Neurosurgery and Psychiatry.* 2001 Feb;70(2):157–64.

[123] Money J, Alexander D, Walker HT. A Standardized Road-map Test of Direction Sense. Baltimore: The Johns Hopkins University Press; 1976.

[124] Flicker C, Ferris SH, Crook T, Reisberg B, Bartus RT. Equivalent spatial-rotation deficits in normal aging and Alzheimer's disease. *J Clin Exp Neuropsychol.* 1988 Aug;10(4):387–99.

[125] Stiles J, Kritchevsky M, Bellugi U. Spatial Cognition. *Psychology Press;* 1988.

[126] Tapley SM, Bryden MP. An investigation of sex differences in spatial ability: mental rotation of three-dimensional objects. *Can J Psychol.* 1977 Sep;31(3):122–30.

[127] Rainville C, Marchand N, Passini R. Performances of patients with a dementia of the Alzheimer type in the Standardized Road-Map test of Direction Sense. *Neuropsychologia.* 2002;40(5):567–73.

[128] Kessels RP, van Zandvoort MJ, Postma A, Kappelle LJ, de Haan EH. The Corsi Block-Tapping Task: standardization and normative data. *Appl Neuropsychol.* 2000;7(4):252–8.

[129] Christensen KJ, Riley BE, Heffernan KA, Love SB, McLaughlin Sta Maria ME. Facial recognition test in the elderly: norms, reliability and premorbid estimation. *Clin Neuropsychol.* 2002 Feb;16(1):51–6.

[130] Benton AL, Van Allen MW, Hamsher K, Levin H. Test of Facial Recognition. Iowa: University of Iowa Hospitals; 1978.

[131] Boyd JL. A validity study of the Hooper Visual Organization Test. *J Consult Clin Psychol.* 1981.

[132] Hooper HE. Hooper Test of Visual Organization. *American Psychologist.* 1952.

[133] Colangelo V, Schurr J, Ball MJ, Pelaez RP, Bazan NG, Lukiw WJ. Gene expression profiling of 12633 genes in Alzheimer hippocampal CA1: transcription and neurotrophic factor down-regulation and up-regulation of apoptotic and pro-inflammatory signaling. *J Neurosci Res.* 2002 Nov 1;70(3):462–73.

[134] Kikuchi M, Hirosawa T, Yokokura M, Yagi S, Mori N, Yoshikawa E, et al. Effects of Brain Amyloid Deposition and Reduced Glucose Metabolism on the Default Mode of Brain Function in Normal Aging. *Journal of Neuroscience.* 2011 Aug 3;31(31):11193–9.

[135] Ginsberg SD, Alldred MJ, Che S. Gene expression levels assessed by CA1 pyramidal neuron and regional hippocampal dissections in Alzheimer's disease. *Neurobiology of Disease.* 2012 Jan;45(1):99–107.

[136] Rizzo M, Anderson SW, Dawson J, Nawrot M. Vision and cognition in Alzheimer's disease. *Neuropsychologia.* 2000;38(8):1157–69.

[137] Lehmann M, Crutch SJ, Ridgway GR, Ridha BH, Barnes J, Warrington EK, et al. Cortical thickness and voxel-based morphometry in posterior cortical atrophy and typical Alzheimer's disease. *Neurobiology of Aging.* 2011 Aug 1;32(8):1466–76.

[138] Geldmacher DS. Visuospatial dysfunction in the neurodegenerative diseases. *Frontiers in Bioscience.* 2003 Sep 1;8:e428–36.

[139] Valenti DA. Alzheimer's disease: Visual system review. Optometry. *Mosby,* Inc; 2010 Jan 1;81(1):12–21.

[140] Tzekov R, Mullan M. Vision function abnormalities in Alzheimer disease. *Surv Ophthalmol.* 2014 Jul;59(4):414–33.

[141] Warren JD, Fletcher PD, Golden HL. The paradox of syndromic diversity in Alzheimer disease. Nature Reviews Neuroscience. *Nature Publishing Group;* 2012 Jul 17;135:1 14.

[142] Au R, Massaro JM, Wolf PA, Young ME, Beiser A, Seshadri S, et al. Association of white matter hyperintensity volume with decreased cognitive functioning: the Framingham Heart Study. *Archives of Neurology.* 2006 Feb;63(2):246–50.

[143] McKee AC, Cabral H. Visual association pathology in pre-clinical Alzheimer disease. *J Neuropathol Exp Neurol.* 2006 Jul 6;65:621–30.

[144] Tang-Wai DF, Graff-Radford NR, Boeve BF, Dickson DW, Parisi JE, Crook R, et al. Clinical, genetic, and neuropathologic characteristics of posterior cortical atrophy. *Neurology.* 2004 Oct 12;63(7):1168–74.

[145] Renner JA, Burns JM, Hou CE, McKeel DW Jr, Storandt M, Morris JC. Progressive posterior cortical dysfunction: a clinicopathologic series. *Neurology.* 2004 Oct 12;63(7):1175–80.

[146] Mendez MF. Posterior Cortical Atrophy. Lecture presented at ANPA Annual Conference. *Lake Buena Vista, FL*; 2015. pp. 1–51.

[147] Singh TD, Josephs KA, Machulda MM, Drubach DA, Apostolova LG, Lowe VJ, et al. Clinical, FDG and amyloid PET imaging in posterior cortical atrophy. *J Neurol. Springer Berlin Heidelberg;* 2015 Apr 13;:1–10.

[148] Ortner M, Kurz A. Posterior cortical atrophy. *Nervenarzt.* 2015 Mar 21.

[149] Borruat F-X. Posterior cortical atrophy: review of the recent literature. *Current Neurology and neuroscience reports.* 2013 Dec;13(12):406.

[150] Levine DN, Lee JM, Fisher CM. The visual variant of Alzheimer's disease: a clinicopathologic case study. *Neurology.* 1993 Feb;43(2):305–13.

[151] Cerami C, Crespi C, Rosa Della PA, Dodich A, Marcone A, Magnani G, et al. Brain changes within the visuo-spatial attentional network in posterior cortical atrophy. *Journal of Alzheimer's Disease.* 2015;43(2):385–95.

[152] Ossenkoppele R, van der Flier WM, Verfaillie SCJ, Vrenken H, Versteeg A, van Schijndel RA, et al. Long-term effects of amyloid, hypometabolism, and atrophy on neuropsychological functions. *Neurology.* 2014 May 20;82(20):1768–75.

[153] Diagnostic and Statistical Manual of Mental Disorders. 5 ed. Arlington, VA: *American Psychological Association* (APA); 2013. 970 p.

[154] Simpson JR. DSM-5 and neurocognitive disorders. *J Am Acad Psychiatry Law.* 2014;42(2):159–64.

[155] McKhann GM II, Knopman DS, Chertkow H, Hyman BT, Jack CR Jr, Kawas CH, et al. The diagnosis of dementia due to Alzheimer's disease: recommendations from the National Institute on Aging-Alzheimer‘s Association workgroups on diagnostic guidelines for Alzheimer's disease. 2011. pp. 263–9.

[156] Vlček K, Laczo J. Neural correlates of spatial navigation changes in mild cognitive impairment and Alzheimer's disease. *Front Behav Neurosci.* 2014;8.

[157] O'Brien HL, Tetewsky SJ, Avery LM. Visual mechanisms of spatial disorientation in Alzheimer's disease. *Cerebral Cortex.* 2001;111:1083–92.

[158] Cherrier MM, Mendez MF, Perryman K. Route learning performance in Alzheimer disease patients. *Neuropsychiatry Neuropsychol Behav Neurol.* 2001 Jul;14(3):159–68.

[159] Mapstone M, Steffenella TM, Duffy CJ. A visuospatial variant of mild cognitive impairment: getting lost between aging and AD. *Neurology.* 2003 Mar 11;60(5):802–8.

[160] Kavcic V, Fernandez R, Logan D, Duffy CJ. Neurophysiological and perceptual correlates of navigational impairment in Alzheimer's disease. *Brain.* 2006 Mar;129(Pt 3):736–46.

[161] Gazova I, Vlček K, Laczó J, Nedelska Z, Hyncicova E, Mokrisova I, et al. Spatial navigation-a unique window into physiological and pathological aging. *Frontiers in aging neuroscience.* 2012;4:16.

[162] Nedelska Z, Andel R, Laczó J, Vlček K, Horinek D, Lisy J, et al. Spatial navigation impairment is proportional to right hippocampal volume. *Proc Natl Acad Sci USA.* 2012 Feb 14;109(7):2590–4.

[163] Hort J, Andel R, Mokrisova I, Gazova I, Amlerova J, Valis M, et al. Effect of Donepezil in Alzheimer Disease Can Be Measured by a Computerized Human Analog of the Morris Water Maze. *Neurodegenerative Dis.* 2014;13(2-3):192–6.

[164] Weniger G, Ruhleder M, Lange C, Wolf S, Irle E. Egocentric and allocentric memory as assessed by virtual reality in individuals with amnestic mild cognitive impairment. *Neuropsychologia.* 2011 Feb;49(3):518–27.

[165] Kalová E, Vlček K, Jarolímová E, Bures J. Allothetic orientation and sequential ordering of places is impaired in early stages of Alzheimer's disease: corresponding results in real space tests and computer tests. *Behavioural Brain Research.* 2005 Apr;159(2):175–86.

[166] Jacobs HIL, Radua J, Lückmann HC, Sack AT. Meta-analysis of functional network alterations in Alzheimer's disease: toward a network biomarker. *Neuroscience and Biobehavioral Reviews.* 2013 Jun;37(5):753–65.

[167] Filippi M, Agosta F. Structural and functional network connectivity breakdown in Alzheimer's disease studied with magnetic resonance imaging techniques. *Journal of Alzheimer's Disease.* 2011;24(3):455–74.

[168] Krajcovicova L, Mikl M, Marecek R, Rektorova I. Disturbed default mode network connectivity patterns in Alzheimer's disease associated with visual processing. *Journal of Alzheimer's Disease.* 2014;41(4):1229–38.

[169] Migliaccio R, Agosta F, Toba MN, Samri D, Corlier F, de Souza LC, et al. Brain networks in posterior cortical atrophy: A single case tractography study and literature review. *CORTEX.* 2012 Nov 12;48(10):1298–309.

[170] Schenk T, Franz V, Bruno N. Vision-for-perception and vision-for-action: which model is compatible with the available psychophysical and neuropsychological data? *Vision Research.* 2011 Apr 22;51(8):812–8.

[171] Thoma V, Henson RN. Object representations in ventral and dorsal visual streams: fMRI repetition effects depend on attention and part–whole configuration. *Neuroimage.* 2011 Jul;57(2):513–25.

[172] Bokde ALW, Karmann M, Born C, Teipel SJ, Omerovic M, Ewers M, et al. Altered brain activation during a verbal working memory task in subjects with amnestic mild cognitive impairment. *Journal of Alzheimer's Disease.* 2010;21(1):103–18.

[173] Prvulovic D, Hubl D, Sack AT, Melillo L, Maurer K, Frölich L, et al. Functional Imaging of Visuospatial Processing in Alzheimer's Disease. *Neuroimage.* 2002 Nov;17(3):1403–14.

[174] Teipel SJ, Bokde ALW, Born C, Meindl T, Reiser M, Moller HJ, et al. Morphological substrate of face matching in healthy ageing and mild cognitive impairment: a combined MRI-fMRI study. *Brain.* 2007 May 29;130(7):1745–58.

[175] Vannini P, Almkvist O, Dierks T, Lehmann C, Wahlund L OO. Reduced neuronal efficacy in progressive mild cognitive impairment: A prospective fMRI study on visuospatial processing. *Psychiatry Research.* 2007 Oct;156(1):43–57.

[176] Jacobs HIL, Gronenschild EHBM, Evers EAT, Ramakers IHGB, Hofman PAM, Backes WH, et al. Visuospatial processing in early Alzheimer's disease: a multimodal neuroimaging study. *CORTEX.* 2015 Mar;64:394–406.

[177] Kennedy KM, Rodrigue KM, Bischof GN, Hebrank AC, Reuter-Lorenz PA, Park DC. Age trajectories of functional activation under conditions of low and high processing demands: An adult lifespan fMRI study of the aging brain. *Human Brain Mapping Journal.* 2014;104(C):1–14.

[178] Dickerson BC, Sperling RA. Functional abnormalities of the medial temporal lobe memory system in mild cognitive impairment and Alzheimer's disease: Insights from functional MRI studies. *Neuropsychologia.* 2008 May;46(6):1624–35.

[179] Maurer K, Prvulovic D. Paintings of an artist with Alzheimer's disease: visuoconstructural deficits during dementia. *J Neural Transm.* 2004 Mar;111(3):235–45.

[180] Bokde ALW, Lopez-Bayo P, Born C, Ewers M, Meindl T, Teipel SJ, et al. Alzheimer disease: functional abnormalities in the dorsal visual pathway. *Radiology.* 2010 Jan;254(1):219–26.

[181] Caterini F, Sala SD, Spinnler H, Stangalino C, Turnbull OH. Object Recognition and Object Orientation in Alzheimer's Disease. *Neuropsychology.* 2002;16(2):146–55.

[182] Kwak YT. "Closing-in" phenomenon in Alzheimer's disease and subcortical vascular dementia. *BMC Neurology.* 2004 Jan 26;4:3.

[183] Yang DW, Kwon S-Y, Lee E-S, Hong YJ, Lim S-C, Shim YS, et al. Anatomical correlate of closing-in phenomenon. *Alzheimer's and Dementia.* 2012 Jul 1;8(S):P43–4.

[184] Lee BH, Chin J, Kang SJ, Kim E-J, Park K-C, Na DL. Mechanism of the closing-in phenomenon in a figure copying task in Alzheimer's disease patients. *Neurocase.* 2004 Oct;10(5):393–7.

[185] Chin J, Lee BH, Seo SW, Kim E-J, Suh MK, Kang SJ, et al. The Closing-in Phenomenon in Alzheimer's Disease and Vascular Dementia. *Journal of Clinical Neurology.* 2005 Oct;1(2):166–73.

[186] Culham JC, Cavina-Pratesi C, Singhal A. The role of parietal cortex in visuomotor control: What have we learned from neuroimaging? *Neuropsychologia.* 2006 Jan;44(13):2668–84.

[187] Gilmore GC, Levy JA. Spatial contrast sensitivity in Alzheimer's disease: a comparison of two methods. *Optometry and Vision Science.* 1991 Oct;68(10):790–4.

[188] Kéri S, Antal A, Kálmán J, Janka Z, Benedek G. Early visual impairment is independent of the visuocognitive and memory disturbances in Alzheimer's disease. *Vision Research.* 1999 Jun;39(13):2261–5.

[189] Lakshminarayanan V, Lagrave J, Kean ML, Dick M, Shankle R. Vision in dementia: contrast effects. *Neurological Research.* 1996 Feb;18(1):9–15.

[190] Vaina LM. Functional segregation of color and motion processing in the human visual cortex: clinical evidence. *Cerebral Cortex.* 1994 Sep;4(5):555–72.

[191] Cronin-Golomb A, Corkin S, Rizzo JF, Cohen JA, Growdon JH, Banks KS. Visual dysfunction in Alzheimer's disease: relation to normal aging. *Annals of Neurology.* 1991 Jan;29(1):41–52.

[192] Kiyosawa M, Bosley TM, Chawluk J, Jamieson D, Schatz NJ, Savino PJ, et al. Alzheimer's disease with prominent visual symptoms. Clinical and metabolic evaluation. *Ophthalmology.* 1989 Jul;96(7):1077–85–discussion1085–6.

[193] Jackson GR, Owsley C. Visual dysfunction, neurodegenerative diseases, and aging. *Neurologic Clinics of NA.* 2003 Aug;21(3):709–28.

[194] Heywood CA, Kentridge RW. Achromatopsia, color vision, and cortex. *Neurology Clinics.* 2003 May;21(2):483–500.

[195] Sala Della S, Kinnear P, Spinnler H. Color-to-figure matching in Alzheimer's disease. *Archives of Clinical Neuropsychology.* 2000;15(7):571–85.

[196] Cronin-Golomb A, Sugiura R, Corkin S, Growdon JH. Incomplete achromatopsia in Alzheimer's disease. *Neurobiology of Aging.* 1993 Jul 6;14(5):471–7.

[197] Lu A, Xu G, Jin H, Mo L, Zhang J, Zhang JX. Electrophysiological evidence for effects of color knowledge in object recognition. *Neuroscience Letters.* 2010 Jan;469(3):405–10.

[198] Tanaka J, Weiskopf D, Williams P. The role of color in high-level vision. *Trends in Cognitive Sciences.* 2001 May 1;5(5):211–5.

[199] Takahashi S, Ohya K, Arakawa K, Ishisaka Y. Perceived Strength of Edge, Depth and Brightness of the Kanizsa Illusion as a Function of the Color Contrast between Figures and Background. *Gestalt Theory.* 2010.

[200] Beglinger LJ, Unverzagt FW, Beristain X, Kareken D. An updated version of the Weigl discriminates adults with dementia from those with mild impairment and healthy controls. *Archives of Clinical Neuropsychology.* 2008 Mar;23(2):149–56.

[201] Lee C-N, Ko D, Suh Y-W, Park K-W. Cognitive Functions and Stereopsis in Patients with Parkinson's Disease and Alzheimer's Disease Using 3-Dimensional Television: A Case Controlled Trial. Jo D-G, editor. *PLoS ONE.* 2015 Mar 30;10(3):e0123229.

[202] Mendez MF, Cherrier MM, Meadows RS. Depth perception in Alzheimer's disease. *Perceptual and Motor Skills.* 1996 Dec;83(3 Pt 1):987–95.

[203] Banks MS, Hooge IT, Backus BT. Perceiving slant about a horizontal axis from stereopsis. *J Vis.* 2001;1(2):55–79.

[204] DeAngelis G. Seeing in three dimensions: the neurophysiology of stereopsis. *Trends in Cognitive Sciences.* 2000 Mar;4(3):80–90.

[205] Tsao DY, Vanduffel W, Sasaki Y, Fize D, Knutsen TA, Mandeville JB, et al. Stereopsis activates V3A and caudal intraparietal areas in macaques and humans. Neuron. 2003 Jul 31;39(3):555–68.

[206] Nishida Y, Hayashi O, Iwami T, Kimura M, Kani K, Ito R, et al. Stereopsis-processing regions in the human parieto-occipital cortex. *NeuroRepo*rt. 2001 Jul 20;12(10):2259–63.

[207] Vishwanath D. Toward a new theory of stereopsis. *Psychol Rev.* 2014;121(2):151–78.

[208] Gilmore GC, Wend HE, Naylor L. Motion perception and Alzheimer's disease. *J Gerontol.* 1994 Jul 6;49:P52–7.

[209] Trick GL, Silverman SE. Visual sensitivity to motion: age-related changes and deficits in senile dementia of the Alzheimer type. *Neurology.* 1991 Sep;41(9):1437–40.

[210] Nestor PG, Parasuraman R, Haxby JV, Grady CL. Divided attention and metabolic brain dysfunction in mild dementia of the Alzheimer's type. *Neuropsychologia.* 1991;29(5):379–87.

[211] Parasuraman R, Greenwood PM, Haxby JV, Grady CL. Visuospatial attention in dementia of the Alzheimer type. *Brain.* 1992 Jun;115 (Pt 3):711–33.

[212] Cronin-Golomb A, Rizzo J, Corkin S. Visual function in Alzheimer's disease and normal aging. *Ann NY Acad Sci.* 1991 Jul 6;640:28–35.

[213] Kurylo DD, Corkin S, Rizzo JF III, Growdon JH. Greater relative impairment of object recognition than of visuospatial abilities in Alzheimer's disease. *Neuropsychology.* 1996;10(1):74–81.

[214] Mendola JD, Cronin-Golomb A, Corkin S, Growdon JH. Prevalence of visual deficits in Alzheimer's disease. *Optom Vis Sci.* 1995 Mar;72(3):155–67.

[215] Tetewsky SJ, Duffy CJ. Visual loss and getting lost in Alzheimer's disease. *Neurology.* 1999;52:958–65.

[216] Tantiwongkosi B, Salamon N. Imaging of Retrochiasmal and Higher Cortical Visual Disorders. *Neurologic Clinics of NA*. 2015 Aug;25(3):411–24.

[217] Pache M, Smeets C, Gasio PF, Savaskan E. Colour vision deficiencies in Alzheimer's disease. *Age and Ageing*. 2003;32(4):422–6.

[218] Wijk H, Sivik L. Some aspects of colour perception among patients with Alzheimer's disease. *Scand J Caring Sci*. 1995;9(1):3–9.

[219] Bassi CJ, Solomon K, Young D. Vision in aging and dementia. *Optom Vis Sci*. 1993 Oct;70(10):809–13.

[220] Kurylo DD, Corkin S, Dolan RP, Rizzo JF, Parker SW, Growdon JH. Broad-band visual capacities are not selectively impaired in Alzheimer's disease. Neurobiology of Aging. 1994;15(3):305–11.

[221] Wijk H, Berg S, Sivik L, Steen B. Colour discrimination, colour naming and colour preferences among individuals with Alzheimer's disease. *Int J Geriat Psychiatry*. 1999;14(12):1000–5.

[222] Gorges M, Pinkhardt EH, Kassubek J. Alterations of Eye Movement Control in Neurodegenerative Movement Disorders. *Journal of Ophthalmology*. 2014;2014(2):1–11.

[223] Ptak R, Müri RM. The parietal cortex and saccade planning: lessons from human lesion studies. *Frontiers in Human Neuroscience*. 2013 Jun 4;:1–11.

[224] Lenoble Q, Bubbico G, Szaffarczyk SB, Pasquier F, Boucart M. Scene Categorization in Alzheimer's Disease: A Saccadic Choice Task. *Dement Geriatr Cogn Dis Extra*. 2015 May 19;5(1):1–12.

[225] Antoniades CA, Kennard C. Oculomotor abnormalities in posterior cortical atrophy: are they different from those in Alzheimer's disease after all? *Brain*. 2015 Jul;138(Pt 7):1773–5.

[226] Shakespeare TJ, Yong KXX, Foxe D, Hodges J, Crutch SJ. Pronounced impairment of everyday skills and self-care in posterior cortical atrophy. *Journal of Alzheimer's Disease*. 2015;43(2):381–4.

[227] Boucart M, Calais G, Lenoble Q, Moroni C. Differential processing of natural scenes in posterior cortical atrophy and in Alzheimer's disease, as measured with a saccade choice task. *Frontiers in Integrative Neuroscience*. 2014;8.

[228] Antoniades CA, Kennard C. Ocular motor abnormalities in neurodegenerative disorders. *Eye* (Lond). 2015 Feb;29(2):200–7.

[229] Fernández G, Castro LR, Schumacher M, Agamennoni OE. Diagnosis of mild Alzheimer disease through the analysis of eye movements during reading. *J Integr Neurosci*. 2015 Mar;14(01):121–33.

[230] Fernández G, Laubrock J, Mandolesi P, Colombo O, Agamennoni O. Registering eye movements during reading in Alzheimer's disease: Difficulties in predicting upcoming words. *Journal of Clinical and Experimental Neuropsychology*. 2014 Feb 17;36(3):302–16.

[231] Lueck KL, Mendez MF, Perryman KM. Eye movement abnormalities during reading in patients with Alzheimer disease. *Neuropsychiatry Neuropsychol Behav Neurol*. 2000 Apr;13(2):77–82.

[232] Parkinson J, Maxner C. Eye Movement Abnormalities in Alzheimer Disease: Case Presentation and Literature Review. *American Orthoptic Journal*. 2005 Jan 1;55(1):90–6.

[233] Mosimann UP, Felblinger J, Ballinari P, Hess CW, Müri RM. Visual exploration behaviour during clock reading in Alzheimer's disease. *Brain.* 2004 Feb;127(Pt 2):431–8.
[234] Hawkins KM, Sergio LE. Visuomotor impairments in older adults at increased Alzheimer's disease risk. *Journal of Alzheimer's Disease* [Internet]. 2014;42(2):607–21.
[235] Mollica MA, Navarra J, Fernández-Prieto I, Olives J, Tort A, Valech N, et al. Subtle visuomotor difficulties in preclinical Alzheimer's disease. *Journal of Neuropsychology.* 2015 Jul 14;
[236] Guariglia CC, Nitrini R. Topographical disorientation in Alzheimer's disease. *Arq Neuropsiquiatr.* 2009 Dec;67(4):967–72.
[237] McShane R, Gedling K, Keene J, Fairburn C, Jacoby R, Hope T. Getting lost in dementia: a longitudinal study of a behavioral symptom. *International Psychogeriatrics.* 1998 Sep;10(3):253–60.
[238] Pai M-C, Jacobs WJ. Topographical disorientation in community-residing patients with Alzheimer's disease. *Int J Geriat Psychiatry.* 2004 Mar 11;19(3):250–5.
[239] Tu M-C, Pai M-C. Getting lost for the first time in patients with Alzheimer's disease. *International Psychogeriatrics.* 2006 Sep;18(3):567–70.
[240] Benke T, Karner E, Petermichl S, Prantner V, Kemmler G. Neuropsychological Deficits Associated With Route Learning in Alzheimer Disease, MCI, and Normal Aging. *Alzheimer Dis Assoc Disord.* 2014;28(2):162–7.
[241] Grady CL. The cognitive neuroscience of ageing. *Nat Rev Neurosci.* 2012 Jun 20;13(7):491–505.
[242] Grady CL, McIntosh AR, Horwitz B, Maisog JM, Ungerleider LG, Mentis MJ, et al. Age-related reductions in human recognition memory due to impaired encoding. *Science.* 1995 Jul 14;269(5221):218–21.
[243] Cogan DG. Visuospatial dysgnosia. *American Journal of Ophthalmology.* 1979 Sep;88(3 Pt 1):361–8.
[244] Gazova I, Laczó J, Rubinova E, Mokrisova I, Hyncicova E, Andel R, et al. Spatial navigation in young versus older adults. *Frontiers in aging neuroscience.* 2013;5:94.
[245] Samadani A-A, Moussavi Z. The effect of aging on human brain spatial processing performance. *Conf Proc IEEE Eng Med Biol Soc.* 2012;2012:6768–71.
[246] Rodgers MK, Sindone JA, Moffat SD. Effects of age on navigation strategy. *Neurobiology of Aging;* 2012 Jan 1;33(1):202.e15–202.e22.
[247] Palermo L, Piccardi L, Bianchini F, Nemmi F, Giorgio V, Incoccia C, et al. Looking for the compass in a case of developmental topographical disorientation: A behavioral and neuroimaging study. *Journal of Clinical and Experimental Neuropsychology.* 2014 Apr 17;36(5):464–81.
[248] Serino S, Riva G. Getting lost in Alzheimer's disease: a break in the mental frame syncing. *Medical Hypotheses.* 2013 Apr;80(4):416–21.
[249] Grossi D, Fasanaro AM, Cecere R, Salzano S, Trojano L. Progressive topographical disorientation: a case of focal Alzheimer's disease. *Neurol Sci.* 2007 Apr;28(2):107–10.
[250] Barrash J, Damasio H, Adolphs R, Tranel D. The neuroanatomical correlates of route learning impairment. *Neuropsychologia.* 2000;38(6):820–36.
[251] Aguirre GK, D'Esposito M. Topographical disorientation: a synthesis and taxonomy. *Brain.* 1999 Sep;122 (Pt 9):1613–28.

[252] delpolyi AR, Rankin KP, Mucke L, Miller BL, Gorno-Tempini ML. Spatial cognition and the human navigation network in AD and MCI. *Neurology.* 2007 Sep 4;69(10):986–97.

[253] Bird CM, Chan D, Hartley T, Pijnenburg YAL, Rossor MN, Burgess N. Topographical short-term memory differentiates Alzheimer's disease from frontotemporal lobar degeneration. *Hippocampus.* 2009 Oct 22;20(10):1154–69.

[254] Pengas G, Patterson K, Arnold RJ, Bird CM. Lost and found: bespoke memory testing for Alzheimer's disease and semantic dementia. *Journal of Alzheimer's Disease.* 2010;21(4).

[255] Pengas G, Williams GB. The relationship of topographical memory performance to regional neurodegeneration in Alzheimer's disease. *Frontiers in aging neuroscience.* 2012 Jul;4(17):1–10.

[256] Serino S, Morganti F, Di Stefano F, Riva G. Detecting early egocentric and allocentric impairments deficits in Alzheimer's disease: an experimental study with virtual reality. *Frontiers in aging neuroscience.* 2015;7:88.

[257] Tangen GG, Engedal K, Bergland A, Moger TA, Hansson O, Mengshoel AM. Spatial navigation measured by the Floor Maze Test in patients with subjective cognitive impairment, mild cognitive impairment, and mild Alzheimer's disease. *International Psychogeriatrics.* 2015 Aug;27(08):1401–9.

[258] Hort J, Laczó J, Vyhnálek M, Bojar M, Bures J, Vlček K. Spatial navigation deficit in amnestic mild cognitive impairment. *Proc Natl Acad Sci USA.* 2007 Mar 6;104(10):4042–7.

[259] Nebes RD, Brady CB. Focused and divided attention in Alzheimer's disease. *CORTEX.* 1989 Jun;25(2):305–15.

[260] Ress D, Backus BT, Heeger DJ. Activity in primary visual cortex predicts performance in a visual detection task. *Nature Neuroscience.* 2000 Sep;3(9):940–5.

[261] Rosler A, Mapstone ME, Hays AK, Mesulam MM, Rademaker A, Gitelman DR, et al. Alterations of visual search strategy in Alzheimer's disease and aging. *Neuropsychology.* 2000 Jul;14(3):398–408.

[262] Bonato M. Neglect and extinction depend greatly on task demands: a review. *Frontiers in Human Neuroscience.* 2012;6.

[263] Rosler A, Mapstone M, HAYSWICKLUND A, GITELMAN D, Weintraub S. The "zoom lens" of focal attention in visual search: Changes in aging and Alzheimer's disease. *CORTEX.* 2005;41(4):512–9.

[264] Cronin-Golomb A, Corkin S, Growdon JH. Visual dysfunction predicts cognitive deficits in Alzheimer's disease. *Optom Vis Sci.* 1995 Mar;72(3):168–76.

[265] Nichelli P, Magherini A. Role of Visuospatial Cognition Assessment in the Diagnosis and Research of Atypical Parkinsonian Disorders. *Atypical Parkinsonian Disorders.* 2005.

[266] Crutch SJ, Lehmann M, Schott JM, Rabinovici GD, Rossor MN, Fox NC. Posterior cortical atrophy. *The Lancet Neurology. Elsevier;* 2012;11(2):170–8.

[267] Giorelli M, Losignore NA, Bagnoli J, Difazio P, Zimatore GB. The progression of posterior cortical atrophy to corticobasal syndrome: lumping or splitting neurodegenerative diseases? *Tremor Other Hyperkinet Mov* (NY). 2014;4:244.

[268] Isella V, Villa G, Mapelli C, Ferri F, Appollonio IM, Ferrarese C. The Neuropsychiatric Profile of Posterior Cortical Atrophy. *J Geriatr Psychiatry Neurol.* 2015 Apr 28;28(2):136–44.
[269] Andrade K, Kas A, Valabregue R, Samri D, Sarazin M, Habert MO, et al. Visuospatial deficits in posterior cortical atrophy: structural and functional correlates. *Journal of Neurology, Neurosurgery and Psychiatry.* 2012 Aug 7;83(9):860–3.
[270] Feldmann A, Trauninger A, Toth L, Kotek G, Kosztolanyi P, Illes E, et al. Atrophy and decreased activation of fronto-parietal attention areas contribute to higher visual dysfunction in posterior cortical atrophy. *Psychiatry Research. Elsevier Ireland Ltd;* 2008 Nov 30;164(2):178–84.
[271] Alves J, Soares JM, Sampaio A, Gonçalves ÓF. Posterior cortical atrophy and Alzheimer's disease: a meta-analytic review of neuropsychological and brain morphometry studies. *Brain Imaging and Behavior.* 2013 May 21;7(3):353–61.
[272] Josephs KA, Whitwell JL, Duffy JR, Vanvoorst WA, Strand EA, Hu WT, et al. Progressive aphasia secondary to Alzheimer disease vs FTLD pathology. *Neurology.* 2007 Dec 31;70(1):25–34.
[273] Alladi S, Xuereb J, Bak T, Nestor P, Knibb J, Patterson K, et al. Focal cortical presentations of Alzheimer's disease. *Brain.* 2007 Oct 1;130(10):2636–45.
[274] Galton CJ, Patterson K, Xuereb JH, Hodges JR. Atypical and typical presentations of Alzheimer's disease: a clinical, neuropsychological, neuroimaging and pathological study of 13 cases. *Brain.* 2000;123:484–98.
[275] Koedam ELGE, Lehmann M, van der Flier WM, Scheltens P, Pijnenburg YAL, Fox N, et al. Visual assessment of posterior atrophy development of a MRI rating scale. *Eur Radiol.* 2011 Dec;21(12):2618–25.
[276] Ishii K, Kawachi T, Sasaki H, Kono AK. Voxel-based morphometric comparison between early-and late-onset mild Alzheimer's disease and assessment of diagnostic performance of z score images. *American Journal of Neuroradiology.* 2005 Feb;26:335–40.
[277] Frisoni GB. Structural correlates of early and late onset Alzheimer's disease: voxel based morphometric study. *Journal of Neurology, Neurosurgery and Psychiatry.* 2005 Jan 1;76(1):112–4.
[278] Carrasquillo MM, Khan QUA, Murray ME, Krishnan S, Aakre J, Pankratz VS, et al. Late-onset Alzheimer disease genetic variants in posterior cortical atrophy and posterior AD. *Neurology.* 2014 Apr 22;82(16):1455–62.
[279] Mendez MF. Visuospatial Deficits with Preserved Reading Ability in a Patient with Posterior Cortical Atrophy. *CORTEX.* 2001 Jan;37(4):535–43.
[280] Yong KXX, Rajdev K, Shakespeare TJ, Leff AP, Crutch SJ. Facilitating text reading in posterior cortical atrophy. *Neurology.* 2015 Jul 2.
[281] McMonagle P, Deering F, Berliner Y, Kertesz A. The cognitive profile of posterior cortical atrophy. *Neurology.* 2006 Feb 14;66(3):331–8.
[282] Rogelet P, Delafosse A, Destée A. Posterior cortical atrophy: Unusual feature of alzheimer's disease. *Neurocase.* 1996 Nov;2(6):495–501.
[283] Tenovuo O, Kemppainen N, Aalto S, Någren K, Rinne JO. Posterior cortical atrophy: a rare form of dementia with in vivo evidence of amyloid-beta accumulation. *Journal of Alzheimer's Disease.* 2008 Nov;15(3):351–5.

[284] Kirshner HS, Lavin PJM. Posterior cortical atrophy: a brief review. *Current Neurology and neuroscience reports.* 2006 Nov;6(6):477–80.

[285] Crutch SJ, Lehmann M, Gorgoraptis N, Kaski D, Ryan N, Husain M, et al. Abnormal visual phenomena in posterior cortical atrophy. *Neurocase.* 2011 Mar 11;17(2):160–77.

[286] Crutch SJ, Schott JM, Rabinovici GD, Boeve BF, Cappa SF, Dickerson BC, et al. Shining a light on posterior cortical atrophy. *Alzheimer's and Dementia. Elsevier Ltd*; 2013 Jan 9;:1–3.

[287] Crutch SJ, Warrington EK. The relationship between visual crowding and letter confusability: Towards an understanding of dyslexia in posterior cortical atrophy. *Cognitive Neuropsychology.* 2009 Jul;26(5):471–98.

[288] Saffran EM. "Attentional Dyslexia" in Alzheimer's Disease: A Case Study. *Cognitive Neuropsychology.* 1996 Mar;13(2):205–28.

[289] Growdon JH, Rossor MN. The Dementias 2. *Elsevier Health Sciences;* 2007.

[290] Yong KXX, Shakespeare TJ, Cash D, Henley SMD, Warren JD, Crutch SJ. (Con)text-specific effects of visual dysfunction on reading in posterior cortical atrophy. *CORTEX.* 2014 Aug 1;57(C):92–106.

[291] Yong KXX, Shakespeare TJ, Cash D, Henley SMD, Nicholas JM, Ridgway GR, et al. Prominent effects and neural correlates of visual crowding in a neurodegenerative disease population. *Brain.* 2014 Nov 19;137(12):3284–99.

[292] Rossor, M., Collinge, J., Fox, N., Howard, R., Mallucci, G., Mummery, C., Warren, J. (2009). Cognitive Impairment and Dementia. In Clarke, C., Howard, R., Rossor, M., Shorvon, S. (Eds.). *Neurology: a Queen Square Textbook* (1st ed. pp.245-288). Chichester: Wiley-Blackwell.

[293] Rosenbloom MH, Alkalay A, Agarwal N, Baker SL, O'Neil JP, Jones JE, et al. Distinct clinical and metabolic deficits in PCA and AD are not related to amyloid distribution. *Neurology.* 2011 May 23;76(21):1789–96.

[294] Beh SC, Muthusamy B, Calabresi P, Hart J, Zee D, Patel V, et al. Hiding in plain sight: a closer look at posterior cortical atrophy. *Practical Neurology.* 2015 Feb;15(1):5–13.

[295] Pariente JJ, Cole SS, Henson RN, Clare LL, Kennedy AA, Rossor MN, et al. Alzheimer's patients engage an alternative network during a memory task. *Annals of Neurology.* 2005 Dec 1;58(6):870–9.

[296] Thiyagesh SN, Farrow TFD, Parks RW, Accosta-Mesa H, Young C, Wilkinson ID, et al. The neural basis of visuospatial perception in Alzheimer's disease and healthy elderly comparison subjects: an fMRI study. *Psychiatry Research.* 2009 May 15;172(2):109–16.

[297] Mishkin M, Ungerleider LG, Macko KA. Object vision and spatial vision: two cortical pathways. *Trends in Neurosciences.* 1983.

[298] Goodale MA, Milner AD. Separate visual pathways for perception and action. *Trends in Neurosciences.* 1992 Jan;15(1):20–5.

[299] Creem SH, Proffitt DR. Defining the cortical visual systems:"what,""where," and "how." *Acta Psychol* (Amst). 2001;(1-3):43–68.

[300] Ross SJ, Graham N, Stuart-Green L, Prins M, Xuereb J, Patterson K, et al. Progressive biparietal atrophy: an atypical presentation of Alzheimer's disease. *Journal of Neurology, Neurosurgery and Psychiatry.* 1996 Oct;61(4):388–95.

[301] Caroppo P, Belin C, Grabli D, Maillet D, De Septenville A, Migliaccio R, et al. Posterior Cortical Atrophy as an Extreme Phenotype of GRN Mutations. *JAMA Neurol.* 2015 Feb 1;72(2):224.

[302] Carrasquillo MM, Barber I, Lincoln SJ, Murray ME, Camsari GB, Khan QUA, et al. Evaluating pathogenic dementia variants in posterior cortical atrophy. *Neurobiology of Aging.* 2015 Oct 24;:1–7.

[303] Murray ME, Cannon A, Graff-Radford NR, Liesinger AM, Rutherford NJ, Ross OA, et al. Differential clinicopathologic and genetic features of late-onset amnestic dementias. *Acta Neuropathologica.* 2014 Jun 5;128(3):411–21.

[304] Ryan NS, Shakespeare TJ, Lehmann M, Keihaninejad S, Nicholas JM, Leung KK, et al. Motor features in posterior cortical atrophy and their imaging correlates. *Neurobiology of Aging.* 2014 Dec;35(12):2845–57.

[305] Muslimovic D, Post B, Speelman JD, Schmand BA. Cognitive profile of patients with newly diagnosed Parkinson disease. *Neurology.* 2005 Oct 25;65(8):1239–45.

[306] Muslimovic D, Schmand BA. Course of cognitive decline in Parkinson's disease: a meta-analysis. *Journal of the ....* 2007.

[307] Hely MA, Reid W, Adena MA. The Sydney multicenter study of Parkinson's disease: the inevitability of dementia at 20 years. *Movement Disorders.* 2008;23(6):837–44.

[308] Buter TC, van den Hout A, Matthews FE, Larsen JP, Brayne C, Aarsland D. Dementia and survival in Parkinson disease: a 12-year population study. *Neurology.* 2008 Mar 25;70(13):1017–22.

[309] Halliday G, Hely M, Reid W, Morris J. The progression of pathology in longitudinally followed patients with Parkinson's disease. *Acta Neuropathologica.* 2008 Apr;115(4):409–15.

[310] Petrou M, Dwamena BA, Foerster BR, MacEachern MP, Bohnen NI, Müller ML, et al. Amyloid deposition in Parkinson's disease and cognitive impairment: A systematic review. *Movement Disorders.* 2015 Apr 16;30(7):928–35.

[311] Villa-Bonomo C, Pagonabarraga J, Martínez-Horta S, Fernandez de Bobadilla R, Garcia-Sanchez C, Campolongo A, et al. Short-lasting episodes of prosopagnosia in Parkinson's disease. *Parkinsonism and Related Disorders.* 2013 Mar;19(3):375–7.

[312] Pagonabarraga J, Kulisevsky J. Cognitive impairment and dementia in Parkinson's disease. *Neurobiology of Disease.* 2012 Jun;46(3):590–6.

[313] Kulisevsky J, Pagonabarraga J. Cognitive impairment in Parkinson's disease: Tools for diagnosis and assessment. *Movement Disorders.* 2009 Jun 15;24(8):1103–10.

[314] Kehagia AA, Barker RA, Robbins TW. Cognitive Impairment in Parkinson's Disease: The Dual Syndrome Hypothesis. *Neurodegenerative Dis.* 2013;11(2):79–92.

[315] Llebaria G, Pagonabarraga J, Martínez-Corral M, García-Sánchez C, Pascual-Sedano B, Gironell A, et al. Neuropsychological correlates of mild to severe hallucinations in Parkinson's disease. *Movement Disorders.* 2010 Oct 19;25(16):2785–91.

[316] Gratwicke J, Jahanshahi M, Foltynie T. Parkinson's disease dementia: a neural networks perspective. *Brain.* 2015 May 26;138(6):1454–76.

[317] Connolly B, Fox SH. Treatment of Cognitive, Psychiatric, and Affective Disorders Associated with Parkinson's Disease. *Neurotherapeutics.* 2013 Nov 28;11(1):78–91.

[318] Davidsdottir S, Cronin-Golomb A, Lee A. Visual and spatial symptoms in Parkinson's disease. *Vision Research.* 2005 May;45(10):1285–96.

[319] Nys GMS, Santens P, Vingerhoets G. Horizontal and vertical attentional orienting in Parkinson's disease. *Brain and Cognition*. 2010 Dec;74(3):179–85.

[320] Young DE, Wagenaar RC, Lin C-C, Chou Y-H, Davidsdottir S, Saltzman E, et al. Visuospatial perception and navigation in Parkinson's disease. *Vision Research*. 2010 Nov 23;50(23):2495–504.

[321] Laudate TM, Neargarder S, Cronin-Golomb A. Line bisection in Parkinson's disease: Investigation of contributions of visual field, retinal vision, and scanning patterns to visuospatial function. *Behavioral Neuroscience*. 2013;127(2):151–63.

[322] Lin C-C, Wagenaar RC, Young D, Saltzman EL, Ren X, Neargarder S, et al. Effects of Parkinson's disease on optic flow perception for heading direction during navigation. *Exp Brain Res*. 2014 Feb 11;232(4):1343–55.

[323] Barber J, Tomer R, Sroka H, Myslobodsky MS. Does unilateral dopamine deficit contribute to depression? *Psychiatry Research*. 1985 May;15(1):17–24.

[324] Gullett JM, Price CC, Nguyen P, Okun MS, Bauer RM, Bowers D. Reliability of Three Benton Judgment of Line Orientation Short Forms in Idiopathic Parkinson's Disease. *Clin Neuropsychol*. 2013 Oct;27(7):1167–78.

[325] Schendan HE, Amick MM, Cronin-Golomb A. Role of a lateralized parietal-basal ganglia circuit in hierarchical pattern perception: Evidence from Parkinson's disease. *Behavioral Neuroscience*. 2009;123(1):125–36.

[326] Cronin-Golomb A. Parkinson's Disease as a Disconnection Syndrome. *Neuropsychol Rev*. 2010 Apr 10;20(2):191–208.

[327] Amick MM, Schendan HE, Ganis G, Cronin-Golomb A. Frontostriatal circuits are necessary for visuomotor transformation: mental rotation in Parkinson's disease. *Neuropsychologia*. 2006;44(3):339–49.

[328] Lee A, Harris J. Problems with perception of space in Parkinson's disease: a questionnaire study. *Neuro-ophthalmology*. 1999;22(1):1–15.

[329] Hipp G, Diederich NJ, Pieria V, Vaillant M. Primary vision and facial emotion recognition in early Parkinson's disease. *Journal of the Neurological Sciences*. 2014 Mar 15;338(1-2):178–82.

[330] Uc EY, Rizzo M, Anderson SW, Qian S, Rodnitzky RL, Dawson JD. Visual dysfunction in Parkinson disease without dementia. *Neurology*. 2005 Dec 27;65(12):1907–13.

[331] Harris JP, Atkinson EA, Lee AC, Nithi K, Fowler MS. Hemispace differences in the visual perception of size in left hemiParkinson's disease. *Neuropsychologia*. 2003 Jan 1;41(7):795–807.

[332] Lee AC, Harris JP, Atkinson EA, Fowler MS. Evidence from a line bisection task for visuospatial neglect in left hemiparkinson's disease. *Vision Research*. 2001 Sep;41(20):2677–86.

[333] Wright WG, Gurfinkel V, King L, Horak F. Parkinson's disease shows perceptuomotor asymmetry unrelated to motor symptoms. *Neuroscience* Letters. 2007 Apr;417(1):10–5.

[334] Norton DJ, Jaywant A, Gallart-Palau X, Cronin-Golomb A. Normal discrimination of spatial frequency and contrast across visual hemifields in left-onset Parkinson's disease: evidence against perceptual hemifield biases. *Vision Research*. 2015 Feb;107:94–100.

[335] Verreyt N, Nys GMS, Santens P, Vingerhoets G. Cognitive Differences Between Patients with Left-sided and Right-sided Parkinson's Disease. A Review. *Neuropsychol Rev*. 2011 Sep 29;21(4):405–24.

[336] Seichepine DR, Neargarder S, Davidsdottir S, Reynolds GO, Cronin-Golomb A. Side and type of initial motor symptom influences visuospatial functioning in Parkinson's disease. *J Parkinsons Dis.* 2015;5(1):75–83.

[337] Ebersbach G, Trottenberg T, Hättig H, Schelosky L, Schrag A, POEWE W. Directional bias of initial visual exploration. A symptom of neglect in Parkinson's disease. *Brain.* 1996 Feb;119 (Pt 1):79–87.

[338] Lee AC, Harris JP, Atkinson EA, Nithi K, Fowler MS. Dopamine and the representation of the upper visual field: evidence from vertical bisection errors in unilateral Parkinson's disease. *Neuropsychologia.* 2002 Jan 1;40(12):2023–9.

[339] Svenningsson P, Westman E, Ballard C, Aarsland D. Cognitive impairment in patients with Parkinson's disease: diagnosis, biomarkers, and treatment. *The Lancet Neurology.* 2012 Jul 11;11(8):697–707.

[340] Johnson DK, Galvin JE. Longitudinal changes in cognition in Parkinson's disease with and without dementia. *Dementia and Geriatric Cognitive Disorders.* 2011;31(2):98–108.

[341] Aarsland D, Andersen K, Larsen JP, Perry R, Wentzel-Larsen T, Lolk A, et al. The rate of cognitive decline in Parkinson disease. *Archives of Neurology.* 2004 Dec;61(12):1906–11.

[342] Bohnen NI, Koeppe RA, Minoshima S, Giordani B, Albin RL, Frey KA, et al. Cerebral glucose metabolic features of Parkinson disease and incident dementia: longitudinal study. *J Nucl Med.* 2011 Jun;52(6):848–55.

[343] Dalrymple-Alford JC, MacAskill MR, Nakas CT, Livingston L, Graham C, Crucian GP, et al. The MoCA: well-suited screen for cognitive impairment in Parkinson disease. *Neurology.* 2010 Nov 9;75(19):1717–25.

[344] Barton BR, Bernard B, Czernecki V, Goldman JG, Stebbins G, Dubois BB, et al. Comparison of the Movement Disorder Society Parkinson's disease dementia criteria with neuropsychological testing. *Movement Disorders.* 2014 May 13;29(10):1252–7.

[345] Palmqvist S, Hansson O, Minthon L, Londos E. Practical suggestions on how to differentiate dementia with Lewy bodies from Alzheimer's disease with common cognitive tests. *Int J Geriat Psychiatry.* 2009 Dec;24(12):1405–12.

[346] Hamilton JM, Salmon DP, Raman R, Hansen LA, Masliah E, Peavy GM, et al. Accounting for functional loss in Alzheimer's disease and dementia with Lewy bodies: Beyond cognition. *Alzheimer's and Dementia. Elsevier Ltd*; 2014 Mar 1;10(2):171–8.

[347] Hamilton JM, Landy KM, Salmon DP, Hansen LA, Masliah E, Galasko D. Early Visuospatial Deficits Predict the Occurrence of Visual Hallucinations in Autopsy-Confirmed Dementia With Lewy Bodies. *The American Journal of Geriatric Psychiatry.* 2012 Sep;20(9):773–81.

[348] Hamilton JM, Salmon DP, Galasko D, Raman R, Emond J, Hansen LA, et al. Visuospatial deficits predict rate of cognitive decline in autopsy-verified dementia with Lewy bodies. *Neuropsychology.* 2008;22(6):729–37.

[349] Goldman JG, Williams-Gray CH, Barker RA, Duda JE, Galvin JE. The spectrum of cognitive impairment in Lewy body diseases. Burn D, Weintraub D, Robbins T, editors. *Movement Disorders.* 2014 Apr 22;29(5):608–21.

[350] Heitz C, Noblet V, Cretin B, Philippi N, Kremer L, Stackfleth M, et al. Neural correlates of visual hallucinations in dementia with Lewy bodies. *Alzheimer's Research and Therapy.* 2015;7(1):6.

[351] Caffarra P, Gardini S, Dieci F, Copelli S, Maset L, Concari L, et al. The qualitative scoring MMSE pentagon test (QSPT): a new method for differentiating dementia with Lewy Body from Alzheimer's disease. *Behav Neurol*. 2013;27(2):213–20.

[352] Mitolo M, Salmon DP, Gardini S, Galasko D, Grossi E, Caffarra P. The new Qualitative Scoring MMSE Pentagon Test (QSPT) as a valid screening tool between autopsy-confirmed dementia with Lewy bodies and Alzheimer's disease. *Journal of Alzheimer's Disease*. 2014;39(4):823–32.

[353] Nasreddine ZS, Phillips NA, Bédirian V, Charbonneau S, Whitehead V, Collin I, et al. The Montreal Cognitive Assessment, MoCA: a brief screening tool for mild cognitive impairment. *Journal of the American Geriatrics Society*. 2005 Apr;53(4):695–9.

[354] Rossetti HC, Lacritz LH, Cullum CM, Weiner MF. Normative data for the Montreal Cognitive Assessment (MoCA) in a population-based sample. *Neurology*. 2011 Sep 26;77(13):1272–5.

[355] Ohta K, Takahashi K, Gotoh J, Yamaguchi K, Seki M, Nihei Y, et al. Screening for impaired cognitive domains in a large Parkinson"s disease population and its application to the diagnostic procedure for Parkinson"s disease dementia. *Dement Geriatr Cogn Dis Extra*. 2014 May;4(2):147–59.

[356] Tiraboschi P, Salmon DP, Hansen LA, Hofstetter RC, Thal LJ, Corey-Bloom J. What best differentiates Lewy body from Alzheimer's disease in early-stage dementia? *Brain*. 2006 Mar;129(Pt 3):729–35.

[357] Gnanalingham KK, Byrne EJ, Thornton A, Sambrook MA, Bannister P. Motor and cognitive function in Lewy body dementia: comparison with Alzheimer"s and Parkinson"s diseases. *Journal of Neurology, Neurosurgery and Psychiatry*. 1997 Mar;62(3):243–52.

[358] O'Brien JT, Ames D, McKeith IG, Chiu E. Dementia with Lewy Bodies. *CRC Press;* 2005.

[359] Ferman TJ, Smith GE, Boeve BF, Graff-Radford NR, Lucas JA, Knopman DS, et al. Neuropsychological differentiation of dementia with Lewy bodies from normal aging and Alzheimer's disease. *Clin Neuropsychol*. 2006 Dec;20(4):623–36.

[360] Misch MR, Mitchell S, Francis PL, Sherborn K, Meradje K, McNeely AA, et al. Differentiating between visual hallucination-free dementia with Lewy bodies and corticobasal syndrome on the basis of neuropsychology and perfusion single-photon emission computed tomography. *Alzheimer's Research and Therapy*. 2014;6(9):71.

[361] Ala TA, Hughes LF, Kyrouac GA, Ghobrial MW, Elble RJ. Pentagon copying is more impaired in dementia with Lewy bodies than in Alzheimer's disease. *Journal of Neurology, Neurosurgery and Psychiatry*. 2001 Apr;70(4):483–8.

[362] Cormack F, Aarsland D, Ballard C, Tovée MJ. Pentagon drawing and neuropsychological performance in Dementia with Lewy Bodies, Alzheimer's disease, Parkinson's disease and Parkinson's disease with dementia. *Int J Geriat Psychiatry*. 2004 Mar 30;19(4):371–7.

[363] Noe E, Marder K, Bell KL, Jacobs DM, Manly JJ, Stern Y. Comparison of dementia with Lewy bodies to Alzheimer"s disease and Parkinson"s disease with dementia. *Movement Disorders*. 2004;19(1):60–7.

[364] Mori E, Shimomura T, Fujimori M, Hirono N, Imamura T, Hashimoto M, et al. Visuoperceptual impairment in dementia with Lewy bodies. *Archives of Neurology*. 2000 Apr 1;57(4):489–93.

[365] Simard M, van Reekum R, Myran D. Visuospatial impairment in dementia with Lewy bodies and Alzheimer's disease: a process analysis approach. *Int J Geriat Psychiatry.* 2003;18(5):387–91.

[366] Mitrushina M. Handbook of Normative Data for Neuropsychological Assessment. *Oxford University Press;* 2005.

[367] Kantarci K, Lowe VJ, Boeve BF, Weigand SD, Senjem ML, Przybelski SA, et al. Multimodality imaging characteristics of dementia with Lewy bodies. *Neurobiology of Aging.* 2012 Sep 1;33(9):2091–105.

[368] Haak KV, Clatworthy P. Assessing visual dysfunction with fMRI. *Advances in Clinical Neuroscience and Rehabilitation.* 2011 Jul 6;:1–2.

[369] Firbank MJ, Lloyd J, O'Brien JT. The relationship between hallucinations and FDG-PET in dementia with Lewy bodies. *Brain Imaging and Behavior.* 2015 Aug 4.

[370] Ramirez-Ruiz B, JunquE C, Martí MJ, Valldeoriola F, Tolosa E. Cognitive changes in Parkinson's disease patients with visual hallucinations. *Dementia and Geriatric Cognitive Disorders.* 2007;23(5):281–8.

[371] Pereira JB, JunquE C, Martí MJ, Ramirez-Ruiz B, BargallO N, Tolosa E. Neuroanatomical substrate of visuospatial and visuoperceptual impairment in Parkinson's disease. *Movement Disorders.* 2009 Jun 15;24(8):1193–9.

[372] Mak E, Su L, Williams GB, O'Brien JT. Neuroimaging characteristics of dementia with Lewy bodies. *Alzheimer's Research and Therapy.* 2014;6(2):18.

[373] Taylor JP, Firbank MJ, He J, Barnett N, Pearce S, Livingstone A, et al. Visual cortex in dementia with Lewy bodies: magnetic resonance imaging study. *The British Journal of Psychiatry.* 2012 Jun 1;200(6):491–8.

[374] Erskine D, Taylor J-P, Firbank MJ, Patterson L, Onofrj M, O'Brien JT, et al. Changes to the lateral geniculate nucleus in Alzheimer's disease but not dementia with Lewy bodies. *Neuropathology and Applied Neurobiology.* 2015 Jul 1;:n/a–n/a.

[375] Katsuse O, Iseki E, Marui W, Kosaka K. Developmental stages of cortical Lewy bodies and their relation to axonal transport blockage in brains of patients with dementia with Lewy bodies. *Journal of the Neurological Sciences.* 2003 Jul;211(1-2):29–35.

[376] Yamamoto R, Iseki E, Murayama N, Minegishi M, Marui W, Togo T, et al. Investigation of Lewy pathology in the visual pathway of brains of dementia with Lewy bodies. *Journal of the Neurological Sciences.* 2006 Jul;246(1-2):95–101.

[377] Iseki E, Marui W, Yamamoto R, Togo T, Katsuse O, Kato M, et al. The nigro-striatal and nigro-amygdaloid pathways undergo different degeneration processes in brains of dementia with Lewy bodies. *Neuroscience Letters.* 2005 May;380(1-2):161–5.

[378] Yamamoto R, Iseki E, Murayama N, Minegishi M, Marui W, Togo T, et al. Correlation in Lewy pathology between the claustrum and visual areas in brains of dementia with Lewy bodies. *Neuroscience Letters.* 2007 Mar;415(3):219–24.

[379] Kenny ER, Blamire AM, Firbank MJ, O'Brien JT. Functional connectivity in cortical regions in dementia with Lewy bodies and Alzheimer's disease. *Brain.* 2012 Feb 17;135(2):569–81.

[380] Harding AJ, Broe GA, Halliday GM. Visual hallucinations in Lewy body disease relate to Lewy bodies in the temporal lobe. *Brain.* 2002;125:391–403.

[381] Onofrj M, Thomas A, D'Andreamatteo G, Iacono D, Luciano AL, Di Rollo A, et al. Incidence of RBD and hallucination in patients affected by Parkinson's disease: 8-year follow-up. *Neurol Sci.* 2002 Sep;23 Suppl 2:S91–4.

[382] Mukaetova-Ladinska EB, Andras A, Milne J, Abdel-All Z, Borr I, Jaros E, et al. Synaptic proteins and choline acetyltransferase loss in visual cortex in dementia with lewy bodies. *J Neuropathol Exp Neurol*. 2013 Jan;72(1):53–60.

[383] Rektorova I, Biundo R, Marecek R, Weis L, Aarsland D, Antonini A. Grey Matter Changes in Cognitively Impaired Parkinson's Disease Patients. Duda J, editor. *PLoS ONE*. 2014 Jan 21;9(1):e85595.

[384] Caproni S, Muti M, Di Renzo A, Principi M, Caputo N, Calabresi P, et al. Subclinical visuospatial impairment in Parkinson's disease: the role of basal ganglia and limbic system. *Frontiers in Neurology*. 2014 Aug 4;5:1–7.

[385] Tessitore A, Amboni M, Cirillo G, Corbo D, Picillo M, Russo A, et al. Regional Gray Matter Atrophy in Patients with Parkinson Disease and Freezing of Gait. *American Journal of Neuroradiology*. 2012 Oct 8;33(9):1804–9.

[386] Watson GS, Leverenz JB. Profile of Cognitive Impairment in Parkinson's Disease. *Brain Pathology*. 2010 May;20(3):640–5.

[387] Auning E, Kjærvik VK, Selnes P, Aarsland D, Haram A, Bjørnerud A, et al. White matter integrity and cognition in Parkinson's disease: a cross-sectional study. *BMJ Open*. 2014;4(1):e003976.

[388] Pizzi SD, Franciotti R, Tartaro A, Caulo M. Structural alteration of the dorsal visual network in DLB patients with visual hallucinations: a cortical thickness MRI study. *PLoS ONE*. 2014.

[389] Delli Pizzi S, Maruotti V, Taylor J-P, Franciotti R, Caulo M, Tartaro A, et al. Relevance of subcortical visual pathways disruption to visual symptoms in dementia with Lewy bodies. *CORTEX*. 2014 Oct;59:12–21.

[390] Crizzle AM, Classen S, Uc EY. Parkinson disease and driving: an evidence-based review. *Neurology*. 2012 Nov 13;79(20):2067–74.

[391] Grace J, Amick MM, D'Abreu A, Festa EK, Heindel WC, Ott BR. Neuropsychological deficits associated with driving performance in Parkinson"s and Alzheimer"s disease. *Journal of the International Neuropsychological Society*. 2005 Oct;11(6):766–75.

[392] Ranchet M, Paire-Ficout L, Uc EY, Bonnard A, Sornette D, Broussolle E. Impact of specific executive functions on driving performance in people with Parkinson's disease. *Movement Disorders*. 2013 Oct 1;28(14):1941–8.

[393] Devos H, Vandenberghe W, Tant M, Akinwuntan AE, De Weerdt W, Nieuwboer A, et al. Driving and off-road impairments underlying failure on road testing in Parkinson's disease. *Movement Disorders*. 2013 Oct 24;28(14):1949–56.

[394] Amick MM, Grace J, Ott BR. Visual and cognitive predictors of driving safety in Parkinson's disease patients. *Archives of Clinical Neuropsychology*. 2007 Nov;22(8):957–67.

[395] Savoiardo M, Grisoli M, Girotti F. Magnetic resonance imaging in CBD, related atypical parkinsonian disorders, and dementias. *Adv Neurol*. 2000;82:197–208.

[396] Kumar R, Bergeron C, Lang AE. Corticobasal Degeneration. In: Jankovic JJ, Tolosa E, editors. Parkinson's disease and movement disorders. *Philadelphia: Lippincott Williams and Wilkins;* 2002. pp. 185–98.

[397] Bak TH, Caine D, Hearn VC, Hodges JR. Visuospatial functions in atypical parkinsonian syndromes. *Journal of Neurology, Neurosurgery and Psychiatry*. 2006 Apr;77(4):454–6.

[398] Murray R, Neumann M, Forman MS, Farmer J, Massimo L, Rice A, et al. Cognitive and motor assessment in autopsy-proven corticobasal degeneration. *Neurology.* 2007 Apr 17;68(16):1274–83.
[399] Zhang Y, Tartaglia MC, Schuff N, Chiang GC, Ching C, Rosen HJ, et al. MRI signatures of brain macrostructural atrophy and microstructural degradation in frontotemporal lobar degeneration subtypes. *Journal of Alzheimer's Disease.* 2013;33(2):431–44.
[400] Peigneux P, Van der Linden M, Garraux G, Laureys S, Degueldre C, Aerts J, et al. Imaging a cognitive model of apraxia: The neural substrate of gesture-specific cognitive processes. *Human Brain Mapping.* 2004;21(3):119–42.
[401] Kertesz A, Martinez-Lage P, Davidson W, Munoz DG. The corticobasal degeneration syndrome overlaps progressive aphasia and frontotemporal dementia. *Neurology.* 2000 Nov 14;55(9):1368–75.
[402] O'Callaghan C, Bertoux M, Hornberger M. Beyond and below the cortex: the contribution of striatal dysfunction to cognition and behaviour in neurodegeneration. *Journal of Neurology, Neurosurgery and Psychiatry.* 2014 Mar 5;85(4):371–8.
[403] Ávila RT, de Paula JJ, Bicalho MA, Moraes EN, Nicolato R, Malloy-Diniz LF, et al. Working Memory and Cognitive Flexibility Mediates Visuoconstructional Abilities in Older Adults with Heterogeneous Cognitive Ability. *Journal of the International Neuropsychological Society.* 2015 May;21(5):392–8.
[404] Blair M, Kertesz A, McMonagle P, Davidson W, Bodi N. Quantitative and qualitative analyses of clock drawing in frontotemporal dementia and Alzheimer's disease. *Journal of the International Neuropsychological Society.* 2006 Mar;12(2):159–65.
[405] Moretti R, Torre P, Antonello RM, Cazzato G, Bava A, Manos PJ. Use of the ten-point clock test to compare executive functioning across 24 months in patients with subcortical vascular dementia. *Perceptual and Motor Skills.* 2005 Feb;100(1):207–16.
[406] Kitabayashi Y, Ueda H, Narumoto J, Nakamura K, Kita H, Fukui K. Qualitative analyses of clock drawings in Alzheimer's disease and vascular dementia. *Psychiatry Clin Neurosci.* 2001 Oct;55(5):485–91.
[407] Zilli EM, Heilman KM. Spatial neglect in a patient with logopenic progressive aphasia. *Neurocase.* 2015 May 26;:1–10.
[408] Chow TW, Hynan LS, Lipton AM. MMSE scores decline at a greater rate in frontotemporal degeneration than in AD. *Dementia and Geriatric Cognitive Disorders.* 2006;22(3):194–9.
[409] Perri RR, Monaco M, Fadda L, Caltagirone C, Carlesimo GA. Neuropsychological correlates of behavioral symptoms in Alzheimer's disease, frontal variant of frontotemporal, subcortical vascular, and lewy body dementias: a comparative study. *Journal of Alzheimer's Disease.* 2014;39(3):669–77.
[410] Paulsen JS, Smith MM, Long JD, the PREDICT HD investigators and coordinators of the Huntington Study Group. Cognitive decline in prodromal Huntington Disease: implications for clinical trials. *Journal of Neurology, Neurosurgery and Psychiatry.* 2013 Oct 9;84(11):1233–9.
[411] Finke K. Parameter-based assessment of spatial and non-spatial attentional deficits in Huntington's disease. *Brain.* 2006 May 1;129(5):1137–51.
[412] Papp KV, Kaplan RF, Snyder PJ. Biological markers of cognition in prodromal Huntington's disease: a review. *Brain and Cognition.* 2011 Nov;77(2):280–91.

[413] Pirogovsky E, Nicoll DR, Challener DM, Breen E, Gluhm S, Corey-Bloom J, et al. The Visual Spatial Learning Test: Differential impairment during the premanifest and manifest stages of Huntington's disease. *Journal of Neuropsychology.* 2013 Dec 11;9(1):77–86.

[414] Ho AK, Nestor PJ, Williams GB, Bradshaw JL. Pseudo-neglect in Huntington's disease correlates with decreased angular gyrus density. *Neuro Report.* 2004 Apr;15(6):1061–4.

[415] Ventura RE, Balcer LJ, Galetta SL. The neuro-ophthalmology of head trauma. *The Lancet Neurology.* 2014 Oct;13(10):1006–16.

[416] Padula WV, Nelson CA, Padula WV, Benabib R, Yilmaz T, Krevisky S. Modifying postural adaptation following a CVA through prismatic shift of visuo-spatial egocenter. *Brain Inj.* 2009 Jan;23(6):566–76.

[417] Padula WV, Munitz R, Magrun WM. Neuro-Visual Processing Rehabilitation. *Optometric Extension Program Foundation;* 2012.

[418] Padula WV, Argyris S. Post trauma vision syndrome and visual midline shift syndrome. *Neurorehabilitation.* 1996;6(3):165–71.

[419] Karnath H-O. Pusher Syndrome – a frequent but little-known disturbance of body orientation perception. *J Neurol.* 2007 Mar 25;254(4):415–24.

[420] Santos-Pontelli TEG, Pontes-Neto OM, Araujo DB de, Santos AC, Leite JP. Persistent pusher behavior after a stroke. *Clinics.* 2011;66(12):2169–71.

[421] Karnath H-O, Broetz D. Understanding and treating "pusher syndrome." *Phys Ther.* 2003.

[422] Armstrong RA. Neuropathological changes in striate and extrastriate visual cortex in variant Creutzfeldt-Jakob disease (vCJD). *Clin Ophthalmol.* 2007 Jun;1(2):119–25.

[423] del Barrio-Manso I, Toribio-García Á, Cordero-Coma M, Tuñón L, Baragaño E. Creutzfeldt - Jakob con debut oftalmológico: la variante Heidenhain. *Archivos de la Sociedad Española de Oftalmología.* 2010 Oct;85(10):341–4.

[424] Verma R, Junewar V, Sahu R. Creutzfeldt-Jakob disease presenting with visual symptoms: a case of the "Heidenhain variant." *BMJ Case Rep.* 2013 Jan 29;2013(jan29 1):bcr2012008006–6.

[425] Cooper SA. Isolated visual symptoms at onset in sporadic Creutzfeldt-Jakob disease: the clinical phenotype of the "Heidenhain variant." *British Journal of Ophthalmology.* 2005 Oct 1;89(10):1341–2.

[426] Prasad S, Lee EB, Woo JH, Alavi A, Galetta SL. MRI and Positron Emission Tomography Findings in Heidenhain Variant Creutzfeldt-Jakob Disease. *J Neuroophthalmol.* 2010 Sep;30(3):260–2.

[427] Jacobs DA, Lesser RL, Mourelatos Z, Galetta SL, Balcer LJ. The Heidenhain variant of Creutzfeldt-Jakob disease: clinical, pathologic, and neuroimaging findings. *J Neuroophthalmol.* 2001 Jun;21(2):99–102.

[428] Kropp S, Schulz-Schaeffer WJ, Finkenstaedt M, Riedemann C, Windl O, Steinhoff BJ, et al. The Heidenhain variant of Creutzfeldt-Jakob disease. *Archives of Neurology.* 1999 Jan;56(1):55–61.

[429] Gooriah R, Dafalla BEA, Tun S, Venugopalan TC, Lwin KK. Visual hallucinations: an unusual manifestation of sporadic Creutzfeldt–Jakob disease termed the "Heidenhain variant." *J Neurol.* 2014 Oct 7;261(11):2228–9.

[430] Armstrong RA. Creutzfeldt-Jakob disease and vision. *Clin Exp Optom.* 2006 Jan;89(1):3–9.

[431] Caselli RJ. Visual syndromes as the presenting feature of degenerative brain disease. *Seminars in Neurology*. 2000;20(1):139–44.

[432] Armstrong RA, Cairns NJ, Ironside JW, Lantos PL. Quantification of vacuolation ("spongiform change"), surviving neurones and prion protein deposition in eleven cases of variant Creutzfeldt-Jakob disease. *Neuropathology and Applied Neurobiology*. 2002 Apr;28(2):129–35.

[433] Fukui T, Lee E. Visuospatial Function is a Significant Contributor to Functional Status in Patients With Alzheimer's Disease. American *Journal of Alzheimer's Disease and Other Dementias*. 2009 Aug 4;24(4):313–21.

[434] Azouvi P, Olivier S, de Montety G, Samuel C, Louis-Dreyfus A, Tesio L. Behavioral assessment of unilateral neglect: study of the psychometric properties of the Catherine Bergego Scale. *YAPMR*. 2003 Jan;84(1):51–7.

[435] Bergego C, Azouvi P, Samuel C, Marchal F, Louis-Dreyfus A, Jokic C, et al. Validation d'une échelle d'évaluation fonctionnelle de l'"hémінégligence dans la vie quotidienne: l"échelle CB. *Annales de Réadaptation et de Médecine Physique*. 1995 Jan;38(4):183–9.

[436] Azouvi P, Samuel C, Louis-Dreyfus A, Bernati T, Bartolomeo P, Beis J-M, et al. Sensitivity of clinical and behavioural tests of spatial neglect after right hemisphere stroke. *J Neurol Neurosurg Psychiatry*. 2002;73:160–6.

[437] Chen P, Hreha K, Fortis P, Goedert KM, Barrett AM. Functional Assessment of Spatial Neglect: A Review of the Catherine Bergego Scale and an Introduction of the Kessler Foundation Neglect Assessment Process. *Topics in Stroke Rehabilitation*. 2012 Sep;19(5):423–35.

[438] van der Putten JJ, Hobart JC, Freeman JA, Thompson AJ. Measuring change in disability after inpatient rehabilitation: comparison of the responsiveness of the Barthel index and the Functional Independence Measure. *Journal of Neurology, Neurosurgery and Psychiatry*. 1999 Apr;66(4):480–4.

[439] Van der Stigchel S, Nijboer TCW. Introduction to the research topic novel insights in rehabilitation of neglect. *Frontiers in Human Neuroscience*. 2014;8:233.

[440] Trauzettel-Klosinski S. Rehabilitative techniques. *Handb Clin Neurol*. 2011;102:263–78.

[441] Cronin-Golomb A, Gilmore GC, Neargarder S, Morrison SR, Laudate TM. Enhanced stimulus strength improves visual cognition in aging and Alzheimer's disease. *CORTEX*. 2007 Oct;43(7):952–66.

[442] Kempler D. Neurocognitive Disorders in Aging. *SAGE*; 2005. 1st edition. 2004.

[443] Baldassarre A, Ramsey L, Hacker CL, Callejas A, Astafiev SV, Metcalf NV, et al. Large-scale changes in network interactions as a physiological signature of spatial neglect. *Brain*. 2014 Nov 19;137(12):3267–83.

[444] Tomer R. Attentional bias as trait: Correlations with novelty seeking. *Neuropsychologia*. 2008 May 15;46(7):2064–70.

[445] Tomer R, Slagter HA, Christian BT, Fox AS, King CR, Murali D, et al. Dopamine Asymmetries Predict Orienting Bias in Healthy Individuals. *Cereb Cortex*. 2013 Nov 14;23(12):2899–904.

[446] Carli M, Evenden JL, Robbins TW. Depletion of unilateral striatal dopamine impairs initiation of contralateral actions and not sensory attention. *Nature*. 1985 Feb;313(6004):679–82.

[447] Marshall JF, Gotthelf T. Sensory inattention in rats with 6-hydroxydopamine-induced degeneration of ascending dopaminergic neurons: apomorphine-induced reversal of deficits. *Experimental Neurology.* 1979 Aug;65(2):398–411.

[448] Ljungberg T, Ungerstedt U. Sensory inattention produced by 6-hydroxydopamine-induced degeneration of ascending dopamine neurons in the brain. *Experimental Neurology.* 1976 Dec;53(3):585–600.

[449] Gorgoraptis N, Mah Y-H, Machner B, Singh-Curry V, Malhotra P, Hadji-Michael M, et al. The effects of the dopamine agonist rotigotine on hemispatial neglect following stroke. *Brain.* 2012 Aug;135(Pt 8):2478–91.

[450] Geminiani G, Bottini G, Sterzi R. Dopaminergic stimulation in unilateral neglect. *Journal of Neurology, Neurosurgery and Psychiatry.* 1998 Sep;65(3):344–7.

[451] Brenneman MM, Hylin MJ, Corwin JV. The time-dependent and persistent effects of amphetamine treatment upon recovery from hemispatial neglect in rats. *Behavioural Brain Research.* 2015 Jul 21;293:153–61.

[452] Manabe Y, Ino T, Yamanaka K, Kosaka K. Increased dosage of donepezil for the management of behavioural and psychological symptoms of dementia in dementia with Lewy bodies. *Psychogeriatrics.* 2015 Jul 16.

[453] Russell C, Li K, Malhotra PA. Harnessing motivation to alleviate neglect. *Frontiers in Human Neuroscience.* 2013;7:230.

[454] Bagurdes LA, Mesulam MM, Gitelman DR, Weintraub S, Small DM. Modulation of the spatial attention network by incentives in healthy aging and mild cognitive impairment. *Neuropsychologia.* 2008 Oct;46(12):2943–8.

[455] Mesulam MM. A cortical network for directed attention and unilateral neglect. *Annals of Neurology.* 1981 Oct;10(4):309–25.

[456] Ishiai S, Sugishita M, Odajima N, Yaginuma M, Gono S, Kamaya T. Improvement of unilateral spatial neglect with numbering. *Neurology.* 1990 Sep;40(9):1395–8.

[457] Small DM. Monetary Incentives Enhance Processing in Brain Regions Mediating Top-down Control of Attention. *Cereb Cortex.* 2005 Mar 2;15(12):1855–65.

[458] Hübner R, Schlösser J. Monetary reward increases attentional effort in the flanker task. *Psychon Bull Rev.* 2010 Dec;17(6):821–6.

[459] Kiss M, Driver J, Eimer M. Reward priority of visual target singletons modulates event-related potential signatures of attentional selection. *Psychological Science.* 2009 Feb;20(2):245–51.

[460] Libera Della C, Perlato A, Chelazzi L. Dissociable Effects of Reward on Attentional Learning: From Passive Associations to Active Monitoring. Herzog MH, editor. *PLoS ONE.* 2011 Apr 29;6(4):e19460.

[461] Chen M-C, Tsai P-L, Huang Y-T, Lin K-C. Pleasant music improves visual attention in patients with unilateral neglect after stroke. *Brain Inj.* 2013 Jan;27(1):75–82.

[462] Domínguez-Borràs J, Armony JL, Maravita A, Driver J, Vuilleumier PO. Partial recovery of visual extinction by pavlovian conditioning in a patient with hemispatial neglect. *CORTEX.* 2013 Mar 1;49(3):891–8.

[463] Riestra AR, Barrett AM. Rehabilitation of spatial neglect. *Handb Clin Neurol.* 2013;110:347–55.

[464] Bowen A, Hazelton C, Pollock A, Lincoln NB. Cognitive rehabilitation for spatial neglect following stroke. *Cochrane database of systematic reviews (Online).* 2013;7:CD003586.

[465] Smania N, Fonte C, Picelli A, Gandolfi M, Varalta V. Effect of eye patching in rehabilitation of hemispatial neglect. *Frontiers in Human Neuroscience*. 2013;7:527.

[466] Nijboer TCW, Olthoff L, Van der Stigchel S, Visser-Meily JMA. Prism adaptation improves postural imbalance in neglect patients. *Neuro Report*. 2014 Jan;25:307–11.

[467] Rabuffetti M, Folegatti A, Spinazzola L, Ricci R, Ferrarin M, Berti A, et al. Long-lasting amelioration of walking trajectory in neglect after prismatic adaptation. *Frontiers in Human Neuroscience*. 2013;7:382.

[468] Barrett AM, Goedert KM, Basso JC. Prism adaptation for spatial neglect after stroke: translational practice gaps. Nature Reviews Neuroscience. *Nature Publishing Group;* 2012 Aug 28;:1–11.

[469] Keane S, Turner C, Sherrington C, Beard JR. Use of Fresnel Prism Glasses to Treat Stroke Patients With Hemispatial Neglect. *Archives of Physical Medicine and Rehabilitation*. 2006 Dec;87(12):1668–72.

[470] Frassinetti F, Angeli V, Meneghello F, Avanzi S, Làdavas E. Long-lasting amelioration of visuospatial neglect by prism adaptation. *Brain*. 2002 Mar;125(Pt 3):608–23.

[471] Rossi PW, Kheyfets S, Reding MJ. Fresnel prisms improve visual perception in stroke patients with homonymous hemianopia or unilateral visual neglect. *Neurology*. 1990 Oct;40(10):1597–9.

[472] Padula WV, Subramanian P, Spurling A, Jenness J. Risk of fall (RoF) intervention by affecting visual egocenter through gait analysis and yoked prisms. *Neurorehabilitation*. 2015 Oct 20;37(2):305–14.

[473] Cappa S, Sterzi R, Vallar G, Bisiach E. Remission of hemineglect and anosognosia during vestibular stimulation. *Neuropsychologia*. 1987;25(5):775–82.

[474] Vallar G, Bottini G, Rusconi ML, Sterzi R. Exploring somatosensory hemineglect by vestibular stimulation. *Brain*. 1993;116(1):71–86.

[475] Bottini G, Gandola M, Sedda A. Caloric vestibular stimulation: interaction between somatosensory system and vestibular apparatus. Frontiers in Integrative *Neuroscience*. 2013 Sep;7(66).

[476] Pizzamiglio L, Vallar G, Doricchi F. Gravitational inputs modulate visuospatial neglect. *Exp Brain Res*. 1997 Nov;117(2):341–5.

[477] Pitzalis S, Spinelli D, Vallar G, Di Russo F. Transcutaneous electrical nerve stimulation effects on neglect: a visual-evoked potential study. *Frontiers in Human Neuroscience*. 2013;7:111.

[478] Vallar G, Rusconi ML, Barozzi S, Bernardini B, Ovadia D, Papagno C, et al. Improvement of left visuo-spatial hemineglect by left-sided transcutaneous electrical stimulation. *Neuropsychologia*. 1995 Jan;33(1):73–82.

[479] Pérennou DA, Leblond C, Amblard B. Transcutaneous electric nerve stimulation reduces neglect-related postural instability after stroke. *Archives of Physical Medicine and Rehabilitation*. 2001 Apr;82(4):440–8.

[480] Guo Y, Shi X, Uchiyama H. A study on the rehabilitation of cognitive function and short-term memory in patients with Alzheimer's disease using transcutaneous electrical nerve stimulation. *Frontiers of Medical and Biological Engineering*. 2001;11(4).

[481] Scherder EJA, Bouma A. Effects of transcutaneous electrical nerve stimulation on memory and behavior in Alzheimer's disease may be stage-dependent. *Biological Psychiatry*. 1999 Mar;45(6):743–9.

[482] Vallar G, Guariglia C, Nico D, Pizzamiglio L. Motor deficits and optokinetic stimulation in patients with left hemineglect. *Neurology.* 1997 Nov;49(5):1364–70.
[483] Vallar G, Guariglia C, Magnotti L, Pizzamiglio L. Optokinetic stimulation affects both vertical and horizontal deficits of position sense in unilateral neglect. *CORTEX.* 1995;31(4).
[484] Sampanis DS, Riddoch J. Motor neglect and future directions for research. *Frontiers in Human Neuroscience.* 2013;7:110.
[485] Borghese NA, Bottini G, Sedda A. Videogame based neglect rehabilitation: a role for spatial remapping and multisensory integration? *Frontiers in Human Neuroscience.* 2013;7:116.
[486] Agosta S, Herpich F, Miceli G, Ferraro F, Battelli L. Contralesional rTMS relieves visual extinction in chronic stroke. *Neuropsychologia.* 2014 Sep;62:269–76.
[487] Kerkhoff G. Neurovisual rehabilitation: recent developments and future directions. *Journal of Neurology, Neurosurgery and Psychiatry.* 2000 Jun;68(6):691–706.
[488] Girkin CA, Miller NR. Central disorders of vision in humans. *Surv Ophthalmol.* 2001 Mar;45(5):379–405.

In: Progressive Cognitive Impairment …
Editor: Gediminas Peter Gliebus

ISBN: 978-1-63485-221-0

Chapter 9

INTRODUCTION TO COMBINED COGNITIVE AND MOVEMENT DISORDERS

Jill M. Farmer*, DO, MPH
Assistant Professor of Neurology
Director, Parkinson's Disease and Movement Disorder Program
Drexel Neurosciences Institute
Drexel University College of Medicine, Philadelphia, PA, US

ABSTRACT

This chapter will focus on the interplay of dopamine and how it functions in the roles of movement disorders and the cognitive symptoms of movement disorders. As Parkinson 's disease is the most common dopamine mediated movement disorder, the bulk of this chapter explores how deficiencies in dopamine alter neurochemistry and neuroanatomy and in turn alter motoric and cognitive planning, processing and function. In this neurochemical context, the chapter will define the terms of mild cognitive impairment in Parkinson's Disease, Parkinson's Disease Dementia and Impulse Control Disorders. The treatment for these disorders is borrowed from the realm of behavioral neurology which is extolled in other chapters of this book and will be mentioned but not highlighted. There will also be a brief discussion of movement disorders in Alzheimer's disease for comparison and completeness as well as hyperkinetic movement disorders such as Huntington's Disease and Tourette's syndrome to offer additional insight into the complex interplay of dopamine and cognition.

INTRODUCTION

When the scientific community thinks of cognitive disorders, acetylcholine is usually the prominent neurotransmitter that comes to mind. It is an important neurotransmitter, but not the only one that significantly impacts cognition. In this chapter we will look at the impact of dopamine on cognition and explore how the specialties devoted to cognition and movement

* Correspondence to: jill.farmer@drexelmed.edu.

disorders overlap. We will also expand the idea of what constitutes cognition and look at how dopamine impacts reward pathways and impulsivity which in turn impacts learning, abstraction and judgment. Cognition is a convoluted and complex concept and can easily trip up the most experienced clinicians. It is our hope by the end of this chapter you will have much more secure footing.

Parkinson's Disease, Dopamine Receptors and Cognition

The world's population is aging, acetylcholine and dopamine decrease with age and if everyone lived long enough, everyone would develop cognitive problems and Parkinson's disease. Our efforts to slow, halt or reverse these events are directly opposed to the natural biological process which is why successfully managing these symptoms has been so limited.

The recognition of cognitive problems in Parkinson's Disease (PD) have gained popularity over the past 30 years and cognitive problems are considered one of the most important symptoms and perhaps the greatest clinical unmet need [1]. Research is exploding from the basic neuroscience pathways to global epidemiologic impact. A recent study from the Parkinson's Progression Marker Initiative noted that at time of diagnosis over 30% of patient present with a cognitive concern [2]. This is important not just for quality of life, but also because other studies have indicated that even mild cognitive impairment can serve as a risk factor for developing Parkinson's Disease Dementia (PDD) and there are some estimates that as many as 90% of patients will develop PDD who have had PD for over 20 years [1].

The types of cognitive deficits seen in PD are different than those seen in Alzheimer's disease (AD). If one thinks of the motor deficits in PD, extrapolating that presentation to how cognitive deficits might manifest in PD is logical. There is bradyphrenia or slowed thinking, cognitive inflexibility or rigidity, perseveration or set shifting difficulties. The way levodopa can help bradykinesia, rigidity and gait stuttering to some extent; it can also impact the cognitive equivalents [1]. This is because not all areas of the basal ganglia respond to dopamine in the same way. The dorsal area which is the main target of the motor pathways is also the area most involved in episodic memory formation which is why this improves with dopaminergic medications. The ventral regions which are less effected by dopamine depletion actually show impairment in cognition with administration of dopaminergic medications [1].

Clinically this is why some patients feel "sharper" with dopaminergic medications while others feel "foggy" with the same medication. Dopamine agonists are a class of medication notorious for highlighting this non linear relationship between dopamine activity and cognition. Bromocriptine, one of the earliest D2 receptor agonists, was shown to improve cognition in patients with low baseline memory capacity but impair it in high performers. This "U" shaped curve is thought to be related to a receptor stimulation threshold [3]. D1 and D2 receptors are often taught as part of the motor pathways of the striatum (a collection of structures receiving input from the cortex, including the caudate, putamen and nucleus accumbens) but dopamine receptors are ubiquitous and are part of the cortex as well and play an important role in cognition. D2 receptor binding in the cortex signals the presence of reward based information and allows the prefrontal cortex to respond to this new information by updating working memory. D1 receptors are more selective in what information they allow to access working memory. D1 system acts as a stabilizer. When there is a hypodopaminergic state cognitive performance is impacted manifesting as impulsivity, poor multitasking and poor working memory. When there is a hyperdopaminergic state this may present with perseverative cognitive performance with reduced cognitive flexibility [3]. Predicting how patients will respond to medication may be based on their motor symptoms at presentation. For example a patient with significant slowness or motoric deficit likely has more involvement of the dorsal striatum which usually respond nicely to dopaminergic therapy and likewise memory impairments may respond as well, where are patients with less motoric deficits likely have more dopamine loss in the ventral striatum which has a less robust response to dopaminergic medications and predictably less cognitive improvement with these medications as well. So for a patient with less motor symptoms, clinical experience and practice may sway treating with a medication whose mechanism effects on the other neurotransmitters involved in cognition before using a dopaminergic medication as this strategy may provide a better clinical outcome and patient satisfaction.

Neurotransmitters: Dopamine, Acetylcholine, Seretonin

The motor symptoms of PD have been mapped to dopamine neuron loss in the dorsal area of the substantia nigra and are intimately related and intertwined with the direct and indirect pathways. The difficulty with comprehending the pathways is that they are not static but always in a state of flux and always interacting with other pathways of the brain, most notably the frontal loops which are equally intimately intertwined when trying to comprehend cognition. The summary in the table adapted from *Neurology Board Review* [4] below can provide a working roadmap.

Table 1.

Circuit	Cortical origin	Striatum	Output	Thalamic nucleus	Function
Motor	Primary motor, SMA, PMA, posterior parietal	Putamen	GPi, SNr	VL, VM, CM	Motor planning and execution
Dorsolateral/ Prefrontal	Dorsolateral/ Prefrontal	Dorsal Caudate	GPi	VA, DM	Behavior/ Executive Tasks
Orbitofrontal	Orbitofrontal	Ventral Caudate	GPi	VA, DM	Social Behavior
Limbic	Anterior Cingulate	Nucleus Accumbens	Ventral Pallidum	DM	Motivation

SMA = supplemental motor area, PMA = primary motor area, GPi = globuspallidusinterna, SNr = substantia nigra pars reticulate, VA = Ventral Anterior, VM = Ventral Medial, CM = Central Medial, DM = Dorsal Medial.

Navigating these pathways and loops is dizzying but it is understandable that medications that modulate dopamine and acetylcholine are the gold standard for management of cognitive problems in PD and PDD [1]. The three main midbrain regions that project send neurons to the basal ganglia, limbic regions and cortical regions also referred to as the nigrostriatal, mesolimbic and mesocortical systems [5]. The dopaminergic projections from the substantia nigra can be divided into vetrolateral projections, ventromedial and ventral tegmental projections. Histopathologic studies have shown that depletion of ventrolateral projections is independent of dementia in PD but medial and ventral tegmental area depletion are related to loss of presynaptic dopamine and decrease in density of post synaptic D1 receptors in the frontal cortex, caudate, nucleus accumbens and hippocampus. Essentially this means that loss of dopamine projections to the mesocortical and mesolimbic systems has a direct impact on cognition and impulsivity [6, 7]. Recalling the role of D1 receptors as selective gait keepers, if they are decreased, the stability of the system is impacted which impacts a patient's ability or multitask, impair recall and increase impulsivity.

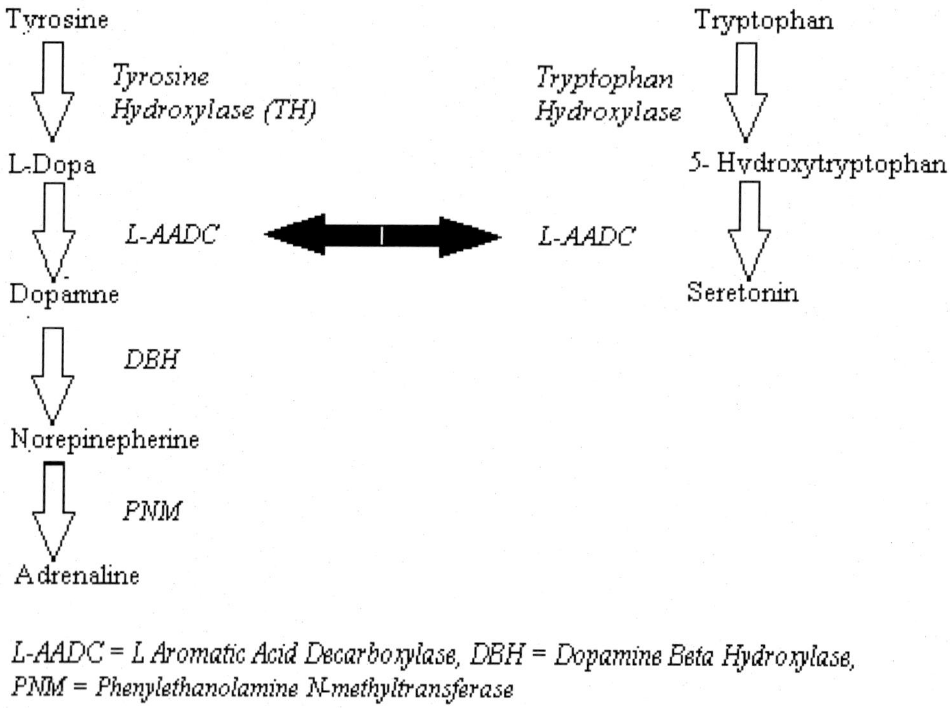

Figure 1.

It is important to discuss not only the interplay of dopamine and its depletion on cognition but also monoamine systems. Monoamines are the neurotransmitters derived from the amino acids tryptophan, tyrosine and phenylalanine and the derivates that this chapter will focus on are dopamine, epinephrine/adrenaline, norepinephrine/noradrenaline and serotonin. [See figure 1] There is a correlation between the loss of the medial and ventral tegmental dopaminergic loss as well loss of noradrenaline locus coerulus neurons and loss of cholinergic neurons in the nucleus basalis in PDD [9]. In early PD there is an up regulation of adrenaline, perhaps for compensation for dopamine depletion, but with a sharp decline with advancing disease. This is portrayed clinically with improvement in cognitive function later in the disease with a noradrenaline reuptake inhibitor such as atomoxetine. While noradrenaline is impacted through histologic studies – the same has not been shown for serotonin and yet clinically selective serotonin reuptake inhibitors (SSRI) are used far more commonly [10].

Lastly, there is a correlation between the loss of cortically projecting acetylcholine (Ch4 and Ch5) neurons. Ch4 nucleus basalis neurons project to the cortex and mesolimbic pathways while Ch5 neurons project from the pedunculopontine nucleus to the thalamus. The Ch4 projections have more impact of cognition and the reduction of cortical choline relates more to cognitive difficulties while the Ch5 neurons relate more to motor difficulties which is why cholinergic medications such as amantadine and trihexyphenidyl can have a positive impact on motor features but a negative impact on cognition [10]. Also, this is why new deep brain stimulation targets have experimented with the nucleus basalis and the pedunculopontine nucleus to impact both cognition and gait/motor function.

Parkinson's Disease Dementia and Mild Cognitive Impairment

While there is debate over the definitions of cognitive impairment and dementia in PD, there is no longer a debate to its role in all stages of PD. It used to be taught that cognitive problems were a late manifestation of PD and that the absence of cognitive problems usually ruled out atypical parkinsonism, such as multiple system atrophy or dementia with Lewy bodies. This is no longer the case and a recent study showed that 30% of newly diagnosed patients had a concern for their cognition at presentation. This is supported by prior works that report a prevalence of 19-38% with mild cognitive impairment (MCI) at time of diagnosis [11]. Also the Pre-motor phase of PD is becoming more appreciated as a valid clinical entity to clue clinicians into PD symptoms and that cognition is impacted in this stage manifesting in deficits in working memory, verbal fluency and attention [12]. Patients will describe this as slowed thinking, inability to multi-task, having words on the tip of their tongue and when under social stressors the recall process grinds to a halt.

To help get a better diagnostic handle of how to categorize these cognitive concerns a task force was assembled to propose diagnostic criteria for MCI in PD and PDD. See Table 2 adapted from Movement Disorder Society Task Force Guidelines for Diagnostic Criteria for MCI in PD [12] and Table 3 from Clinical Diagnostic Criteria for dementia associated with PD [13]. The criteria for both MCI and PDD are not far from similar criteria for MCI and AD in behavioral neurology. Most importantly is a diagnosis of PD provides the context for these cognitive changes in the absence of reversible or comorbid medical conditions and the deficits need to be appreciated in one or more cognitive domain (Attention, Executive function, visuo-spatial, memory and language). In PDD these deficits have to interfere with daily function and behavioral deficits are also appreciated such as apathy, changes in personality, hallucination, delusions and excessive daytime somnolence.

Important tools in establishing the diagnosis of PD-MCI and PDD are global assessment scales, whether they be abbreviated scales such as the Montreal Cognitive Assessment(MoCA) or formal neuropsychological testing. These scales look at the different domains of cognition and the most common area of cognition impacted when tested is executive function. Frontal dysfunction tests include tests of planning, spatial working memory and set shifting and problems with trail making, cube copying and clock drawing reveal dopaminergic dysfunction in the frontal striatal loops [14]. When examined, those with

PD describe a global cognitive deficit, but it is not that all areas of cognition are impacted, this may be more a result of the umbrella of executive dysfunction having impact on attention and memory as well. This is evident clinically by cueing. Cueing in PD disease suggests a problem of information retrieval rather than storage and is a phenomena that can improve memory and mobility [1]. There are a number of studies which look at the impact of cueing on gait freezing in PD. The exact mechanism is unknown but, "it is believed to be that during motor planning a timed external cue can trigger motor planning in the premotor cortex and this increased activation suppresses the pathologic activity in the subthalamic nucleus through direct pathways leading to motor facilitation." [15] Cueing can be valuable in "jogging" one's memory as well. If one looks at the 5 word recall task on the MoCA there are areas which allow for category or multiple choice clues. Clues are equivalent to cues and in patients with dopaminergic dysfunction, often these cues can facilitate recall of the word or phrase in question.

Table 2.

Clinical PD-MCI **Inclusion**
• Diagnosis of Parkinson's disease as based on the UK PD Brain Bank Criteria
• Gradual decline, in the context of established PD, in cognitive ability reported by patien, informant, *or* observed by the clinician
• Documented deficits by validated clinical scale or neuropsychological testing
• Cognitive deficits are not sufficient to interfere significantly with functional independence
Exclusion
• Preexisting established diagnosis of Dementia
• Comorbidexplanations for cognitive impairment that are not first addressed such as delirium, stroke, psychiatric disease, metabolic derangement
Specific guidelines for PD-MCI level I and level II categories
A. Level I (abbreviated assessment)
• Impairment on a scale of global cognitive abilities validated for use in PD
• Impairment on at least two tests, when a limited battery of neuropsychological tests is performed (i.e., the battery includes less than two tests within each of the five cognitive domains, or less than five cognitive domains are assessed)
B. Level II (comprehensive assessment)
• Neuropsychological testing involving two tests within each of the five cognitive domains
• Impairment on at least two neuropsychological tests, represented by either two impaired tests in one cognitive domain or one impaired test in two different cognitive domains
• Impairment on neuropsychological tests may be demonstrated by performance 1 to 2 SD below the mean or decline noted on serial testing

Risk Factors for Cognitive Impairment and Progression in Parkinson's Disease

Gaining a better understanding and appreciation of early cognitive impairment in PD is not only important for proper clinical diagnosis and treatment but also for patient prognosis because the inevitable question that is asked once a diagnosis of PD is given is, "will I develop Alzheimer's disease or dementia?" It is recognized from epidemiologic studies that in patients with PD for over 20 years, up to 90% may develop dementia, but does having MCI early on increase the risk? More fundamentally is there is there a reason some patients develop MCI and others do not? This is an active area of research. An ongoing longitudinal trial, the CamPaIGN (Cambridgeshire Parkinson's Incidence from GP to Neurologist) study recently reported a 10 year follow and cognitive measures of age greater than 72, semantic fluency of less than 20 words in 90 seconds and inability to copy intersecting pentagons were significant predictors for the development of dementia, whereas phonemic fluency and other frontally based tasks were not associated with dementia [16].

Table 3.

Probable PD-D	**Possible PD-D**
Core features: Both must be present Supportive clinical features: 1. Typical profile of cognitive deficits with impairment in at least two of the four core cognitive domains 2. The presence of at least one behavioral symptom (apathy, depressed or anxious mood, hallucinations, delusions, excessive daytime sleepiness) supports the diagnosis of Probable PD-D, lack of behavioral symptoms, however, does not exclude the diagnosis	Core features: Both must be present Associated clinical features 1. Atypical profile of cognitive impairment in one or more domains, such as prominent or receptive-type (fluent) aphasia, or pure storage-failure type amnesia (memory does not improve with cueing or in recognition tasks) with preserved attention 2. Behavioral symptoms may or may not be present
Core features 1. Diagnosis of Parkinson's disease according to Queen Square Brain Bank criteria 2. A dementia syndrome with insidious onset and slow progression, developing within the context of established Parkinson's disease and diagnosed by history, clinical, and neuropsychological examination, with Impairment in more than one cognitive domain, a decline from premorbid level and deficits severe enough to impair daily life.	

As far as inherent risks, as with all aspects of medicine, genetics and biomarkers in PD is also an active area of research. Thus far the chapter has highlighted the complexities of the neurotransmitters and the pathways they regulate and their symptomatic impact on motor and cognition. Replacing, degrading, blocking and mimicking the activity of these neurotransmitters has been the pharmacologic focus but research is looking at manipulating the genetic foundation of the synthesis of these transmitters to better understand the varied phenotype of PD and cognition. Research investigating the catabolism of dopamine in the cortex has found that it primarily happens through monoamine oxidase (MAO) on mitochondrial membranes and catechol-o-methyl transferase (COMT) in extrasynaptic spaces, though of the two COMT appears to be more significant in modulating fronto-striatal networks [3]. It has been discovered that COMT has a genotype resulting from a single nucleotide polymorphism swapping a valine (Val) with methionine (Met). The COMT-Val is the normal high functioning enzyme with retained ability to clear the cortex of extrasynaptic dopamine. The COMT-Met variant is unstable at body temperature and is far less effective [3].

The hypothesis of how small change impacts cognition again implicates the delicate D1 and D2 receptor balance. COMT-Val is efficient in removing the extrasynaptic dopamine from the frontal cortex shifting the balance to binding of the intrasynaptic D2 receptors which would result in decreased ability to maintain information in working memory whereas COMT-Met leads to decreased cognitive flexibility and recall because of excessive D1 stimulation since more dopamine is available extrasynaptically [3]. Should genetic testing in the future be available to determine which patients carry COMT-Val gene or COMT-Met gene we can better select cognitive medications. Studies have shown that patient with COMT-Val resulting in suboptimal D1 activation respond wonderfully to amphetamine stimulant medications. These medications block dopamine uptake and allow for more extrasynaptic dopamine and show an improvement in cognitive function where as COMT-Met have an adverse effect. Likewise antipsychotics which block dopamine receptors showed a better cognitive performance in COMT-Met individuals than COMT-Val individuals [3]. One might think that identifying this genetic mutation would serve as a biomarker of risk for developing dementia because of its strong association with cognitive impairment. The CamPaIGN study looked at the COMT genotype, and despite its well documented impact on dopamine metabolism and cognition, the genotype had no effect dementia risk [16]. This supports the idea that in one can have symptomatic cognitive impairment but not progress to dementia.

Other genetic testing has looked at the impact of tau in Lewy body diseases of the brain and the Microtubule Associated Protein (MAPT) H1/H1 genotype was an independent predictor of dementia. This supports that the dementing process in PD is related to tau while frontal-executive cognitive dysfunction is more related to dopamine with a better prognosis as those followed in the CamPaIGN study did not progress after almost 4 years [16]. The implication of tau is logical given its common association with alpha-synuclein, neurodegenerative diseases, but it is important to note that tau when associated with AD is not the H1 haplotype. These serum findings were confirmed by a recent CSF biomarker study which looked at the levels of amyloid and tau in the spinal fluid of PD patients which showed that after initiation of levodopa therapy patient with higher CSF hyperphosphorylated-tau/amyloid beta42 levels predicted subsequent cognitive decline on cognitive tasks [17]. Amyloid imaging studies have also been explored in PD as they have in the AD literature and findings suggest that amyloid beta may play a similar role. Amyloid's impact in PD may in fact even be greater since PD by pathology is synucleinopathy and amyloid and alpha-synuclein have a synergistic and magnifying effect together [18].

While genetic testing is still not standard of care when diagnosing PD, commercially available laboratory studies now have panels more readily available. The vast majority of PD cases are sporadic but it is worth noting that the most prevalent genetic mutation, leucine rich repeat kinase 2 (LRRK2) actually show lower rates of cognitive dysfunction and dementia whereas PARK1 and PARK4 and glucocerebrocidase (GBA) genes have shown an increased risk in developing dementia [19]. These associations, while appreciated to be associated with increased risk of developing dementia, again have little clinical impact as management with the medications currently available does not change.

A Side Step Worth Taking: Movement Disorders in Alzheimer's Disease

A discussion of cognition and movement disorders would be remiss if it did not mention the concepts of pyramidal and extrapyramidal symptoms. These terms are still often used despite the recognition that they are inadequate. As AD progresses, rigidity, slowness and gait impairment are commonly observed. These motor symptoms are classically described as "extrapyramidal." Extrapyramidal initially described the non-pyramidal descending pathways of the spinal cord (the pyramidal tracts are the corticospinal tract and corticobulbar tract) but its definition was expanded to currently encompass all subcortical pathways which impact automatic/involuntary motor control [20]. Attempts to identify an anatomic or physiologic separation of the pyramidal and extrapyramidal systems have failed but non the less the term is vestigial vocabulary that is still used and equated with parkinsonian features.

The presence of parkinsonism in patients with AD is well described and estimated to be on the order of 30-60% [21]. And of these symptoms rigidity, gait and slowing are most noted with resting tremor rarely observed. It is in the details of the description that the vocabulary is important and movement disorders is built on the shaky world of semantics. For example, use of the clinical terms spasticity and rigidity can be debated but when examining a stiff patient, the classic definitions are often blurred but the underlying pathology resulting in the increased tone is quite different. In PD the rigidity is often referred to as "lead pipe" and this is from disruption of subcortical pathways where as in AD the rigidity is more paratonic or "gegenhalten" and this is more from a cortical disruption. Gegenhalten, like spasticity, is speed dependent – the faster a limb is moved the more resistance will be felt. Lead pipe is independent of speed. Also the concept of "mitgehen"or when the patient assists the examiner and can't relax during the movement exam is also more consistent with cortical findings [20] Likewise when assessing gait, shuffling is present for both PD and AD. In PD the shuffling is related to hypokinesia and difficulty initiating movement whereas in AD shuffling is related to a cortical apraxia. Clinically, if a behavioral neurologist and a movement disorder specialists were observing an AD and PD patient walking side by side down a hallway it might be hard to tell the difference between them, but both clinicians would agree the patients should be using a walker! To help distinguish apraxic gait seen in AD from hypokinetic gait seen in PD, they should really be tested sitting in a chair. The apraxic patient is able to perform the act of walking while seated but when asked to stand and walk they cannot, whereas the hypokinetic patient has difficulty with lifting and tapping foot both seated and standing [20].

When parkinsonism is present in patients with AD, the patient should have an evaluation for apathy, as patients with AD and apathy had more parkinsonism than those without. There is a practical implication for recognizing AD patients with motor signs as those with motor signs have a more rapid rate of progression and a higher annual total cost of care [21]. The presence of bradykinesia is associated with an increased risk for functional decline, and the presence of gait and postural impairment was associated with an increased risk of institutionalization and death [22]. Another abnormal movement that happens more commonly in AD then PD is myoclonus. Myoclonus is also more associated with cortical dysfunction and electrodiagnostic studies can be used to confirm this origin [23].

Cognitive Dysfunction Is More than Memory: Impulsivity Disorders in PD

How good is your memory? Can you recall about 2000 words ago the discussion of the cortical loops? Remember that the loops were intimately dependent on dopamine as well as other neurotransmitters? As much as memory is impacted, impulsivity is also impacted by disruptions in these circuits. Functional connectivity in the brain is what maintains cognitive function and there have been many studies exploring this in AD, but the literature is far more limited in PD. In 2014 a longitudinal study was published and was unique in that it looked at whole brain resting state functional connectivity and followed PD patients over 3 years. It revealed that there is progressive loss of resting state connectivity over multiple brain regions which correlates strongly with decreasing global cognitive performance [24]. It did not look into specific pathways. In 2015 a similar study explored specific corticostriatal functional connectivity in patients with impulse control disorders and found an association with disconnection between the left anterior putamen, left inferior gyrus and left anterior cingulated gyrus [25]. This biological decrease in neural networks is an example of the increasing evidence that PD patients are at increased risk of developing one or more of the four major impulse control disorders (ICD's) and impulse control behaviors (ICB's) [26].

ICD's include pathologic gambling, buying, sexual and eating behaviors that are performed repetitively, excessively and compulsively to an extent that interferes with daily function [26]. ICB's include phenomena such as punding, hobbyism, walkabouts and hoarding. Exploring impulsivity in PD is like trying to answer the riddle, "which came first, the chicken or the egg?" Does having PD predispose patients to impulsivity or do patients become impulsive because of the medications used to treat PD? In the large DOMINION trial which looked at medicated patients, one or more ICD was identified in 13.6% of patients [27]. In one of the few prospective studies looking a patients without ICD at baseline when treated with dopamine agonist, 39% developed one over 2 years [26]. Understanding neuroanatomy and neurochemistry can help better explain why PD patients are so affected by these disorders.

Gambling is the most studied compulsive disorder and in the general population impulsive subjects show larger amphetamine-induced release of dopamine in the striatum, and in patients with pathologic gambling positron emission tomography (PET) studies have shown that when presented with any reward there is an increased dopamine release and reduction of dopamine transporter in the ventral striatum [29]. When dopamine is not rapidly cleared from the synapses of the striatum, it is considered "extrastriatal" and binds to D2/D3 receptors which may play a role in the pathogenesis of ICD's in PD patients as dopamine receptor abnormalities and reduction in transporter proteins have been implicated to predispose PD patients [29]. Again, PET studies have demonstrated that impulsive choices and risk taking in PD fire mainly in the ventral striatal, orbitofrontal and anterior cingulated and this activity is enhanced in patients taking dopamine agonists [30]. The connections of the ventral striatum and prefrontal cortex play critical roles in directing behavior toward rewards and reinforcement learning [28].

Executive function and working memory are also implicated with changes in the dorsolateral prefrontal cortex in patients with PD and comorbid ICD. In patients with both, whether "on" or 'off' medication, their ability to recall a digit span is reduced implicating an imbalance in the dopaminergic system due to elevated extrasynaptic dopaminergic levels [28]. Impulsivity and difficulty in the mentioned cognitive domains have been studied in newly diagnosed and not yet medically treated patients and abnormalities are appreciated in terms of choice impulsivity, reflection impulsivity (not utilizing available data before making a decision appropriately) and impairment of motor inhibition (No-Go/Stop-signal tasks). It is hypothesized that this is because of depletions in noradrenaline, serotonin and white matter changes in the prefrontal/striatal tracts [28].

The cortico-ventral basal ganglia circuit is the central network at assessing reward value and the rational decision making to direct behavior. This circuit includes the orbitofrontal cortex, anterior cingulated gyrus, ventral striatum (nucleus accumbens, caudate and putamen), ventral pallidum (output fibers to thalamus) and the midbrain dopamine neurons [31]. What has become more apparent as more research has been conducted on the neuroanatomical and neurochemical basis of behavior is that these are integrated pathways that do not run in parallel but can transfer input between components of the circuit and interface with pathways that mediate cognition and motor planning. When the cortical-nigro-striatal circuit is interrupted, information transfer for instrumental learning does not take place [31].

TREATING DISORDERS OF COGNITION IN PARKINSON'S DISEASE

The medications that are used to treat dementia of Alzheimer's type are borrowed by the movement disorder specialists to treat dementia in their patients, but there is only one FDA approved therapy for the treatment of PDD and that is the rivastigmine patch. The pivotal trial that was integral in gaining this approval looked at 410 patients meeting the clinical criteria for dementia in PD which were randomized to placebo or 3 to 12 mg of rivastigmine patch for 24 weeks and it was found that those t using the patch had a statistically significant improvement on the ADAS-cog primary endpoint [32]. There are currently no medications approved for the treatment of MCI in PD given it's unclear predictive value of progressing to dementia despite its impact on quality of life. A recent study looked at using rivastigmine patch in MCI for PD. 28 patients were enrolled in a 6 month randomized, placebo controlled trial with the Alzheimer's Disease Cooperative Study-Clinical Global Impression of Change scale as the primary measure with the MoCA, the Everyday Cognition Battery (ECB) and Parkinson's Disease Questioniare-8 (PDQ-8) as secondary outcomes. No effect was seen on any cognitive measures but, and perhaps more importantly, there was a significant improvement on ECB and PDQ-8 quality of life measures [33].

The management of ICD's also lack a magic bullet. The first step is to reduce the offending agent and lower or remove the dopamine agonist completely as they are usually the most culpable, but levodopa and MAO-B-inhibitors can also play a role and should be reduced when possible. There is no clear evidence to support the use of antidepressants of any class (tricyclic antidepressants, SSRI, serotonin norepinephrine reuptake inhibitors), anxiolytics and anticonvulsants to improve the symptoms of ICD's. There is also little evidence to support the use of atypical antipsychotics and dopamine blockade in reducing the symptoms of ICD and these medications can clearly worsen motor symptoms in PD. One area of research is looking at the opioid antagonist naltrexone 50mg to 100mg daily. A small study with 50 patients did not show a statistically significant change in the primary measure, it did show a significant reduction in the questionnaire for impulsive-compulsive disorders rating scale which supports further investigation [34].

It is important to mention in this section treatment of psychosis in PDD since it is this symptom that is most bothersome to patient and caregivers. Psychotic symptoms occur in up to 40% of patients with PD [35]. When behavioral modifications and redirection are no longer effective, currently patient, families and practitioners are stuck between two ineffective therapies – sedative medications and antipsychotics – and the known side effects they bring. Currently quetiapine used because it is felt that this will have the least motoric complications compared to other antipsychotics but its efficacy is lacking and three randomized studies it failed to show superiority over placebo [35]. Clozapine is efficacious and tolerated but caries a black box warning of agranulocytosis and prescribers must become part of a registry to prescribe it, hurdles which have impeded more wide spread clinical practice [36]. Clozapine and quetiapine's mechanism in PD psychosis set the stage for development of other drugs which looked to mechanisms besides dopamine modulation. In studying their mechanism of action it was discovered that their effectiveness was not so much their D2 receptor blockade but rather serotonin blockade. This finding has been further supported by research in which cortical 5HT2 receptors were stimulated resulting in hallucinations [35]. At the time of writing this chapter, pimavanserin, a drug with a novel mechanist just obtained FDA approval for treatment of psychosis in PD through serotonergic blockade instead of dopaminergic blockade which will alleviate the motoric side effects that come with antipsychotics. In a 6 week randomized phase III trial industry sponsored trial, 200 patients were randomized and those receiving pimavanserin showed a statistically significant decrease in the primary outcome measure of Schedule for Assessment of Positive Symptoms -PD [37]. It is anticipated that this drug will be available for clinical use in late 2016.

Hyperkinetic Disorders and Cognition

If one thinks of PD as difficulty with starting movement, then hyperkinetic disorders can be thought of as disorders with difficulty stopping movement. The most infamous of these disorders is Huntington's Disease, but other disorders such as Tourette's syndrome, Tics, Ataxia and Wilson's Disease, to name a few, all fall under this umbrella term and all have cognitive symptoms included in their clinical phenotype. Books have been dedicated to each of these disorders and they are recognized in this chapter so that their impact on cognition can be appreciated and propel those readers interested to seek out more detailed explanations in the references provided.

Huntington's Disease (HD) is an ungraceful spiral into motor and cognitive decline. HD is an autosomal dominant genetic disorder resulting in expansion of a trinucleotide, CAG, repeat on chromosome 4. With each generation this repeat length grows, ie: anticipates, which results in worsening symptoms in subsequent generations. As with the shift in the PD literature, there is an appreciation that non-motor symptoms such as cognitive symptoms can be detectable in patients with in 10 years of clinical diagnosis and that annual cognitive decline is a robust marker of disease progression [38, 39]. The anatomy which is impacted in Huntington's is the same area of the brain, the same circuits and pathways are impacted in PD, it again falls to the balance of neurotransmitters that cause such a different presentation.

If one appreciates that this is a disorder with difficulty stopping spontaneous movement then intuitively one thinks that the problem must lie in the neurotransmitters and areas of the brain that excite and that these somehow are functioning unchecked. The main inhibitory neurotransmitter of the brain is gamma-aminobutyric acid (GABA) and the main excitatory neurotransmitter of the brain is glutamate (GLU), The striatum, the collection of deep nuclei composed of the caudate and putamen, has neuronal connections which are dominated by GABA (inhibitory) transmission. These neurons are disproportionately affected in HD causing them to loose function and atrophy, resulting in the blunting of the caudate and shrinking of the cortical projections that is seen on magnetic resonance imaging (MRI) studies and which correlate to a reduction in the inhibition usually provided to keep the excitatory neurons of the cortex in check. This anatomical volume loss that is seen on MRI has been found to highly correlate with cognitive and behavioral symptoms and is being looked into as a predictive biomarker [39]. Without the balance of GABA, glutamate becomes more readily available to have an excitatory impact on the striatum which drives the direct and indirect pathways and also increases dopamine release. This influx of dopamine again shifts the balance of D1 and D2 receptors which again result in motor and cognitive derangements [38].

The cognitive deficits that are seen in early HD present in visuomotor integration, psychomotor and cognitive processing speed, executive function and emotional recognition (this should trigger thoughts of the frontal loops). Of these, the earliest presenting symptoms is usually the processing speed where routine mental tasks seem more "effortful" this observation is not without basis, the reason it takes longer to process is that alternate areas of the brain are being recruited for task completion [40]. More cortical domains that do not rely on subcortical inputs such as semantic memory, language comprehension, spatial awareness and orientation are usually well preserved [38]. The cognitive decline, as with those in other neurodegenerative diseases, are often the most burdensome for patient's and families' and are the greatest predictor of nursing home placement [40].

Another hyperkinetic disorder that emphasizes the interplay between motor and cognitive deficits is Tourette's Syndrome (TS). TS is more than vocal and motor tics and when acknowledging that cognition is more than memory, TS again highlights the recognition that non-motor cognitive changes, learning deficits, impulsivity, etc, can predate a motor symptom presentation and diagnosis. The pathophysiology of TS is unknown for both the cognitive and motor phenomena, but again dopaminergic systems are highly suspect. It is hypothesized and widely accepted that TS have defective inhibitory mechanism of the basal ganglia and functional MRI studies show decreased neuronal activity during periods of suppression in the ventral globus pallidus, putamen and thalamus and increased activity in the right caudate and frontal cortex and other cortical areas that are involved in impulse inhibition [41]. Dopamine Active Transporter (DAT) imaging in TS patients found increased DAT, D2 and D1 receptors suggesting a supradopaminergic response in the frontal lobes leading to impulsivity and poor mental flexibility through disruption of the dorsolateral prefrontal loop and the orbitofrontal loop [41].

Lastly a word on the cerebellum as this small structure is becoming more recognized for its role in movement and cognition as symptoms manifest in essential tremor, cerebellar type of multiple system atrophy (MSA-C) and genetic ataxias. Because MSA is on the spectrum of parkinsonism, and genetic ataxias such as spinal cerebellar ataxias, Friedreich's ataxia or fragile X syndrome have an association with degenerative diseases, considering cognitive impairment as one aspect of a complex clinical phenotype is not difficult. Thinking of cognitive changes as part of the presentation of Essential tremor (ET) however may be a novel idea. ET is the most common movement disorder and it is often confused with PD but historical teaching differentiated the two not only by the type of tremor (action vs. rest) but also the presence of neurodegeneration and non-motor symptoms completing the PD picture. This is no longer the case and ET is now considered a neurodegenerative condition with a constellation of non-motor symptoms, among which, cognition is a factor [42]. The pathophysiology of ET is still debated, but the role of the cerebellum has emerged as critical. MRI Imaging studies have shown microstructural abnormalities in the dentate nucleus and superior cerebellar peduncle and PET studies have shown over-activity on the cerebellar-rubral-thalamic-cortical connections corresponding to a tremor generator centered in the cerebellum [41]. As the appreciation of the cerebellum's impact on motor function became better understood and the pathways were more discretely mapped, more evidence began to emerge that there is a connection between the cerebellum and cortex. By comparing the topography of the dentatothalamic and thalamocortical projections, they deduced that the output channel from the cerebellum contains substantial projections to the cerebral association areas including those within the prefrontal cortex [43]. These connections lay the anatomical foundation for recognizing that ET does in fact present with cognitive changes and while there is not a discrete pattern of impairment that has emerged, global cognitive function and domains of attention, working memory, verbal fluency, set shifting, visuospatial function and naming all appear to be impacted [44].

Conclusion

The purpose of this chapter was to provide a more secure foundation of the impact of dopamine on cognition. This was by no means all inclusive and there are many movement disorders mentioned but not discussed in detail or some omitted completely which also have cognitive symptoms, such as Wilson's disease, acanthocytosis, spinal cerebellar ataxias, dystonias, and many more. Going forward, appreciating, and understanding the delicate choreography of dopamine, cognition, movement and memory has hopefully helped with the transition from a clumsy clinician to a graceful diagnostician.

References

[1] Robbins T, Cools R. Cognitive Deficits in Parkinson's Disease: A Cognitive Perspective. *Movement Disorders* 2014;30:597-607.

[2] De la Riva P, Smith K, Xie SX, et al. Course of psychiatric symptoms and global cognition in early Parkinson's disease. *Neurology* 2014; Epub 2014 Aug. 15.

[3] Savitz J, Solms M, Ramesar R. The molecular genetics of cognition: dopamine, COMT, and BDNF. *Genes, Brain and Behavior* 2006;5:311-328.

[4] Mowzoon N, Flemming K, editors. *Neurology Board Review An Illustrated Guide.* Mayo Clinic Scientific Press; 2007.

[5] Roeper J. Dissecting the diversity of midbrain dopamine neurons. *Trends Neuroscience* 2013;36:336-342.
[6] Ito K, Nagano-Saito A, Kato T, et al. Striatal and extrastriatal dysfunction in Parkinson's disease with dementia: a 6-[18F]flouro-L-Dopa PET Study. *Brain* 2002;125;1358-1365.
[7] Mattila PM, Roytta M, Lonnberg P, Marjamaki, et al. Choline acetyltransferase activity and striatal dopamine receptors in Parkinsons disease in relation to cognitive impairment. *ActaNeuropathol* 2001;102;160-166.
[8] Goridis C, Rohrer H. Specification of catecholaminergic and sertonergic neurons. *Nature Reviews Neuroscience:*3;531-541.
[9] Gaspar P, Gray F. Dementia in idiopathic Parkinson's disease. A neuropathological study of 32 cases. *ActaNeuropathol* 1984;64:43-52.
[10]Halliday G, Leverenz J, Schneider J, Adler C. *The Neurobiology of Cognitive Impairment in Parkinson's Disease.*
[11]Elgh E, Domellof M, Linder J, et al. Cognitive Function in early Parkinson's Disease: a population based study. *Eur J Neurol* 2009;16:1278-1284.
[12]Litvan I, Goldman JG, Troster A, et al. Diagnostic Criteria for mild cognitive impairment in Parkinson's disease: Movement Disorder Society Task Force guidelines. *MovDisord* 2012:27;349-356.
[13]13 Emre M, et al. Clinical Diagnostic Criteria for Dementia Associated with Parkinson's Disease. *Move Disord* 2012;27:1689-1707.
[14]Owen AM, James M, Leigh PN, et al. Fronto-striatal cognitive deficits at different stages of parkinson's disease. *Brain* 1992;115:1727-1751.
[15]Sarma S, Ming C, Eden U, et al. The effects of cues on neurons in the basal ganglia in Parkinson's disease. *Frontiers in integrative Neuroscience* 2012;6:40 1-12.
[16]Williams-Gray C, Evans J, Goris, A, et al. The distinct cognitive syndromes of Parkinson's Disease: 5 year follow-up of the CamPaIGN cohort. *Brain* 2009;132:2958-2969.
[17]Liu C, Cholerton B, Shi M, Ginghina C, et al. CSF tau and tau/AB42 predict cognitive decline in Parkinson's Disease. *Parkinsonsism and RelatDisord* 2015;3:271-276.
[18]Gomperts S, et al. Amyloid is linked to cognitive decline in patients with Parkinson's Disease without dementia. *Neurology* 2013;80:85-91.
[19]Romo-Gutierrez D, Yescas P, Lopez-Lopez M, et al. Genetic Factors associated with dementia in Parkinson's Disease. *GacetaMedica de Mexico* 2015;151:110-118.
[20]Kurlan R, Richard IH, Papka M, et al. Movement Disorders in Alzheimer's Disease: More Rigidity of Definitions Is Needed. *Move Disord* 2000;15(1):24-29.
[21]Starkstein S, Merello M. Movement Disorders In Alzheimer's Disease Scarmeas N, Albert M, et al. Motor signs predict poor outcomes in Alzheimer's Disease. *Neuology* 2005;64:1696-1703.
[22]Wilkins D, Hallet M, et al. Physiologic analysis of the myoclonus of Alzheimer's disease. *Neurology* 1984;34:898-904.
[23]Olde K, Schoonheim, Deijen J, et al. Functional connectivity and cognitive decline over 3 years in Parkinson Disease. *Neurology* 2014;83:2046-2053.
[24]Carriere N, Lopes R, et al. Impaired corticostriatal connectivity in impulse control disorders in Parkinson disease. *Neurology* 2015.
[25]Weintraub D, David A, Evans A, et al. Clinical Spectrum of Impulse Control Disorders in Parkinson's Disease. *Movement Disorders* 2015;30:121-127.

[26]Hassan A, Bower JH, et al. Dopamine Agonist Triggered Pathological Behaviors: Surveillance in the PD clinic reveals high frequencies. *Parkinsonism Related Disord* 2011;17:260-264.

[27]Napier T, Corvol J, Grace A, et al. Linking Neuroscience with Modern Concept of Impulse Control Disorders in Parkinson's Disease. *Movement Disorders* 2015;30:141-149.

[28]Vreind C, Nordbeck AH, et al. Reduced dopamine transporter binding predates impulse control disorders in Parkinson's disease. *Movement Disorders* 2014;29:904-911.

[29]Buckholtz JW, Treadway MT, et al. Dopaminergic network differences in human impulsivity. *Science* 2010;329:532.

[30]Haber S. Neuroanatomy of Reward: A View from the vetral striatum. In: Gottfried J, editor. *Neurobiology of Sensation and Reward.* Boca Raton(FL): CRC Press:2011. Chapter 11.

[31]Emre M, Aarsland D, Albanese A, et at. Rivastigmine for Dementia Associated with Parkinson's Disease. *The New England Journal Of Medicine* 2004;351:2509-18.

[32]Mamikonyan E, Xie S, Melvin E, Weintraub D. Rivastigmine for Mild Cognitive Impairment in Parkinson Disease: A Placebo Controlled Study. *Movement Disorders* 2015;30:912-918.

[33]Papay K, Xie SX, Stern M, et al. Naltrexone for impulse control disorders in Parkinson disease: a placebo-controlled study. *Neurology* 2014;83:826-833.

[34]Meltzer H, Mills R, Revell S, et al. Pimavanserin, a Serotonin 2A Recepter Inverse Agonist, for the Treatment of Parkinson's Disease Psychosis. *Neuropsycho-pharmacology* 2010;35:881-892.

[35]Weintraub D, Stern M. Psychiatric Complications in Parkinson's Disease. *American Journal Geriatric Psychiatry* 2005;13:844-851.

[36]Cummings J, Isaacson S, Mills R, et al. Pimavanserin for patients with Parkinson's disease psychosis: a randomized, placebo-controlled phase III trial. *The Lancet* 2013;DOI.

[37] Papoutsi M, Labuschagne I, et al. The Cognitive Burden in Huntington's Disease: Pathology, Phenotype, and Mechanisms of Compensation. *Movement Disoders* 2014;29:673-683.

[38]Paulsen JS, Long JD. Onset of Huntington's Disease: Can it be purely cognitive? *Movement Disorders* 2014;29:1342-50.

[39]Paulson JS. Cognitive Impairment in Huntington Disease: Diagnosis and Treatment. *Curr Neurol Neurosci Rep* 2011;11:474-483.

[40]Fahn S, Jankovich J, Hallet M. *Principles and Practice of Movement Disorders.* Saunders 2011.

[41]Jhunjhunwala K, Pal P. The Non-motor Features of Essential Tremor: A Primary Disease or Just Secondary Phenomenon? *Tremor and Other Hyperkinetic Movements* 2014;4.DOI.

[42]Buckner R. The Cerebellum and Cognitive Function: 25 Years of Insight from Anatomy and Neuroimaging. *Neuron* 2013;80:807-815.

[43]Walterfang M, van de Warrenburg B. Cognitive Impairment in "other" Movement disorders: Hidden Deficits and Valuable Clues. *Movement Disorders* 2014;29:694-703.

About the Editor

Gediminas Peter Gliebus, MD
Assistant Professor of Neurology
Drexel Neurosciences Institute / Drexel University College of Medicine
Philadelphia, PA, US

Dr. G. Peter Gliebus received his medical degree from Vilnius University in Vilnius, Lithuania. After completing the neurology residency at Drexel University College of Medicine in Philadelphia, PA, where he was named a chief resident, Dr. Gliebus completed the J. Rosentone Behavioral Neurology and Neuropsychiatry Fellowship at the Cognitive Neurology and Alzheimer's Disease Center in Northwestern University in Chicago, IL. Currently Dr. Gliebus is a faculty member at Drexel Neurosciences Institute of Drexel University, where he serves as a Co-Director of the Alzheimer's Disease and Cognitive Disorders program and is actively involved in clinical, educational and research activities.

INDEX

#

^{11}C-PIB-PET, 28, 29
^{123}I-2β-carbometoxy-3β-(4-iodophenyl)-*N*-(3-fluoropropyl) nortropane, 18, 30
^{123}I-2β-carbometoxy-3β-(4-iodophenyl)-*N*-(3-fluoropropyl) nortropane (^{123}I-FP-CIT), 30
^{123}I-FP-CIT, 18, 30, 31, 45
^{123}I-β-carbomethoxy-3ss-(4-iodophenyl) tropane SPECT, 28
^{123}I-β-carbomethoxy-3ss-(4-iodophenyl) tropane SPECT (^{123}I-β-CIT-SPECT), 28
^{123}I-β-CIT-SPECT, 28
^{18}F-FDG, 18, 28, 42
^{18}F-labelled fluorodeoxyglucose radiotracer, 28
^{18}F-labelled fluorodeoxyglucose radiotracer (^{18}F-FDG), 28
^{1}H-MRS, 18, 31
20th century, 109
3R, 2, 7, 8
3-repeat, 2, 6
3-repeat (3R), 2
4R, 2, 7, 8, 9
4-repeat, 2, 8, 14, 139
4-repeat (4R), 2
^{99m}Tc-ECD, 18, 30
^{99m}Tc-ethyl cysteinate dimer, 18, 30, 32
^{99m}Tc-ethyl cysteinate dimer (^{99m}Tc-ECD), 30, 32
^{99m}Tc-hexamethylpropyleneamineoxime, 18, 30
^{99m}Tc-hexamethylpropyleneamineoxime (^{99m}Tc-HMPAO), 30
^{99m}Tc-HMPAO, 18, 30

A

abstract thinking, 57, 59
abstraction, 58, 94, 262
abulia, 59, 60, 67, 71, 79, 97
Abulia, 71
abuse, 119
acanthocytosis, 274
ACC, 53, 54, 55, 59, 62, 96, 97, 99, 102, 103, 107, 108
access, 58, 132, 160, 161, 164, 168, 206, 207, 262
accessibility, 35
accounting, 105
acetylcholine, 30, 96, 146, 149, 261, 262, 263, 265
Acetylcholine Esterase Activity, 29
acetylcholinesterase, 44, 230
acetylcholinesterase inhibitor, 230
achromatopsia, 197, 199, 215, 219, 242
acid, 14, 273
acquisition, 27, 129, 131, 134, 147, 153, 194
action initiation, 69, 70, 71
Action Termination, 71
action-intentional disorders, 69, 73, 79
actuality, 86, 89
adaptation, 85, 145, 195, 217, 218, 231, 233, 256, 259
ADC, 18, 27
adenine, 95
adherence disorders, 73, 74
adrenaline, 264
adults, 2, 108, 122, 149, 152, 176, 194, 209, 210, 211, 216, 218, 223, 243, 245
advancements, ix
adynamic aphasia, 76
age, ix, 4, 6, 7, 14, 25, 66, 105, 109, 115, 134, 136, 138, 150, 161, 168, 176, 184, 194, 196, 205, 206, 210, 211, 216, 226, 231, 238, 243, 245, 262, 267
aggregation, 29, 136
aggression, 89
aging population, ix, 14
agnosia, 93, 165, 168, 199, 201, 202, 204, 206, 211, 213, 219, 235
agonist, 79, 230
agrammatism, 162, 165, 186

agranulocytosis, 272
AIDS, 62
akinesia, 71, 72, 73, 74, 76, 77, 78, 79, 83
Akinesia, 71, 83
Akinesia Paradoxica, 71
akinetic mutism, 59, 60, 79, 80, 82, 97
alcoholics, 140
alertness, 20, 96, 134
alexia, 163, 199, 219, 228
alexithymia, 102
algorithm, 4
allele, 18, 24, 179
ALS, 7, 16, 109, 115, 227
Alzheimer disease neuropathologic change, 2
Alzheimer Disease Neuropathologic Change, 2, 4
American Neurological Association, 185
American Psychological Association, 240
amine, 172
amino, 82, 264
amino acid, 82, 264
amino acids, 82, 264
amnesia, 123, 135, 139, 140, 141, 149, 151, 152, 197, 267
amphetamines, 230
amplitude, 149, 224
amygdala, 2, 3, 4, 7, 13, 22, 38, 76, 87, 89, 90, 91, 92, 93, 94, 96, 98, 99, 102, 103, 105, 107, 108, 118, 119, 120, 123, 125, 126, 130, 132, 139, 145, 146, 150, 153
Amygdala, 6, 89, 90, 93, 122, 130, 145, 153
Amygdala Predominant type, 6
amyloid beta, 49, 268
amyloid deposits, 4, 211
Amyloid PET, 28, 43, 176, 180, 181
Amyloid PET scan, 176
Amyloid precursor protein, 18, 34
Amyloid precursor protein (APP), 34
amyloid-beta (Aβ) plaques, 20
amyloid-beta plaques, 20
amyloidosis, 34, 138
amyotrophic lateral sclerosis, 7, 15, 109, 115
anatomy, x, 2, 45, 108, 119, 125, 147, 156, 170, 185, 186, 197, 272
ANC, 130
ancestors, 156
aneurysm, 97, 151
anger, 85, 88, 90, 93, 95, 98, 100, 101
anisotropy, 19, 27
anomic PPA, 163
anorexia, 140
anorexia nervosa, 140
anoxia, 196
anterior cingulate cortex, 32, 53, 54, 96, 98, 103, 107, 108, 114, 116, 120, 121, 123
anterior insula, 96, 99, 102, 103, 105, 120, 165
anterior limb of the internal capsule, 77
anterior temporal lobe, 93, 102, 115, 118, 124, 159, 161, 165, 172, 185
anterior temporal lobe (ATL), 159, 172
anterograde amnesia, 135, 151
Anterograde memory, 128, 132
anthropologists, 156
antibody, 10
antidepressants, 147, 271
anxiety, 85, 100
anxious mood, 267
APA, 240
apathy, 59, 60, 62, 63, 67, 71, 80, 97, 114, 116, 265, 267, 269
Apathy Evaluation Scale, 59, 72, 80
aphasia, 2, 6, 11, 14, 76, 81, 104, 115, 123, 155, 157, 161, 162, 163, 164, 165, 167, 169, 173, 179, 181, 182, 183, 184, 185, 186, 187, 188, 189, 190, 191, 202, 213, 226, 227, 235, 247, 255, 267
APP, 18, 179
appetite, 60, 99
appraisal, 86, 89, 91, 93, 99, 102, 103, 106, 107, 108, 114, 116
Appraisal, 89
appraisals, 89
apraxia, 74, 162, 165, 168, 169, 183, 191, 203, 213, 221, 226, 228, 255, 269
arcuate fasciculi, 77
arcuate fasciculus, 157, 158, 165, 184
Argyrophilic grain disease, 139, 151
arousal, 86, 88, 97, 120, 132, 134
ARS, 80
arteries, 139
artery, 97, 139, 151, 163
aspartate, 19, 31, 129
aspiration, 116
aspiration pneumonia, 116
assessment, 1, 2, 14, 47, 51, 56, 58, 59, 60, 61, 66, 91, 134, 149, 153, 165, 186, 194, 203, 206, 208, 209, 220, 224, 228, 247, 249, 255, 257, 265, 266
astrocytes, 8, 9, 115
astrocytic plaque, 9, 10, 115, 226
asymmetry, 117, 124, 156, 221, 226, 235, 250
asymptomatic, 136
ataxia, 144, 197, 203, 273
Ataxia, 202, 272
atherosclerosis, 1
ATL, 159, 160, 163, 171, 172, 176
atomoxetine, 79, 264

atrophy, 1, 3, 4, 5, 6, 8, 9, 10, 11, 12, 13, 14, 18, 19, 22, 23, 27, 32, 34, 37, 38, 39, 40, 41, 47, 48, 62, 63, 95, 110, 115, 120, 121, 124, 137, 142, 144, 146, 150, 163, 164, 165, 170, 171, 172, 173, 174, 175, 176, 188, 189, 203, 213, 216, 218, 219, 220, 221, 226, 227, 228, 235, 238, 239, 240, 241, 244, 246, 247, 248, 249, 255, 265, 273
attention deficit disorder, 94, 147
attentional disorder, 72, 79
attitudes, 106, 107
atypical FTLD-U, 6
Atypical Parkinsonian Disorders, 226, 246
auditory cortex, 104, 118
auditory stimuli, 128
autism, 102, 105, 233
autobiographical memory, 131
autoimmune disease, 104, 124
autonomic nervous system, 95, 98, 99, 121
autopsy, 1, 2, 23, 45, 106, 139, 173, 212, 224, 251, 252, 255
autosomal dominant, 272
avoidance, 20, 88
avoidance behavior, 88
awareness, 71, 103, 117, 120, 122, 194, 198, 202, 234, 273
Awareness, 70, 231
axons, 194
Aβ plaques, 22
$A\beta_{40}$, 2, 4, 18, 34, 35, 48
$A\beta_{42}$, 2, 4, 18, 34, 35, 48

B

Balint/Holmes Syndrome, 195, 196
basal forebrain, 89, 132, 138, 151
basal ganglia, 2, 3, 4, 9, 25, 33, 60, 76, 77, 78, 92, 95, 97, 101, 104, 107, 115, 121, 142, 165, 195, 201, 250, 254, 262, 263, 271, 273, 275
Basophilic Inclusion Body Disease, 6, 12
batteries, 59, 78
BEA, 256
Beck Depression Inventory, 119
behavior therapy, 147
behavioral assessment, 193
behavioral change, 171, 194
behavioral problems, 105
behavioral variant, 6, 68, 97, 99, 105, 109, 110, 115, 121, 123, 125, 161, 181
behavioral variant (bvFTD), 6, 109
behaviors, 71, 78, 88, 114, 116, 124, 165, 194, 197, 215, 228, 229, 270
Behavioural Variant Frontotemporal Dementia, 62
Behavioural Variant Frontotemporal Dementia (bvFTD), 62
Benton Judgment of Line Orientation, 205, 225, 236, 250
beta amyloid, 2, 212
bias, 96, 223, 227, 251, 257
bilateral, 2, 27, 28, 32, 33, 76, 77, 79, 100, 104, 110, 123, 124, 137, 139, 146, 151, 195, 202, 203, 214, 226
biochemistry, ix
biological systems, 88, 95, 135
biomarkers, x, 18, 21, 26, 30, 31, 32, 34, 35, 37, 48, 49, 136, 155, 170, 173, 174, 176, 177, 178, 179, 180, 181, 190, 213, 223, 251, 267
biopsy, 139
bipedal, 156
bleeding, 232
blindness, 93, 103, 194, 202, 228
blood, 19, 30, 31, 99, 138, 139, 140, 173, 224, 225
blood flow, 19, 31, 138, 140, 224, 225
blood oxygen level dependent, 31
blood oxygen level dependent (BOLD), 31
blood pressure, 99
blood supply, 139
Boas, 156
body weight, 99
BOLD, 18, 31, 32, 33, 122
bonding, 99
bone, 16, 69, 115
bones, 156
bottom-up, 89, 203, 226
bradycardia, 121
bradyphrenia, 262
brain, vii, ix, x, 1, 2, 3, 4, 14, 20, 22, 25, 27, 28, 30, 31, 32, 33, 34, 35, 37, 38, 39, 40, 44, 45, 46, 47, 48, 55, 56, 58, 60, 61, 62, 63, 64, 66, 70, 71, 76, 78, 82, 86, 89, 94, 96, 97, 98, 100, 102, 104, 106, 107, 109, 110, 116, 117, 118, 119, 120, 121, 122, 123, 124, 127, 128, 129, 130, 131, 132, 134, 136, 137, 138, 139, 140, 141, 142, 143, 144, 146, 150, 151, 156, 157, 170, 171, 172, 173, 174, 176, 177, 182, 184, 188, 189, 194, 195, 196, 197, 198, 200, 201, 205, 210, 211, 213, 214, 215, 218, 219, 226, 231, 232, 233, 235, 237, 241, 243, 247, 255, 257, 258, 263, 268, 270, 272, 273
brain activity, 64
brain damage, 66, 124, 140, 197, 201, 205
brain functions, ix, 134, 196
brain stem, 20, 232
brain structure, 89, 127, 196
brainstem, 1, 4, 5, 6, 8, 54, 92, 94, 96, 98, 99, 109, 138, 142, 196
breakdown, 30, 214, 241

breast cancer, 140
bromocriptine, 79, 82, 181, 191, 230
Bromocriptine, 82, 181, 262
building blocks, 195
bvFTD, 11, 60, 61, 62, 63, 64, 68, 97, 99, 104, 109, 110, 114, 115, 116, 146, 179, 181

C

CA1, 19, 20, 23, 25, 39, 129, 139, 140, 212, 239
CAA, 4, 19, 20, 29
cancellation task, 75, 81
cancer, 140
capsule, 77, 158, 159
cardiovascular disease, 33
cardiovascular diseases, 33
caregivers, 60, 101, 116, 229, 272
caries, 272
case study, 182, 191, 240
catabolism, 267
catechol-o-methyl transferase, 267
catechol-o-methyl transferase (COMT), 267
categorization, 6, 15, 58, 160
caudate, 2, 3, 6, 10, 13, 25, 30, 39, 40, 55, 94, 95, 104, 106, 115, 262, 264, 271, 273
causality, 96
CBD, 6, 7, 9, 10, 115, 139, 202, 220, 226, 227, 254
CBS, 115, 227, 229
C-C, 250
cell biology, 14
cell body, 24
cell death, 136, 137
cell surface, 140
central executive, 132
central nervous system, 92, 194
cerebellar disorders, 233
cerebellum, 1, 4, 13, 14, 115, 196, 232, 233, 273
cerebral akinetopsia, 198
cerebral amyloid angiopathy, 4, 20
cerebral amyloid angiopathy (CAA), 20
cerebral blood flow, 30, 77, 152, 172, 188
cerebral cortex, 8, 132
cerebral function, 27
cerebral hematoma, 151
cerebral hemisphere, 122, 149
cerebral hypoxia, 195, 196
cerebrospinal fluid, 21, 48, 49, 136, 150, 155, 170, 221
Cerebrospinal Fluid Biomarkers, v, 17, 177, 190
cerebrum, 1, 14
challenges, 165, 180
changing environment, 85
Chicago, 1, 155
chicken, 270
children, 79, 210, 233
chimpanzee, 67
choline, 30, 254, 265
cholinergic deficit, 20, 29
cholinergic medications, 265
cholinesterase, 181, 230
chorea, 68, 95
chromosome, 7, 11, 16, 95, 115, 138, 178, 190, 272
chronic traumatic encephalopathy, 7
Cingulate Island Sign, 28
circumlocutions, 163, 164
CIS, 19, 28
citalopram, 95
clarity, 86, 109, 213
classification, 10, 15, 127, 128, 132, 135, 186, 188
cleavage, 2, 34
clinical application, 45
clinical assessment, 60
Clinical Assessment of Prefrontal Functions, 55
clinical diagnosis, 2, 30, 34, 45, 164, 165, 166, 176, 194, 266, 272
clinical presentation, x, 6, 10, 63, 138, 142, 161, 172, 220
clinical symptoms, 20, 142
clinical syndrome, x, xi, 6, 93, 96, 109, 155, 164, 170, 197, 218
clinical trials, 17, 22, 24, 26, 33, 104, 177, 255
Clock Drawing Task, 206, 207, 223
clock drawing test, 58, 237
Clock Reading Test, 203, 229, 236
clock-drawing task, 203
closure, 210
clothing, 209
C-N, 243
CNS, 45, 120, 151
cocaine, 90, 118
codon, 179, 190
cognition, 33, 43, 47, 117, 142, 146, 162, 181, 194, 230, 231, 237, 239, 246, 251, 254, 255, 257, 261, 262, 263, 264, 265, 267, 268, 269, 271, 272, 273, 274
cognitive abilities, 266
cognitive ability, 266
cognitive deficit, 61, 146, 168, 213, 216, 227, 246, 262, 266, 267, 273, 275
cognitive deficits, 61, 146, 213, 216, 246, 262, 267, 273, 275
cognitive domains, vii, 20, 139, 142, 144, 145, 157, 161, 165, 196, 211, 213, 227, 252, 266, 267, 271
cognitive dysfunction, 109, 268
cognitive flexibility, 263, 268

cognitive function, vii, x, 52, 53, 54, 56, 60, 64, 143, 161, 195, 196, 204, 206, 216, 223, 227, 239, 252, 259, 264, 268, 270, 274
cognitive impairment, viii, x, 1, 5, 14, 15, 19, 25, 26, 29, 38, 40, 41, 42, 46, 47, 49, 62, 66, 67, 78, 82, 125, 127, 136, 137, 138, 139, 140, 142, 143, 144, 145, 146, 147, 150, 154, 164, 189, 206, 207, 212, 216, 217, 222, 237, 240, 241, 246, 249, 251, 252, 258, 261, 262, 265, 266, 267, 268, 274, 275
cognitive inflexibility, 262
cognitive map, 213, 216
cognitive performance, 137, 262, 268, 270
cognitive perspective, 106, 125
cognitive process, 52, 54, 97, 106, 194, 196, 217, 234, 255, 273
cognitive processing, 234, 273
cognitive profile, vii, x, 49, 142, 247
cognitive representations, 161
cognitive skills, 193, 208
cognitive system, 85
cognitive tasks, 56, 60, 232, 268
cognitive testing, 51, 64, 162, 229
coherence, 214
coiled bodies, 8, 9, 139
collaboration, 92
color, iv, 2, 77, 130, 198, 199, 201, 212, 215, 221, 223, 242, 243
commissure, 2, 3
common findings, 223
communication, 102, 122, 156, 180, 182, 183, 187, 215, 230
communication abilities, 180
community, 106, 150, 196, 216, 229, 245, 261
comparative analysis, 232
compensation, 214, 236, 264
competition, 96
complexity, vii, 89, 128, 167, 169, 197, 211, 217
complications, 272
compounds, 31
comprehension, 14, 71, 93, 101, 104, 106, 155, 157, 159, 160, 161, 162, 163, 164, 165, 166, 176, 185, 187, 273
compression, 202, 223
compulsive behavior, 114
computed tomography, 18, 19, 30, 32, 45, 137, 138, 150, 170, 252
computer, 61, 71, 183, 241
COMT, 267, 268, 274
conditioned stimulus, 94, 107
conditioning, 89, 118, 128, 258
configuration, 8, 241
conflict, 97
confrontation, 203
Congo, 4
Congress, iv
connectivity, 19, 27, 31, 33, 46, 52, 53, 54, 55, 82, 96, 98, 108, 120, 127, 129, 138, 143, 148, 149, 160, 173, 174, 185, 188, 189, 214, 232, 237, 241, 253, 270, 275
connectivity patterns, 54, 241
conscious awareness, 92, 96
conscious perception, 102
consciousness, 109, 119, 127, 131
consensus, 31, 162, 185
Consensus, 4, 15, 48, 189
consolidation, 96, 129, 131, 135, 145, 149
construction, 88, 134, 143, 160, 207, 222
context memory, 120, 153
Continental, 167
continuous perseveration, 75, 78
contour, 59
contrast sensitivity, 193, 215, 224, 242
control condition, 31
control group, 29
Controlled Oral Word Association Test, 76
convention, 110
convergence, 25, 172
Convergent fusion, 195
coordination, 95, 131, 203
cornu ammonis-1, 23
cornu ammonis-1 (CA1), 23
corona radiata, 77
corpus callosum, 6, 9, 27
correlation, 39, 104, 157, 207, 228, 264, 265
correlations, 40, 151, 157, 187, 226
cortex, 2, 3, 5, 7, 10, 11, 13, 19, 25, 27, 28, 39, 41, 46, 51, 53, 54, 55, 76, 77, 87, 92, 94, 95, 96, 97, 99, 100, 103, 104, 105, 106, 107, 111, 112, 113, 114, 115, 118, 119, 120, 121, 122, 123, 125, 129, 130, 131, 132, 136, 137, 139, 141, 146, 148, 149, 153, 157, 158, 159, 161, 165, 168, 172, 173, 177, 185, 191, 194, 199, 200, 211, 214, 216, 217, 221, 223, 224, 225, 228, 232, 242, 253, 254, 255, 256, 262, 265, 266, 267, 271, 273, 274
cortical neurons, 5, 121, 129, 142
cortical pathway, 91, 93, 248
corticobasal degeneration, viii, x, 7, 34, 78, 81, 97, 110, 115, 169, 255
Corticobasal degeneration, 9, 111
Corticobasal Degeneration, 6, 9, 78, 219, 254
corticobasal ganglionic degeneration, 226
Corticobasal Ganglionic Degeneration, 226
Cortico-Striato-Pallido-Thalamo-Cortical Loops, 53
cost, 269
cough, 221
coughing, 108

covering, 98
Cr, 19, 31, 150
cranial nerve, 100
craving, 90, 95, 118
creatine, 31
creatine (Cr), 31
creativity, 191
Creutzfeldt-Jakob disease, 6, 16, 228, 256, 257
Creutzfeldt-Jakob Disease, 13, 228, 256
criteria for the diagnosis of PPA, 162
cross-sectional study, 24, 254
cryopreservation, 1
CSF, 17, 19, 21, 22, 34, 35, 48, 49, 136, 137, 140, 144, 150, 170, 173, 176, 177, 178, 179, 180, 181, 190, 268, 275
CSF biomarkers, 18, 34, 49, 178, 190
CT scan, 170, 171
cues, 103, 104, 105, 122, 124, 182, 217, 230, 266, 275
current limit, 68
cytoplasm, 7, 10
cytosine, 95

D

D1, 79, 262, 264, 268, 273
D2 receptors, 262, 268, 273
daily living, 162, 180, 218, 219, 230
damages, iv, 164
Darwin, Charles, 101
database, 258
decay, 136
decision task, 210
declarative, 76, 127, 129, 132, 135, 136, 139, 141, 143, 146, 148, 149
declarative memory, 127, 129, 132, 135, 139, 143, 149
deep brain stimulation, 120, 265
default mode network, x, 31, 46, 47, 106, 131, 132, 241
default mode network (DMN), 32, 131
defective response inhibition, 69, 71, 73, 74, 75, 76, 77, 78, 79
defects, 66, 213, 221, 228
deficiencies, 57, 59, 64, 135, 142, 244, 261
deficiency, 136, 139, 146, 151, 215
deficit, 29, 56, 57, 74, 75, 94, 95, 106, 114, 119, 139, 147, 157, 159, 165, 168, 169, 184, 218, 220, 225, 227, 246, 250, 263
degenerate, 97
degenerative conditions, 127
degenerative dementia, 47, 213
degradation, 35, 255
delirium, 266
delusions, 32, 115, 194, 265, 267
dementia, vii, 2, 4, 6, 7, 11, 13, 14, 15, 16, 19, 20, 22, 23, 25, 26, 28, 29, 32, 33, 34, 36, 37, 38, 39, 40, 41, 42, 43, 44, 45, 46, 47, 48, 49, 60, 61, 62, 63, 64, 66, 67, 68, 78, 79, 82, 97, 99, 102, 105, 106, 109, 110, 114, 115, 116, 117, 119, 121, 123, 124, 125, 139, 142, 146, 148, 149, 150, 151, 152, 160, 161, 163, 164, 165, 176, 179, 181, 185, 188, 189, 190, 191, 193, 194, 195, 196, 198, 202, 203, 204, 207, 208, 210, 213, 215, 216, 217, 218, 220, 221, 222, 223, 227, 228, 229, 230, 231, 236, 237, 238, 240, 242, 243, 244, 245, 246, 247, 249, 250, 251, 252, 253, 254, 255, 258, 264, 265, 267, 268, 271, 275
dementia with Lewy bodies, 15, 20, 36, 37, 38, 39, 40, 41, 42, 44, 45, 46, 47, 48, 49, 139, 142, 152, 215, 230, 238, 251, 252, 253, 254, 258, 265
Dementia with Lewy Bodies, 5, 37, 39, 219, 224, 252
Demyelinating diseases, 78
dendrites, 5, 10
dentate gyrus, 2, 3, 7, 8, 11, 129, 139
deoxyribonucleic acid, 110
deoxyribose, 7
deposition, 14, 22, 23, 29, 42, 43, 63, 136, 138, 139, 149, 189, 228, 249, 257
deposits, 28, 104, 115, 136
depression, vii, 62, 85, 95, 115, 147, 180, 181, 206, 219, 250
depressive symptoms, 237
deprivation, 194
depth, ix, 109, 195, 196, 199, 203, 214, 218, 228
depth perception, 195, 218, 228
depth perception (stereopsis), 218
deregulation, 85
Design fluency, 58, 66
destruction, 140, 149
detectable, 213, 272
detection, ix, 1, 32, 170, 175, 217, 234, 236, 246
Diagnostic and Statistical Manual of Mental Disorders, 240
diagnostic criteria, 23, 38, 162, 185, 187, 265
diagnostic markers, 48
dichotomy, 89
dietary habits, 202
differential diagnosis, xi, 18, 21, 31, 33, 34, 35, 44, 45, 49, 127, 217
diffuse plaques, 4, 29
diffusion, 18, 27, 40, 41, 92, 138, 157, 185
Diffusion Tensor Imaging, 27, 157
Diffusion Tensor Imaging (DTI), 27, 157
diffusivities, 27

diffusivity, 19, 27
digestion, 99
Digit span, 57
dilation, 153
dinosaurs, 107, 108
diplopia, 228
direct, 30, 55, 77, 79, 91, 102, 105, 130, 136, 138, 145, 156, 166, 182, 191, 215, 229, 263, 264, 266, 271, 273
direct observation, 229
Directional Akinesia, 72
Directional impersistence, 75
disability, 80, 162, 185, 216, 224, 228, 257
discomfort, 108, 114
discordance, 109
discrimination, 116, 190, 203, 210, 212, 223, 244, 250
discrimination tasks, 212
disease gene, 247
disease progression, 18, 22, 26, 35, 38, 121, 174, 183, 212, 216, 221, 272
diseases, xi, 1, 5, 6, 13, 14, 43, 61, 64, 68, 69, 78, 85, 99, 101, 102, 104, 108, 116, 138, 139, 140, 142, 169, 177, 189, 224, 251, 252, 268, 273
disgust, 88, 99, 100, 105, 106, 114, 121
disorder, 5, 8, 9, 37, 69, 72, 73, 74, 75, 76, 77, 94, 95, 104, 108, 109, 119, 138, 139, 140, 142, 143, 145, 147, 162, 202, 219, 226, 261, 269, 270, 271, 272, 273, 274
Disorders of Emotional Regulation, 108
Disorders of Prefrontal Functions, 61
displacement, 27
dissociation, 118, 146, 148
distinctness, 55
distortions, 143, 233
distress, 100, 165
distribution, 13, 14, 15, 143, 172, 176, 177, 189, 213, 219, 248
diversity, 239, 275
DLPFC, 51, 53, 54, 55, 56, 57, 58, 59, 60, 62, 63, 64, 182
DMN, 19, 32, 33, 131, 136, 138, 141, 214
DNA, 6, 9, 10, 104, 110, 115
dogs, 107
DOI, 276
dominance, 100, 156, 157, 205
dopamine, 25, 30, 31, 44, 79, 82, 94, 95, 96, 119, 120, 142, 152, 224, 250, 257, 258, 261, 262, 263, 264, 267, 268, 270, 271, 272, 273, 274, 275, 276
dopamine agonist, 82, 120, 258, 270, 271
dopamine transporter, 25, 30, 44, 152, 270, 276
dopaminergic, 30, 44, 79, 82, 89, 94, 95, 101, 142, 147, 230, 258, 262, 263, 264, 265, 271, 272, 273
Dopaminergic Reward Pathway, 94
dorsal area of the substantia nigra, 263
Dorsal Language Pathway, 158
dorsal visual-stream, 198
dorsolateral prefrontal cortex, 51, 53, 54, 77, 97, 106, 107, 114, 132, 165, 174, 270
Dorsolateral Prefrontal Functions, 56
dosage, 258
DOT, 208, 238
double-pentagon copy, 207
Down syndrome, 233
down-regulation, 239
drainage, 144
drawing, 57, 58, 66, 75, 203, 204, 205, 207, 209, 221, 227, 237, 252, 255, 265
drug abuse, 94
drug discovery, 37
drugs, 17, 29, 35, 119, 147, 181, 272
DTI, 19, 27, 124
dual-route model, 161
durability, 176
dysarthria, 62, 162
dysfluent, 162, 164
dysgraphia, 163, 164, 219, 220, 221
dyslexia, 162, 163, 164, 169, 173, 189, 220, 248
dysphagia, 139
dysphoria, 88
dystonia, 226

E

Echopraxia, 74
ECTF, 207
edema, 1
editors, 64, 68, 184, 232, 236, 251, 254, 274
education, 66, 150, 168, 180, 183, 189, 238
EEG, 117, 175, 184
egg, 270
elaboration, 53
elderly population, 238
electric current, 147
electrodes, 94
Electroencephalography, 170, 175
Electroencephalography (EEG), 175
electromyography, 125
elephants, 63
elucidation, 27
emboli, 116
emergency, 144, 229
emission, 18, 19, 27, 30, 32, 42, 45, 138, 141, 150, 188, 252
emotion, 60, 76, 85, 86, 87, 88, 89, 90, 91, 92, 95, 96, 97, 98, 100, 101, 102, 103, 104, 105, 106,

108, 109, 116, 117, 118, 119, 120, 121, 123, 125, 126, 145, 148, 223, 250
emotion recognition, 86, 95, 96, 103, 104, 223, 250
Emotion Recognition, 102
emotion regulation, 86, 106, 125, 126
Emotion Type Hypothesis, 88
emotional and behavioural self-regulation, 54
emotional disorder, 116, 146
emotional enhancement of memories, 130, 145
emotional experience, 76, 85, 86, 90, 102, 107, 109
Emotional Expression, 100
emotional information, 102, 104
emotional or behavioural self-regulation, 51, 53
emotional processes, 54, 85
Emotional Processing, v, 85, 86, 88
emotional reactions, 86, 93, 98, 146
emotional reactivity, 86, 96, 97, 98, 99, 102, 116, 117, 121
Emotional Reactivity, 95, 97
Emotional Reappraisal, 107
emotional responses, 55, 97
emotional self-regulation, 53
emotional state, 61, 97, 100
emotional stimuli, 89, 91, 104, 145, 146, 153
Emotional Suppression, 108
emotional understanding, 86, 102, 103
emotional valence, 89
empathy, 61, 63, 64, 85, 105, 106, 114, 125
Empathy, 106, 123
EN, 63, 64, 190, 255
encephalitis, 93, 140, 151, 196, 202
encephalopathy, 7, 14, 93, 140, 202, 228
encoding, 32, 46, 62, 95, 96, 129, 130, 131, 133, 134, 135, 140, 141, 142, 143, 144, 145, 148, 149, 152, 187, 234, 245
endocrine, 69, 98
endocrine system, 98
endogenously evoked activities, 76
energization, 51, 53, 54, 55, 58, 59, 62, 64
energy, 88
England, 238
entorhinal cortex, 2, 3, 4, 6, 22, 25, 27, 39, 92, 93, 129, 130, 136, 137, 139, 145, 150, 164, 211
environment, 61, 69, 70, 74, 77, 89, 96, 129, 195, 203, 216, 217, 229, 236
environmental change, 95
environmental stimuli, 71
environments, 216
enzyme, 2, 49, 178, 267
enzymes, 2
EOG, 224
epidemiologic, 262, 267
epidemiologic studies, 267
epidemiology, 120
epidermoid cyst, 80
epinephrine, 264
episodic, 32, 128, 132, 135, 148, 149, 152, 153, 262
episodic memory, 32, 132, 135, 148, 149, 152, 153, 262
episodic memory tasks, 32
EPS, 224
equipment, 55
essential tremor, 273
Essential tremor, 274
Etiologic or State Biomarkers, 176
etiology, 25, 99, 101, 141, 162, 170, 218, 227
euphoria, 88
Europe, 15
event-related potential, 258
everyday life, 194, 229
evidence, 32, 34, 41, 46, 49, 54, 68, 72, 77, 81, 97, 104, 114, 117, 120, 125, 143, 146, 151, 153, 156, 160, 165, 170, 173, 175, 187, 189, 196, 199, 212, 213, 215, 218, 221, 222, 224, 230, 231, 233, 237, 242, 243, 247, 250, 251, 254, 270, 271, 274
evoked potential, 72, 224, 259
exclusion, 93
execution, x, 125, 159, 169, 196, 208, 263
Executive and Social Cognition Battery, 61
executive control network, 55
executive function, vii, 25, 40, 52, 53, 56, 57, 58, 63, 64, 76, 97, 107, 116, 134, 143, 165, 206, 213, 222, 226, 227, 254, 255, 265, 273
executive functioning, 116, 143, 213, 255
executive functions, 25, 52, 53, 57, 76, 107, 134, 165, 254
Executive Interview, 59
exercise, 204
exertion, 82
EXIT-25, 59, 67
explicit, 104, 107, 127
explicit memory, 127
exposure, 107, 108, 128, 147
expressivity, 101
extinction, 73, 81, 107, 227, 231, 246, 258, 260
extinction phase, 107
extraction, 37, 116
extrasylvian areas, 158, 161
eye fixations, 218
eye movement, 199, 203, 215, 234, 244

F

facial expression, 72, 100, 101, 104, 105, 106, 108, 122, 123, 124, 125
facial grasp, 74, 81

facial muscles, 103
factual knowledge, 132
false belief, 61
false belief tasks, 61
false positive, 56, 58
families, 183, 190, 272, 273
family history, 138, 162, 178, 179
family members, 163, 183
FAS, 58, 66, 168
FAS test, 58, 168
fatal sporadic insomnia, 13
FBI, 60
FC, 19, 32, 33, 94, 131, 153
FDA, 176, 271, 272
FDA approval, 272
FDG-PET Scan, 172
fear, 85, 88, 89, 90, 93, 94, 101, 107, 117, 118, 120
fear response, 90, 118, 120
feelings, 101, 106, 122, 123
fiber, 158, 159
fiber bundles, 158
fibers, 99, 100, 194, 200, 271
fight or flight, 97
figure-ground, 210, 225
filament, 7, 115
films, 96, 117
Finger Response Inhibition, 74
fixation, 1, 195, 196, 222
flame, 93
flatulence, 114
flawed perseveration, 75
flexibility, 273
flight, 88, 97
fluctuations, 20, 104, 222
Fluency, 66, 166, 168
fluid, 18, 19, 21, 25, 36, 49, 177, 190, 268
flying marks, 75
fMRI, 19, 31, 32, 33, 45, 46, 67, 105, 124, 149, 153, 157, 160, 173, 174, 182, 185, 214, 232, 233, 237, 241, 248, 253
food, 60, 94, 105
Food and Drug Administration, 176
force, 37, 70, 75, 78, 82, 108, 265
forebrain, 94, 95, 99
formation, 25, 34, 39, 45, 48, 81, 94, 99, 108, 122, 127, 128, 129, 132, 135, 141, 220, 262
FPs, 53, 55, 61, 64
fractional anisotropy, 27
free recall, 143, 152
freezing, 100, 121, 223, 266
frontal, 2, 3, 4, 6, 7, 9, 12, 20, 22, 27, 28, 29, 30, 33, 39, 47, 51, 52, 53, 54, 55, 56, 57, 58, 59, 60, 61, 62, 63, 64, 66, 67, 68, 76, 77, 78, 79, 81, 82, 92, 97, 101, 102, 103, 104, 105, 107, 109, 110, 112, 114, 115, 116, 117, 124, 125, 132, 134, 137, 143, 152, 153, 163, 168, 170, 171, 172, 173, 186, 196, 199, 202, 206, 209, 214, 215, 216, 226, 255, 263, 264, 265, 268, 273
Frontal Assessment Battery, 59, 67
Frontal Behavioral Inventory, 60
frontal cortex, 12, 62, 76, 103, 109, 112, 116, 124, 173, 264, 268, 273
frontal dysfunction, 60, 76, 226
frontal functions, 52
frontal lobe, 22, 39, 47, 51, 52, 53, 54, 56, 59, 61, 63, 64, 66, 67, 76, 77, 78, 79, 81, 82, 101, 102, 103, 109, 115, 125, 152, 153, 172, 214, 216, 273
Frontal Networks, 55
Frontal Polar Functions, 61
frontal pole, 52, 53, 55
frontal poles, 52, 53
frontal-subcortical, 53, 55, 60, 62, 76, 77, 134
Frontal-Subcortical Circuits, 54
fronto-subcortical dementia, 62
Frontotemporal dementia, 78, 146, 190, 227
Frontotemporal Dementia, 12, 65, 67, 68, 109, 110, 111, 112, 113, 115
Frontotemporal dementia (FTD), 78
frontotemporal lobar degeneration, 2, 7, 15, 16, 62, 124, 162, 217, 246, 255
Frontotemporal Lobar Degeneration, 6, 9, 11, 12, 194
frontotemporal lobar degenerations, 15, 162
frontotemporal lobar degenerations (FTLDs), 162
fruits, 163, 166
FTD, 6, 7, 8, 9, 16, 78, 81, 105, 109, 115, 178, 179, 181, 190, 227
FTLDs, 6, 178
functional activation, 241
functional architecture, 40, 118, 125
functional changes, 28, 138
functional connectivity, 31, 46, 82, 96, 108, 174, 214, 270
functional connectivity (FC), 31
functional imaging, 77, 105, 136, 141, 149, 159, 170, 172, 173, 174
Functional imaging, 77, 141, 146, 173
functional Magnetic Resonance Imaging, 157
Functional Magnetic Resonance Imaging, 31
functional Magnetic Resonance Imaging (fMRI), 157
Functional Magnetic Resonance Imaging (fMRI), 31
functional MRI, 18, 46, 47, 55, 125, 160, 173, 198, 214, 241, 273
FUS, 2, 6, 7, 12, 13, 110, 115
fused in sarcoma, 6, 7, 110, 115
fusion, 195

G

GABA, 273
gait, 25, 223, 228, 259, 262, 264, 265, 266, 269
Galantamine, 181
gambling, 270
ganglion, 194
gastrointestinal tract, 102
gender differences, 211
gene expression, 129, 211
genes, 62, 138, 239, 268
Genetic Biomarkers, 178
genetic mutations, 6, 7
genetic predisposition, 180
genetic testing, 268
genetics, 16, 267, 274
genotype, 43, 190, 267, 268
Gestalt, 197, 201, 207, 243
Gestalt psychology, 197
gestures, 100, 102
glasses, 201, 214, 230
glaucoma, 194
glia, 8, 10
globose tangles, 8, 115
Globular Glial Tauopathies, 6
globus, 2, 3, 8, 53, 54, 104, 273
glucose, 18, 28, 42, 138, 188, 224, 251
glutamate, 96, 119, 273
gnosis, 164, 201
go no-go paradigm, 74
goal-setting, 52
grades, 207
grading, 4, 237
Grammaticality, 166, 167
Graphemes, 156
Grasp Reflex, 73
gray matter, 8, 13, 14, 22, 43, 100, 111, 177, 219, 226
Greece, 156
grouping, 58
growth, 181
growth factor, 181
Grumose degeneration, 8
guanine, 95
guidance, vii, 202, 216, 231, 234
guidelines, 4, 14, 15, 37, 186, 208, 240, 266, 275

H

Habituation, 71
hair, 209, 229
half-life, 176
hallucinations, 20, 32, 115, 142, 194, 211, 222, 224, 225, 226, 228, 249, 251, 253, 254, 256, 267, 272
handedness, 162
handwriting, 221
happiness, 88
head injuries, 67
head injury, 135, 195
head trauma, 256
health, vii, x, 17, 20, 31, 122
health care, x
hearing loss, 105
heart rate, 97, 99, 100, 102, 103
Heidenhain variant, 219, 228, 256
hemianopsia, 199, 219
hemiparesis, 72, 227
hemiplegia, 72, 80
Hemispatial Neglect, 199, 259
hemisphere, 2, 73, 76, 77, 81, 104, 117, 169, 198, 199, 216, 231
hemorrhage, 139, 140
herpes, 93, 141
heterogeneity, 14, 17, 21, 29, 36, 186
hippocampal sclerosis, 2, 4, 138, 150, 151
hippocampus, 2, 3, 4, 5, 6, 7, 20, 22, 23, 27, 28, 31, 32, 38, 45, 87, 90, 92, 93, 96, 99, 129, 130, 131, 137, 139, 145, 148, 149, 150, 164, 189, 212, 216, 217, 219, 264
histology, 7
history, 32, 52, 59, 60, 61, 64, 100, 116, 145, 161, 172, 184, 196, 210, 212, 224, 267
HIV, 153
homeostasis, 76
homes, 229
Homonymous visual field disorders, 195
hormones, 99, 145
hub, 55, 103
human, 18, 48, 53, 60, 68, 70, 88, 103, 104, 105, 116, 117, 118, 119, 120, 122, 123, 124, 125, 136, 145, 147, 149, 150, 156, 181, 189, 193, 195, 198, 232, 242, 243, 244, 245, 246, 276
human animal, 60
human behavior, 193
human body, 105, 125
human brain, 18, 48, 68, 70, 116, 117, 118, 147, 149, 189, 198, 232, 245
human immunodeficiency virus, 145
hydrocephalus, 4, 144, 153
Hydrocephalus, 144, 190
hygiene, 114
hyperactivity, 119, 199
hyperkinesia, 81
Hyperkinetic Disorders, 272
hypokinesia, 72, 77, 78, 79, 80, 81, 205, 269

Hypokinesia, 72
hypoperfusion, 22, 30, 31, 32, 34, 38, 141, 142, 152, 226
hypotension, 47, 202
hypothalamic, 79, 82, 98, 99, 120, 121
hypothalamus, 22, 54, 76, 87, 92, 93, 95, 96, 98, 99, 130
Hypothalamus, 98
hypothesis, 29, 53, 80, 88, 198, 230, 231, 268
Hypoxic brain injury, 140

I

IBD, 115
ideal, 180
identification, x, 21, 103, 117, 170, 195, 208, 211, 220
identification problem, 211
identity, 86, 123, 220
idiopathic, 62, 140, 144, 153, 190, 211, 275
illumination, 166
image, 24, 93, 144, 170, 203, 235, 237
imagery, 235
images, 25, 26, 32, 36, 37, 89, 90, 98, 104, 108, 170, 172, 219, 247
Imaging biomarkers, 18
imaging modalities, 142, 143
imbalances, 227
imitation, 105, 125, 214, 233
immune reaction, 140
immunity, 211
immunohistochemistry, 7, 13
immunoreactivity, 151
impairments, x, 64, 69, 115, 124, 153, 168, 169, 187, 193, 194, 206, 215, 217, 219, 223, 224, 226, 228, 231, 245, 246, 254, 263
impersistence, 69, 71, 74, 77, 78, 79, 81, 82
implicit, 107, 126, 127, 128
implicit memory, 127
improvements, 30, 230
impulsive, 270, 272
impulsivity, 262, 264, 270, 271, 273, 276
Impulsivity Disorders, 270
in vivo, 27, 28, 41, 136, 189, 247
inattention, 71, 72, 199, 210, 218, 230, 232, 258
incidence, 95, 164, 179, 220
independence, 216, 230, 266
Independence, 257
India, 156
indirect measure, 27
indirect pathways, 263, 273
individuals, xi, 6, 25, 31, 79, 115, 122, 134, 136, 139, 150, 157, 161, 163, 167, 176, 177, 182, 184, 213, 216, 223, 227, 240, 244, 268
industry, 37, 272
inefficiency, 218
inertia, 63, 116
inevitability, 249
infarction, 79, 82, 139, 151, 202
inferior frontal gyrus, 77, 81, 105, 106, 157, 172
inferior parietal region, 32
inflammation, 178
information processing, 25, 40, 124, 215, 232
information processing speed, 25, 40
information retrieval, 266
infundibulum, 98
inhibition, 44, 54, 58, 69, 70, 71, 73, 74, 75, 76, 77, 78, 79, 81, 199, 231, 271, 273
inhibitor, 79, 181, 230, 264
initiation, 69, 70, 71, 78, 79, 218, 257, 268
Initiation, 70, 71
injure, 78
injuries, 53, 140, 143, 210
injury, iv, 2, 18, 27, 35, 61, 72, 82, 128, 132, 140, 143, 200
insomnia, 13
integration, 83, 90, 104, 196, 197, 208, 209, 211, 212, 219, 234, 260, 273
integrity, 18, 27, 30, 31, 33, 41, 133, 254
intelligence, 40
interface, 157, 158, 271
interference, 163, 187, 220
interpersonal relations, 101
interpersonal relationships, 101
intervention, 21, 141, 155, 174, 180, 181, 182, 183, 259
intonation, 187
intracranial pressure, 144
intrusions, 215
inversion, 19, 25, 26
inversion recovery, 19, 25, 26
Iowa, 239
ipsilateral, 72, 73, 100
Ireland, 247
iron, 106
irritability, 62, 119
ischemia, 140
isolation, 144, 201, 206, 220, 221
isomers, 2

J

Jakob-Creutzfeldt disease, 187
joints, 69, 70

Judgment of Line Orientation test, 203

K

Karl Wernicke, 157
Kinsey, 233
Kluver-Bucy Syndrome, 93
Klüver-Bucy syndrome, 118, 202
Korsakoff syndrome, 139

L

labeling, 160
laboratory studies, 268
laminar, 13
Language Disorders, v, 155, 187
language impairment, 161, 162, 163, 173, 186
language processing, 157, 163, 173
languages, 104
latency, 224
Late-onset hippocampal sclerosis, 138
lateral sclerosis, 109
laterality, 200, 226
lead, 20, 34, 62, 74, 78, 88, 90, 92, 96, 97, 99, 107, 114, 165, 198, 202, 203, 212, 219, 231, 269
leakage, 35
learning, vii, 53, 56, 57, 92, 94, 98, 120, 126, 127, 128, 129, 134, 149, 162, 185, 197, 211, 213, 216, 217, 233, 240, 245, 262, 271, 273
learning difficulties, 211
learning process, 128
learning task, 56, 134
left DLPFC, 51, 53, 57, 58, 174
left hemisphere, 2, 11, 76, 77, 81, 88, 101, 117, 130, 157, 169, 170, 172, 175, 176, 182
left visual field, 223
lens, 211, 218, 246
lesions, x, 2, 20, 25, 40, 43, 51, 56, 57, 58, 59, 61, 66, 72, 75, 76, 77, 79, 80, 81, 85, 89, 90, 96, 102, 103, 106, 109, 118, 119, 136, 139, 140, 141, 143, 144, 146, 148, 152, 153, 195, 196, 201, 208, 215, 216, 233
leucine, 268
Lewy bodies, 2, 19, 20, 21, 29, 35, 36, 37, 38, 42, 44, 45, 142, 152, 187, 196, 253
Lewy body, 2, 5, 6, 15, 17, 19, 20, 21, 38, 43, 44, 47, 78, 99, 138, 139, 142, 152, 169, 222, 232, 251, 252, 253, 268
Lewy Body Dementia, 78, 194
Lewy body disease, 2, 6, 43, 47, 99, 139, 152, 232, 251, 253, 268
Lewy Body Disease, 4, 5, 6
Lewy body spectrum disorders, 17, 19, 20, 142
Lewy Body spectrum disorders, 142
Lewy neurites, 5, 21, 142
Lexical/semantics, 156
Lichtheim, 157
life expectancy, ix
ligand, 44, 142, 176, 177, 178, 179
Ligand-Based PET Biomarkers, 176
light, ix, 33, 74, 193, 214, 248
Lille Apathy Rating Scale, 72
Limb Akinesia, 72
limb rigidity, 221
Limb-hand impersistence, 75
limbic encephalitis, 140
limbic system, 5, 6, 76, 77, 86, 89, 95, 129, 130, 132, 135, 136, 140, 141, 143, 149, 211, 254
Limbic System, 86, 119
Line bisection, 204, 232, 236, 250
line cancellation, 81, 204
Line extension task, 205
Line orientation task, 205
linguistic task, 173
linguistics, 156
localization, 33, 164, 165, 170, 172, 173, 195, 196, 215, 219
locus, 2, 3, 4, 5, 6, 8, 10, 100, 142, 264
locus coerulus, 264
logopenia, 165
Logopenic PPA, 164
Logopenic PPA (PPA-L), 164
longitudinal study, 223, 245, 251, 270
long-term memory, 23, 129, 132, 133, 148
long-term potentiation, 129
loss of consciousness, 143
lumbar puncture, 144
Luo, 189
Luria hand sequences, 57, 59

M

macular degeneration, 194
magnetic field, 147
magnetic fields, 147
magnetic resonance, 18, 19, 21, 26, 31, 38, 39, 40, 41, 45, 47, 124, 137, 138, 148, 151, 170, 232, 233, 241, 253, 273
magnetic resonance image, 21, 26
magnetic resonance imaging, 18, 19, 21, 31, 38, 39, 40, 41, 47, 124, 137, 138, 148, 151, 170, 232, 233, 241, 253, 273
magnetic resonance spectroscopy, 18, 31, 45
magnitude, 34, 199
majority, ix, 20, 56, 135, 136, 175, 268

malnutrition, 140
mammals, 194
management, vii, 15, 17, 20, 35, 36, 67, 120, 155, 177, 180, 183, 208, 231, 258, 263, 268, 271
Management of Progressive Aphasias, 180
manipulation, 62, 209, 226
MAO, 271
mapping, 44, 123, 159, 160
masking, 108
materials, 55, 56
matrix, 58
matter, iv, 8, 13, 19, 25, 26, 37, 40, 41, 62, 77, 78, 112, 143, 152, 189, 254
mean diffusivity, 27
mean length of utterance, 164, 167
measurement, 18, 36, 44, 117, 172, 173
measurements, 21, 105, 122, 172
Medial Prefrontal Functions, 59
medial temporal lobe, x, 18, 20, 23, 39, 45, 128, 129, 130, 131, 134, 136, 138, 151, 199, 202, 214, 216, 220, 241
Medial temporal tauopathy without amyloidosis, 138
median, 98
mediastinum, 19, 33
mediation, 89
medical, vii, 91, 106, 109, 144, 265
medication, 79, 146, 177, 222, 262, 270
medicine, vii, ix, 34, 35, 267
medulla, 2, 3, 6
melody, 101
Memantine, 181
membranes, 47, 267
memory, vii, x, 20, 23, 32, 33, 39, 40, 45, 46, 47, 57, 58, 62, 67, 68, 75, 90, 96, 97, 106, 108, 114, 115, 117, 120, 123, 127, 128, 129, 130, 131, 132, 133, 134, 135, 137, 139, 140, 141, 143, 144, 145, 146, 147, 148, 149, 150, 152, 153, 154, 157, 159, 164, 168,뗄182, 183, 188, 189, 194, 196, 206, 207, 209, 210, 211, 212, 213, 216, 217, 219, 221, 222, 223, 225, 226, 227, 232, 233, 235, 237, 238, 240, 241, 242, 245, 246, 248, 259, 262, 265, 266, 267, 268, 270, 273, 274
memory capacity, 147, 262
memory formation, 96, 127, 128, 129, 130, 132, 135, 141, 145
memory function, x, 39, 129, 130, 132, 134, 135, 143, 147, 152, 182
memory loss, 20, 211
memory performance, 146, 150, 246
memory retrieval, 96, 131, 148
meningitis, 202
mental image, 207, 237
mental imagery, 207, 237
mental model, 123
mental state, 61, 237
mental states, 61
mesial frontal, 76, 79
mesocortical systems, 263
mesolimbic, 94, 119, 120, 263, 265
meta-analysis, 23, 26, 35, 38, 40, 49, 122, 149, 185, 219, 232, 235, 249
Metabolic, 41
metabolic change, 223
metabolic changes, 223
metabolism, 18, 28, 42, 45, 110, 138, 140, 141, 143, 150, 172, 173, 188, 189, 224, 268
metabolites, 30, 31, 45
metacognition, 53
metacognitive functions, 52, 53
methylphenidate, 79
Mexico, 275
Miami, 190
microexpressions, 101
midbrain, 2, 3, 6, 13, 22, 76, 79, 100, 115, 195, 263, 271, 275
middle temporal gyrus, 158, 214, 219
mixing, 221
models, 53, 86, 88, 104, 105, 225
models of prefrontal function, 53
modifications, 166, 272
molecules, 27
monitoring, 22, 45, 51, 52, 53, 54, 55, 56, 57, 58, 59, 94, 97, 144, 216, 224
monoamine oxidase, 267
monoamine oxidase (MAO), 267
morphemes, 163, 169
Morphemes, 156
morphology, 10, 185
morphometric, 247
motion perception, 198, 218
motivation, 67, 97, 114, 126, 183, 258
motor actions, 57
motor activity, 94
motor behavior, 198, 199
motor control, 120, 269
Motor Extinction, 73
motor neuron disease, 11, 178
motor task, 33, 57, 70
motor tic, 273
movement disorders, x, 45, 102, 165, 196, 254, 261, 262, 269, 274
movement programs, 70
MP4A, 19, 44
MRI, 18, 19, 21, 22, 23, 25, 26, 31, 32, 33, 37, 38, 39, 40, 41, 43, 46, 47, 55, 100, 110, 125, 137, 138, 142, 144, 150, 152, 160, 170, 172, 173, 174,

175, 187, 188, 198, 214, 220, 221, 227, 237, 241, 247, 254, 255, 256, 273, 274
MRI scans, 170
multidimensional, 233
multiple sclerosis, 62, 67, 78, 108, 145, 153, 227
Multiple sclerosis, 145
multiple system atrophy, 5, 34, 47, 48, 265, 273
Multisystem Atrophy, 78
muscles, 69, 122
music, 183, 191, 258
music therapy, 191
mutant, 16
mutation, 6, 11, 178, 179, 268
mutations, 11, 12, 16, 62, 138, 177, 178, 179, 180, 190, 221
Myocardial Scintigraphy, 33
myoclonus, 221, 269, 275
myopathy, 16, 115
mythology, 91

N

N-[^{11}C]-methyl-4-piperidyl acetate, 19, 30
N-[^{11}C]-methyl-4-piperidyl acetate (MP4A), 30
NAA, 19, 31
N-acetyl aspartate, 19, 31
N-acetyl aspartate (NAA), 31
naming, 59, 103, 155, 157, 159, 163, 164, 165, 168, 174, 176, 181, 182, 187, 191, 206, 208, 210, 215, 235, 244, 274
Naom Chomsky, 156
NAP, 229
narratives, 187
National Academy of Sciences, 125
negative affectivity, 117
negative emotions, 117, 123, 124
negative experiences, 108
neglect, 72, 75, 77, 80, 121, 197, 199, 200, 201, 203, 204, 205, 210, 220, 223, 227, 229, 230, 231, 232, 235, 236, 250, 251, 255, 256, 257, 258, 259, 260
neocortex, 4, 6, 8, 9, 95, 119, 120, 149, 191, 212
neoplasm, 162
nerve, ix, 33, 105, 127, 137, 140, 172, 231, 259
nervous system, 89, 184
neural network, 85, 89, 107, 109, 129, 156, 183, 213, 234, 249, 270
neural networks, 85, 89, 107, 129, 234, 249, 270
neural system, 126
neural systems, 126
neuritic plaques, 3, 4, 29, 213, 219
neurobiology, 45, 121, 185
neurodegeneration, ix, 16, 29, 34, 62, 64, 109, 114, 116, 137, 138, 150, 178, 194, 212, 213, 217, 222, 246, 255, 274
neurodegenerative dementia, 20, 21, 27, 109, 193, 201, 230
neurodegenerative diseases, ix, 1, 33, 35, 61, 62, 85, 101, 106, 161, 164, 169, 194, 215, 228, 231, 239, 242, 246, 268, 273
neurodegenerative disorders, 139, 244
neurofibrillary tangles, x, 3, 9, 20, 136, 138, 212, 213, 219
Neurofibrillary tangles, 4, 19
neurofibrillary tangles (NFTs), 20
neuroimaging, 21, 27, 40, 55, 63, 68, 96, 106, 122, 155, 162, 170, 175, 183, 184, 185, 214, 218, 221, 222, 226, 232, 237, 241, 242, 245, 247, 256
neuroleptics, 142
neurological disease, 60, 78, 79, 80, 102, 105, 116
neurologist, 269
Neuromodulatory Intervention, 182
neuron response, 125
Neuronal Intermediate Filament Inclusion Disease, 6, 12
neurons, x, 4, 5, 7, 8, 9, 10, 33, 63, 68, 79, 95, 97, 99, 105, 114, 115, 119, 120, 121, 123, 129, 136, 139, 149, 151, 180, 196, 226, 258, 263, 264, 265, 271, 273, 275
neuropathologies, 34
neurophysiology, 243
neuropil threads, 8
neuropsychological tests, 55, 134, 194, 266
neuropsychology, 149, 184, 197, 233, 236, 237, 252
neuroscience, 85, 122, 197, 234, 235, 240, 245, 246, 248, 262
neurotransmission, 20
neurotransmitter, 20, 44, 76, 94, 261, 273
neurotransmitters, 95, 263, 264, 267, 270, 272
Neurotransmitters, 263
neurovisual impairment, 193
neutral, 86, 108, 128, 145, 204
neutral stimulus, 128
New England, 276
NFTs, 4, 19, 20, 34, 136, 137
nigrostriatal, 25, 263
NMDA receptors, 129, 146, 151
Nobel Prize, 196
nodes, 62, 159
nondeclarative, 127, 148
Nonfluent/Agrammatic PPA, 162
Nonfluent/Agrammatic PPA (PPA-G), 162
non-primary progressive aphasia, 161
non-primary progressive aphasia (nPPA), 161
norepinephrine, 33, 79, 96, 264, 271

norepinephrine agonists, 79
normal aging, 40, 224, 238, 242, 243, 252
normal pressure hydrocephalus, 62, 153, 190
Norman Geschwind, 157
North America, 191
novel stimuli, 132
novelty seeking, 257
nPPA, 164
nuclei, 6, 10, 29, 87, 92, 94, 96, 97, 98, 99, 129, 130, 136, 139, 232, 273
nucleic acid, 7
nucleus, 2, 3, 4, 6, 8, 9, 10, 13, 25, 39, 40, 46, 55, 60, 87, 91, 92, 93, 94, 95, 96, 98, 99, 102, 119, 120, 122, 130, 132, 136, 200, 253, 262, 263, 264, 265, 266, 271, 274
nucleus accumbens, 60, 87, 92, 94, 95, 99, 119, 130, 262, 264, 271
nucleus basalis, 2, 3, 4, 13, 92, 132, 264, 265
null, 88
null hypothesis, 88
nursing, 229, 273
nursing home, 229, 273

O

object alternation test, 60
Object/Picture Naming, 168
observational learning, 197
observed behavior, 105
obsessive-compulsive disorder, 94, 119
obstruction, 144
occipital cortex, 2, 3, 28, 93, 243
occipital hypometabolism, 22
occipital lobe, 4, 13, 22, 27, 45, 137, 142, 198, 207, 213, 224, 225, 226
occipital regions, 27, 32
occlusion, 139, 151
oculomotor, 195, 215, 226, 234
Oculomotor Function, 215
OFC, 53, 54, 55, 60, 61, 63, 64, 94, 99, 107, 207
Oklahoma, 85
oligodendrocytes, 9, 139
oligomers, 34, 48, 178
omentum, 181
Omentum transposition surgery, 181
Omentum transposition surgery (OT), 181
ophthalmologist, 201
optic chiasm, 98
optic nerve, 194
orbitofrontal, 54, 55, 60, 67, 76, 77, 82, 87, 92, 94, 106, 107, 114, 115, 130, 146, 153, 165, 214, 270, 271, 273
Orbitofrontal Functions, 60
orchestration, 109
organ, 96
organism, 89
organize, 92
organs, vii, 76
oscillatory activity, 233
OT, 181, 210
outpatient, vii
outpatients, 216
overlap, 105, 136, 142, 161, 222, 227, 262
overlay, 98
overproduction, 144
oxygen, 18, 31, 140, 173
oxyhemoglobin, 31

P

pacemaker, 170
pain, 90, 96, 100, 101, 102, 114, 118
pallor, 4, 5, 10
Panini, 156
Papez circuit, 129
parahippocampal gyrus, 22, 129, 219
parallel, 53, 74, 76, 86, 89, 109, 164, 169, 204, 234, 236, 271
paralysis, 197
parasympathetic nervous system, 89
parietal cortex, 131, 147, 158, 214, 218, 232, 242, 244
parietal lobe, 7, 22, 27, 28, 31, 77, 81, 106, 115, 137, 201, 202, 207, 212, 216, 220, 226, 231
parietal lobes, 7, 22, 27, 28, 77, 106, 115, 137, 207, 212, 216, 220, 226
Parkinson 's disease, 261
Parkinson Disease, 5, 254, 275, 276
Parkinson Disease Dementia, 5
parkinsonism, 8, 9, 20, 22, 82, 122, 226, 265, 269, 273
Parkinsons disease, 222, 230, 275
Parkinsons Disease, 222, 226
Parkinsons Disease Dementia, 222
partial seizure, 138
participants, 21, 48, 77, 206, 217
pathogenesis, 146, 270
pathologic diagnosis, 15, 238
pathological aging, 240
pathologist, 164, 166, 182
pathology, ix, x, 2, 4, 6, 8, 10, 14, 15, 20, 21, 22, 23, 29, 31, 34, 43, 48, 49, 62, 64, 67, 97, 99, 110, 121, 137, 138, 139, 141, 142, 143, 147, 149, 150, 156, 169, 170, 176, 177, 180, 181, 186, 189, 196, 211, 212, 213, 218, 221, 226, 227, 228, 231, 239, 247, 249, 253, 268, 269

pathophysiological, viii, 27, 47, 228
pathophysiology, 35, 69, 80, 138, 157, 165, 173, 181, 273, 274
pathway, 34, 62, 92, 93, 95, 97, 98, 99, 103, 104, 119, 129, 130, 158, 159, 160, 161, 163, 164, 165, 169, 186, 198, 199, 214, 216, 242, 253
pathways, 14, 34, 77, 78, 79, 85, 89, 92, 93, 94, 95, 99, 103, 104, 108, 109, 121, 132, 149, 155, 158, 161, 195, 200, 214, 226, 248, 253, 254, 262, 263, 265, 266, 267, 269, 270, 271, 272, 274
patient care, vii
Paul Broca, 157
PCA, 140, 195, 196, 203, 212, 213, 215, 218, 219, 220, 221, 226, 248
PCC, 19, 27, 28, 32, 33, 46, 174
Peabody Picture Vocabulary Test, 166
Peabody Picture Vocabulary Test (PPVT), 166
pedal, 53
Pentagon, 224, 252
peptidase, 178
peptide, 18, 34, 177
peptides, 2, 34, 43, 49
perceptual learning, 233
perceptual processing, 224
performers, 262
perfusion, 18, 32, 45, 48, 141, 187, 252
pergolide, 79
peripheral blood, 35
permission, iv, 11, 12, 128, 206
permit, 69, 91
perseverance, 70, 183
perseveration, 67, 69, 75, 76, 77, 78, 79, 81, 82, 202, 215, 262
Persistence, 70, 82, 123
personality, 60, 62, 123, 141, 265
PET, 19, 22, 27, 28, 29, 34, 41, 42, 43, 44, 58, 77, 110, 136, 138, 142, 149, 150, 151, 152, 155, 157, 172, 173, 175, 176, 177, 178, 179, 180, 181, 188, 189, 190, 221, 240, 253, 270, 274, 275
PET scan, 58, 138, 173, 176, 177, 178, 179
Pharmacological Interventions, 181
pharmacological treatment, 33, 176, 231
pharmacology, 276
pharmacotherapy, 230
phenotype, 16, 62, 155, 170, 179, 256, 267, 272, 274
phenotypes, 62, 162, 179, 194, 218
phenylalanine, 264
Philadelphia, vii, viii, ix, 127, 149, 186, 187, 254, 261
phonemes, 167
Phonemes, 156
phonemic paraphasias, 163, 164, 168
phosphorylated-tau, 21, 34
phosphorylated-tau (p-tau), 34
phosphorylation, 137, 177, 178
physicians, vii, ix, x, 48, 55, 78
physiology, 95, 117, 157, 173
physiopathology, 225
pia mater, 90
Pick Disease, 6
pitch, 101, 104
Pittsburgh compound-B, 18, 28
pituitary gland, 98, 99
placebo, 181, 230, 271, 272, 276
planum temporale, 159
plaque, 4, 9, 22, 29, 34, 43, 48, 177
plasticity, 129
Plato, 156
plausibility, 160
playing, 109, 130
pleasure, 89, 90, 94, 107, 118, 119
PM, 39, 45, 186, 189, 243, 275
PNFA, 11
polar, 139, 151
polymorphism, 267
pons, 2, 3, 6, 94, 100
poor performance, 207, 224
population, 40, 97, 140, 152, 186, 207, 248, 249, 252, 262, 270, 275
positron, 22, 38, 42, 43, 110, 136, 138, 141, 151, 155, 188, 270
positron emission tomography, 22, 38, 42, 43, 110, 136, 138, 141, 151, 155, 188, 270
Positron Emission Tomography, 27, 66, 114, 157, 172, 256
Positron Emission Tomography (PET), 27, 157, 172
posterior cingulate cortex, 27, 136, 223
posterior cortex, 218
posterior cortical atrophy, 164, 203, 213, 221, 228, 235, 238, 239, 240, 241, 244, 246, 247, 248, 249
Posterior Cortical Atrophy, 201, 213, 218, 219, 220, 221, 226, 228, 239, 247, 249
posterior insula, 92, 96, 102
PPA, 155, 160, 161, 162, 163, 164, 165, 166, 167, 168, 169, 170, 171, 172, 173, 174, 175, 176, 177, 179, 180, 181, 182, 183, 188, 191, 199
PPA+, 171, 180
PPA-G, 162, 163, 164, 165, 166, 167, 168, 169, 170, 171, 172, 173, 174, 176, 179, 181, 182
PPA-L, 164, 165, 166, 167, 168, 169, 170, 171, 172, 173, 174, 175, 176, 177, 182
PPAOS, 162
PPA-plus, 165
PPA-plus (PPA+), 165
PPA-S, 163, 164, 165, 166, 167, 168, 169, 170, 171, 172, 173, 176, 182

praxis, 62, 70, 102, 115, 164, 169, 213, 224, 227
precuneus, 28, 29, 32, 33, 136, 207, 220
prednisone, 181
prefrontal cortex, 32, 51, 53, 54, 63, 77, 92, 94, 95, 103, 106, 107, 121, 126, 130, 131, 141, 143, 262, 270, 274
prefrontal function, 51, 52, 55, 56, 64
prefrontal lobe functions, 52
preparation, iv, 100
preservation, 22, 23, 28, 108, 142, 206, 227, 228
prevention, 14
primary age-related tauopathy, 7
primary function, 108
primary progressive aphasia, 2, 6, 14, 104, 115, 123, 155, 161, 169, 185, 186, 187, 188, 189, 190, 191
primary progressive aphasia (PPA), 6, 155, 161, 185, 187
primary progressive apraxia of speech, 162
primary progressive apraxia of speech (PPAOS), 162
primary visual cortex, 212, 217, 222, 224, 225, 234, 246
primate, 119, 120, 122
priming, 117, 128
principles, 55, 133, 180, 194
Prion Disease, 13, 219
prions, 16
proactive interference, 148
probe, 55
procedural memory, 128
processing deficits, 212, 226
professionals, vii, 122
prognosis, 140, 266, 268
programming, 156, 215
Progressive Non-fluent Aphasia, 162
Progressive Non-fluent Aphasia (PNFA), 162
progressive supranuclear palsy, viii, 7, 61, 62, 68, 97, 102, 109, 115, 165
Progressive Supranuclear Palsy, 6, 8, 78, 194
pro-inflammatory, 211, 239
project, 54, 129, 132, 237, 263, 265
propagation, 14, 85
prosopagnosia, 103, 123, 199, 219, 228, 249
proteasome, 6, 7
proteins, vii, 2, 6, 13, 35, 62, 254, 270
Proton Magnetic Resonance Spectroscopy, 31
proverbs, 58
Pseudobulbar affect, 108
pseudobulbar palsy, 108
psychiatric diagnosis, 114
psychiatric disorder, 69, 235
psychiatric disorders, 69, 235
psychiatry, vii
psychology, 56, 61, 89, 232
psychometric properties, 236, 257
psychomotor speed, 59, 60
psychosis, 202, 272, 276
Psychosocial Interventions, 183
Psychosocial Interventions and Quality of Life Programs, 183
psychosocial remediations, 155
psychotherapy, 147
psychotic symptoms, 142
p-tau, 19, 35, 177, 178
Puerto Rico, 193
punishment, 76, 78, 90, 94, 97, 114
putamen, 2, 3, 25, 30, 33, 39, 94, 95, 201, 262, 270, 271, 273

Q

quality of life, 69, 85, 180, 182, 183, 216, 218, 230, 262, 271
quantification, 22, 30, 176
questionnaire, 222, 250, 272
quetiapine, 272

R

rapid eye movement sleep, 142
rating scale, 59, 60, 80, 220, 247, 272
reaction time, 72, 74, 79, 80, 81, 83, 215
reactions, 20, 85, 92, 95, 98, 99, 102, 108, 116, 153
reactivity, 86, 96, 97, 98, 99, 102, 108, 116, 117, 121
reading, 70, 115, 155, 157, 161, 163, 164, 169, 182, 195, 196, 199, 203, 207, 214, 215, 219, 220, 227, 229, 230, 244, 245, 247, 248
Reading, 67, 122, 161, 169, 195, 207, 209, 220, 247
reading difficulties, 195
reading skills, 220
reality, 109, 194, 230, 240, 246
reasoning, 212, 222, 227
recall, 96, 108, 133, 134, 135, 141, 143, 145, 146, 149, 207, 210, 264, 265, 266, 268, 270
recalling, 56, 135
receptor, 30, 79, 95, 97, 230, 262, 268, 270, 272
receptors, 29, 91, 94, 129, 199, 262, 264, 268, 270, 272, 273, 275
recognition, 61, 86, 95, 96, 102, 103, 104, 105, 116, 119, 123, 124, 125, 133, 134, 143, 146, 163, 164, 166, 193, 194, 195, 196, 199, 201, 206, 208, 210, 212, 214, 215, 216, 217, 220, 222, 223, 224, 228, 234, 239, 243, 245, 250, 262, 267, 269, 273
recognition test, 224, 239
recommendations, iv, 37, 48, 240
reconstruction, 131, 141, 234

recovery, 231, 258
recurrent perseveration, 75
redistribution, 145
reference frame, 236
reflex action, 96
regional, ix, x, 22, 23, 24, 30, 32, 39, 41, 45, 131, 138, 150, 172, 213, 214, 239, 246
Registry, 4
Regulation of Emotion, 106
rehabilitation, 147, 156, 164, 193, 217, 229, 230, 231, 257, 258, 259, 260
reinforcement, 119, 270
reinforcement learning, 270
reinforcers, 94
relative impairment, 243
relatives, 185
relativity, 194
relevance, 15, 45, 96
reliability, 208, 239
remediation, 155
repetition effect, 241
repetitive behavior, 204
Repetitive transcranial magnetic stimulation, 147, 182, 231
repression, 117
reproduction, 134
requirement, 57
requirements, 75, 230
researchers, 53, 94, 104
resection, 118
residue, 18
residues, 34
resistance, 269
resolution, 24, 25, 29, 33, 39, 215
resources, 70, 86, 89, 96, 97, 103
response, 7, 32, 42, 45, 51, 53, 57, 59, 60, 64, 68, 69, 71, 73, 74, 75, 76, 77, 78, 79, 81, 88, 90, 92, 97, 101, 102, 103, 104, 106, 107, 117, 120, 140, 144, 173, 218, 221, 222, 235, 263, 273
response time, 77
responsiveness, 21, 257
resting state fMRI, 46, 174
resting state fMRI (rs-fMRI), 174
retention, 29, 34, 35, 129, 134, 135, 136, 139, 140, 141, 142, 143
reticular activating system, 96
retina, 199, 200, 211, 212, 224
retrieval, iv, 14, 23, 58, 62, 96, 127, 129, 130, 131, 134, 135, 140, 141, 142, 143, 144, 145, 148, 149, 152, 153, 157, 159, 160, 162, 163, 168, 182, 207, 266
retrograde amnesia, 135, 139
Retrograde memory, 128, 132
reward pathways, 94, 95, 262
rewards, 54, 60, 94, 107, 270
Rey-Osterreith Complex-Figure Test, 207
rhythm, 101
right dorsolateral prefrontal cortex, 51, 53, 77
right dorsolateral prefrontal cortex (DLPFC), 51, 53
right hemisphere, 11, 54, 72, 75, 76, 77, 80, 81, 88, 100, 101, 103, 122, 175, 182, 257
right hemisphere hypothesis, 88
Right Hemisphere Hypothesis, 88
rights, iv
rigidity, 221, 226, 262, 269
risk, 26, 29, 31, 32, 35, 44, 95, 104, 161, 179, 213, 215, 216, 228, 231, 245, 262, 267, 268, 269, 270
risk factors, 26, 161
risk taking, 270
risks, 26, 267
RNA, 10
RNA processing, 10
rodents, 94
ROI, 19, 22, 23, 27
Romania, 184
root, 88, 220
routes, 216, 217
rs-fMRI, 160, 174, 182
rules, 56

S

saccades, 196, 222
sadness, 88
safety, 216, 254
salience network, 55, 96, 103, 114
Sapir, 156
sarcoidosis, 169
Saussure, 156
scaling, 233
Scene Description, 205
science, 116, 118
sclerosis, 2, 4, 138, 145, 150, 151
scope, 56, 87, 98, 102, 133, 144
sedative, 272
sedative medication, 272
seed, 33, 174
segregation, 225, 242
seizure, 108
selective attention, 96, 107, 108, 234
Selective Attention, 107
selective serotonin reuptake inhibitor, 109, 264
selectivity, 109, 218
self-awareness, 53
self-presentation, 122
self-regulation, 51, 53, 54

semantic, 11, 58, 59, 81, 101, 104, 115, 124, 128, 132, 149, 159, 160, 161, 162, 163, 164, 165, 168, 174, 176, 179, 182, 185, 186, 187, 189, 196, 201, 206, 207, 208, 221, 225, 237, 246, 267, 273
semantic dementia, 11, 124, 160, 163, 165, 176, 179, 189, 221, 246
semantic memory, 58, 128, 132, 149, 206, 207, 225, 273
semantic paraphasias, 163
Semantic PPA, 163
Semantic PPA (PPA-S), 163
semantic processing, 159, 160
Semantic processing, 159
semantics, 156, 269
semicircle, 209
senile dementia, 243
sensation, 70, 90, 96, 103, 108, 201
sensations, 85, 96, 102
senses, 129
sensitivity, 18, 23, 28, 29, 30, 34, 37, 56, 58, 114, 138, 170, 176, 177, 204, 214, 215, 217, 224, 227, 243
sensory experience, 198
sensory extinction, 73
Sensory Extinction, 71
Sensory memory, 128
sensory modalities, 54, 128, 198
sensory modality, 202
sensory system, 70, 130
sensory systems, 70, 130
sentence comprehension, 159, 160, 163
sequencing, 57, 133, 220
Seretonin, 263
serine, 34
serotonin, 95, 96, 181, 264, 271, 272
serum, 140, 268
services, iv, 149
set shifting difficulties, 262
sex, 238
sex differences, 238
sexual behavior, 93
sexuality, 202
sham, 98
shape, 22, 23, 59, 132, 198, 207, 220
shock, 107
short-term memory, 128, 135, 217, 246, 259
showing, 20, 21, 27, 33, 101, 167, 174, 177, 207, 225
side effects, 79, 95, 272
signals, 31, 104, 108, 262
signs, 60, 63, 69, 78, 80, 82, 169, 195, 214, 221, 230, 269, 275
silhouette, 208
silver, 2, 7, 13
similarities test, 57
simulation, 86
simultanagnosia, 198, 203, 204, 213
Sinai, 51
single test, 144
Single-Photon Emission Computed Tomography, 30
Single-Photon Emission Computed Tomography (SPECT), 30
SMPFC, 55, 59, 60, 62, 63, 64
SN, 43, 55, 62, 63, 64, 248
social behavior, 118
social cognition, 60, 121, 213
social consequences, 101
social context, 103
social group, 93, 96
social interaction, 88
social interactions, 88
social rules, 116
social stress, 265
society, 37, 85, 116
somnolence, 265
spasticity, 269
spatial ability, 238
Spatial Akinesia, 72
spatial cognition, 194, 216, 236
spatial frequency, 212, 250
spatial information, 216
spatial learning, 227
spatial location, 71
spatial memory, 216
spatial neglect, 75, 210, 227, 229, 235, 257, 258, 259
spatial processing, 196, 245
specialists, 269, 271
specialization, 117, 131
species, 14, 88, 116, 127, 145
SPECT, 19, 28, 30, 31, 32, 34, 38, 42, 44, 45, 48, 138, 142, 151, 172, 175, 181, 187, 188, 226
SPECT Scan, 172
spectroscopy, 45
speculation, 105
speech, 62, 76, 79, 101, 122, 124, 155, 156, 159, 162, 163, 164, 165, 166, 167, 168, 170, 172, 173, 176, 180, 182, 183, 191
Speech, 124, 156, 159, 164, 182, 184, 187, 191, 235, 237
Speech and Language Interventions, 182
speech perception, 124
speech-language therapy, 155
spelling, 169, 186, 221
spin, 138, 150
spin labeling, 138, 150
spinal cord, 2, 13, 100, 269
Spontaneous Speech, 166, 236

Spring, 46, 151, 232
stability, 264
stabilization, 34, 131
standardization, 238
stars, 204
state, 18, 28, 31, 32, 33, 46, 47, 54, 55, 61, 89, 96, 120, 132, 149, 155, 160, 173, 174, 181, 184, 189, 214, 237, 262, 263, 270
states, ix, 51, 55, 59, 61, 85, 88, 114, 231
stereopsis, 195, 215, 218, 243
Stereopsis, 195, 243
Stereopsis and depth perception, 195
stereotypes, 106
Steroid, 181, 191
stimulant, 268
stimulation, 79, 81, 83, 94, 99, 119, 131, 147, 148, 154, 173, 182, 191, 199, 229, 230, 231, 233, 235, 258, 259, 260, 262, 268
stimulus, 53, 57, 59, 70, 71, 73, 76, 86, 89, 90, 93, 94, 95, 102, 103, 104, 107, 108, 117, 128, 131, 132, 149, 187, 195, 198, 199, 202, 227, 230, 235, 257
stimulus cards, 57
storage, 23, 117, 127, 129, 130, 131, 133, 134, 145, 148, 266, 267
strategy use, 108
stress, 57, 145, 214
striae, 92
striatum, 13, 53, 54, 60, 76, 77, 82, 87, 92, 94, 95, 126, 130, 262, 270, 271, 273, 276
stroke, 26, 80, 81, 101, 117, 121, 122, 139, 157, 162, 165, 173, 182, 185, 186, 201, 203, 228, 229, 256, 257, 258, 259, 260, 266
structural changes, 22, 28, 131
Structural Magnetic Resonance Imaging, 22
Structural Magnetic Resonance Imaging (MRI), 22
structure, 23, 46, 52, 69, 94, 98, 129, 156, 160, 162, 167, 184, 211, 273
Subcortical Dementias, 61
subcortical nuclei, 136
subcortical vascular mild cognitive impairment, 78
subgroups, 23
subiculum, 23, 92, 139
subjective experience, 107, 109
sublexical route, 161
substitution, 168
substrate, viii, 93, 106, 161, 241, 253, 255
substrates, 43, 64, 161
sucrose, 1
superior longitudinal fascicle, 158
superior longitudinal fasciculus, 77
superior medial prefrontal regions, 51, 53
superior medial prefrontal regions (SMPFC), 53
superior temporal gyrus, 157, 158, 214
Supervisory System model, 53
supplementation, 140
suppression, 88, 97, 108, 121, 125, 273
survival, 100, 145, 249
susceptibility, 25, 35, 162
Switzerland, 184
sympathetic denervation, 47, 143
sympathetic nervous system, 89, 121
sympathetic system, 97
sympathy, 114
symptoms, viii, x, 20, 29, 63, 67, 69, 78, 80, 93, 115, 119, 123, 138, 139, 141, 142, 143, 144, 162, 165, 170, 180, 181, 213, 214, 216, 218, 221, 222, 223, 224, 226, 228, 229, 230, 231, 242, 249, 250, 254, 255, 256, 258, 261, 262, 263, 265, 267, 269, 271, 272, 273, 274
synapse, 4, 15, 100, 150
synaptic plasticity, 129, 149
synaptic transmission, 148
synchronization, 95
syndrome, x, xi, 36, 51, 59, 62, 63, 64, 67, 80, 81, 93, 101, 108, 109, 114, 115, 118, 119, 120, 136, 138, 139, 140, 141, 142, 146, 151, 153, 161, 163, 164, 165, 168, 169, 170, 171, 179, 180, 181, 183, 197, 198, 202, 203, 205, 213, 218, 219, 221, 222, 223, 224, 228, 238, 246, 252, 255, 256, 261, 267, 272, 273
Syntactic processing, 160, 184
Syntax, 156
synthesis, 88, 194, 211, 245, 267

T

tachycardia, 103
Tactile Adherence Disorders, 73
Tactile Defective Response Inhibition, 73
Tactile Mitgehen, 73
tangles, 3, 4, 8, 19, 115
TAR DNA binding protein of 43 kD, 6
target, 57, 68, 75, 76, 104, 116, 131, 189, 197, 202, 209, 210, 215, 217, 218, 220, 223, 230, 258, 262
target response, 57
target stimuli, 223
task demands, 215, 235, 246
Task Force, 265, 275
task performance, 149
task setting, 51, 53, 54, 56, 57, 58, 59
tau, vii, 2, 4, 6, 7, 8, 9, 10, 14, 15, 16, 19, 20, 21, 34, 35, 43, 48, 49, 62, 111, 112, 115, 136, 137, 139, 142, 150, 170, 177, 178, 180, 190, 191, 211, 226, 268, 275
taxonomy, 245

TBI, 79, 143, 227
TDP-43, 2, 4, 6, 7, 9, 10, 11, 14, 15, 62, 110, 112, 113, 115, 124, 139, 151
techniques, ix, 18, 22, 24, 33, 36, 106, 138, 147, 157, 198, 229, 241, 257
technology, 106, 193
TEG, 256
telencephalon, 129
temperature, 96, 267
tempo, 101
temporal lobe, x, 4, 6, 7, 9, 18, 19, 20, 23, 27, 38, 39, 45, 46, 62, 77, 90, 92, 93, 102, 103, 104, 115, 118, 119, 124, 125, 128, 129, 130, 131, 132, 134, 136, 138, 139, 141, 148, 151, 153, 159, 161, 165, 168, 172, 185, 199, 202, 207, 208, 212, 214, 216, 220, 241, 253
temporal lobes, 6, 7, 9, 62, 77, 93, 103, 132, 202, 207
terminal motor perseveration, 75
terminals, 8
territory, 163
testing, xi, 38, 55, 58, 60, 69, 72, 73, 75, 132, 133, 136, 144, 147, 166, 188, 193, 201, 203, 204, 205, 208, 210, 216, 217, 223, 246, 251, 254, 265, 266
tests of prefrontal functions, 56
textbook, vii
texture, 2
TGA, 141
thalamus, 2, 3, 6, 13, 53, 55, 76, 77, 78, 91, 92, 96, 97, 98, 115, 118, 129, 130, 140, 200, 201, 265, 271, 273
The Three Words Three Shapes test, 133
theory of mind, 53, 61, 67, 124
therapeutic effect, 22, 33
therapeutic effects, 22, 33
therapeutic interventions, 21, 172, 173, 180
therapist, 229
therapy, 99, 146, 155, 173, 186, 187, 191, 229, 230, 263, 268, 271
therapy interventions, 173
thinning, 8, 9, 22, 150, 226
thoughts, 106, 273
threonine, 34
thymoma, 140
Tics, 272
timbre, 101
time frame, x
tissue, 2, 4, 14, 16, 18, 22, 27, 28, 31, 34, 41, 86, 116, 140, 172
TMC, 232
Togo, 151, 253
ToM, 53, 61
tones, 101
tonic, 196
top-down, 77, 89, 97, 203, 226, 234
Topographic Disorientation, 216
Topographical or Progression Biomarkers, 170
Total-tau, 19, 34
Total-tau (t-tau), 34
tracks, 189
Trail-making Test, 58
training, vii, 182
trajectory, 165, 211, 231, 259
Transcranial direct current stimulation, 79
Transcranial magnetic stimulation, 79
transcription, 239
transection, 151
transformation, 250
Transient global amnesia, 141, 151
translation, 194
transmission, 273
transport, 14, 33, 253
transverse section, 1
trauma, 101, 122, 196, 256
traumatic brain injury, vii, 60, 72, 79, 143, 148, 153, 227
Traumatic brain injury, 140, 143
treatment, 1, 21, 26, 28, 31, 33, 38, 44, 69, 79, 82, 109, 120, 140, 144, 146, 170, 173, 174, 180, 182, 183, 189, 191, 222, 230, 231, 251, 258, 261, 266, 271, 272
Treatments, 79
tremor, 269, 274
trial, 42, 180, 181, 191, 267, 270, 271, 272, 276
tricyclic antidepressant, 109, 271
tricyclic antidepressants, 109, 271
triple loops, 75
tryptophan, 264
t-tau, 19, 35
tumors, 141, 169
tyrosine, 264

U

ubiquitin, 2, 6, 7, 12, 13, 15, 16, 115
uncinate fasciculi, 77
uniform, 135
unilateral spatial neglect, 258
United States, 2, 125
updating, 54, 55, 58, 215, 262
USA, 148, 235, 236, 240, 246
Utilization Behavior, 74

V

vagus, 2, 3, 6, 99
vagus nerve, 6
valence, 88, 89, 90, 94, 97, 107, 117
valence hypothesis, 88
Valence Hypothesis, 88
validation, 80, 137, 189, 236
valine, 179, 267
valuation, 55
variations, 33, 108, 204
varieties, 228
Vascular cognitive impairment, 139
vascular dementia, 23, 38, 39, 40, 52, 78, 82, 152, 227, 242, 255
Vascular dementia, 19, 78, 220
vasculitides, 169
vasectomy, 161, 181
vasodilation, 97
vasopressin, 99
vector, 235
vegetables, 163, 166, 168
vehicles, 196
vein, 93
ventral object-recognition stream of vision, 199
ventral striatum, 54, 60, 76, 77, 94, 126, 130, 263, 270, 271
ventricle, 80, 90, 92, 144, 171
ventromedial prefrontal cortex, 51, 53, 107
verbal fluency, 56, 66, 167, 181, 186, 221, 265, 274
Vermeer, 40
victims, 63
Vigilance, 70
vision, 194, 195, 196, 198, 199, 203, 211, 214, 215, 216, 219, 222, 227, 228, 241, 242, 243, 244, 248, 250, 256, 260
visual acuity, 193, 201, 203, 212
Visual Acuity, 195
Visual Adherence Disorders, 74
visual agnosia, 93, 168, 199, 206, 211, 219, 224
Visual Agnosia, 201, 202, 236
visual area, 118, 125, 213, 226, 228, 253
visual attention, 203, 215, 258
Visual Cognitive Assessment Test, 204, 236
Visual disorientation, 202
visual environment, 203
visual field, 73, 74, 139, 195, 203, 213, 217, 220, 224, 228, 231, 250, 251
visual grasp, 74
visual images, 195, 203
Visual object and face recognition, 196
visual processing, 125, 156, 194, 197, 200, 210, 214, 222, 223, 226, 228, 234, 241
Visual Search, 217
visual stimuli, 105, 128, 194, 195, 198, 202, 224
visual stimulus, 202, 217
visual system, 103, 105, 198, 211, 248
visual word form area, 161
visualization, 198
Visual-Ocular Response Inhibition, 74
Visual-spatial perception, 195
visuoconstructive deficits, 194
Visuoconstructive Function, 206
visuoperceptual, 194, 205, 219, 224, 225, 226, 227, 253
visuospatial, 20, 58, 114, 134, 139, 183, 194, 195, 196, 198, 199, 200, 203, 206, 207, 208, 209, 211, 212, 213, 214, 216, 218, 219, 222, 223, 224, 225, 226, 227, 228, 230, 231, 232, 235, 236, 237, 240, 241, 243, 248, 250, 251, 253, 254, 259, 274
visuospatial function, 20, 58, 203, 206, 222, 224, 230, 231, 232, 250, 251, 274
Visuospatial function, 194, 197, 237, 254
visuospatial processing, 195, 198, 204, 212, 214, 241
vocabulary, 269
vocalizations, 105, 124
volumetric changes, 22, 23, 95
von Economo neurons, 63, 68, 114, 123
vulnerability, x, 41, 151, 162

W

WAIS, 208, 210, 238
walking, 203, 214, 217, 219, 231, 259, 269
Washington, 65
water, 27, 31, 72, 214, 217
WCST, 56
weakness, 71, 72
Wechsler Adult Intelligence Scale, 66, 238
well-being, 125
Wernicke-Geschwind model, 157
Wernicke-Lichtheim model, 157
White House, 101
white matter, 2, 4, 7, 8, 9, 10, 18, 22, 25, 26, 40, 41, 62, 77, 78, 79, 108, 111, 112, 115, 132, 143, 169, 177, 185, 239, 271
White Matter Hyperintensities, 25
whole-brain volumetric changes, 22
Wisconsin, 56, 65, 77
Wisconsin Card Sorting Task, 77
Wisconsin Card Sorting Test, 56, 65
withdrawal, 88
word recognition, 163, 165
word-list generation, 58
words per minute, 162, 164, 167

working memory, 33, 57, 68, 75, 97, 128, 131, 132, 133, 134, 135, 148, 149, 159, 164, 168, 196, 211, 232, 238, 241, 262, 265, 268, 270, 274
Working memory, 62, 128, 132, 133, 144, 148
Writing, 161, 169, 220, 221
writing to dictation, 161

Y

yes/no, 169
yield, 179, 203
young adults, 108

α

α-synuclein, 5, 6, 19, 20, 21, 49, 142